When Your Child
Has a Disability

When Your Child Has a Disability

The Complete Sourcebook of Daily and Medical Care

Revised Edition

edited by

Mark L. Batshaw, M.D.

"Fight for Children" Chair of Academic Medicine
Chief Academic Officer
Director, Children's Research Institute
Children's National Medical Center

Chairman, Department of Pediatrics
The George Washington University
School of Medicine and Health Sciences

Washington, D.C.

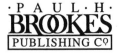

Baltimore • London • Toronto • Sydney

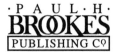

Paul H. Brookes Publishing Co., Inc.
Post Office Box 10624
Baltimore, Maryland 21285-0624

www.brookespublishing.com

Typeset by A.W. Bennett, Inc., Hartland, Vermont.
Manufactured in the United States of America by The Maple Press Co., York, PA

First printing of second revised edition: November 2000.
10   9   8   7   6   5   4   3   2   1

Library of Congress Cataloging-in-Publication Data

Batshaw, Mark L., 1945–
    When your child has a disability : the complete sourcebook of daily and medical care /
edited by Mark L. Batshaw.—2nd rev. ed.
      p.   cm.
    Previous ed. published under the title: Your child has a disability.
    Includes bibliographical references and index.
    ISBN 1-55766-472-2
    1. Developmentally disabled children—Medical care.   2. Developmentally disabled
children—Care.   3. Developmentally disabled children—Education.   4. Developmentally
disabled children—Legal status, laws, etc.   I. Batshaw, Mark L., 1945– Your child has a
disability.   II. Title.

RJ506.D47 B37   2001
649'.15—dc21

00-058540

British Library Cataloguing in Publication data are available from the British Library.

To Andrew, Christian, Debbie, Katie, Narayan, Sarah, Sonny,
and all of the other children
and their families I have had the honor to care for

Contents

About the Editor

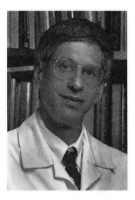 Dr. Mark L. Batshaw, a developmental pediatrician, has treated children with developmental disabilities for 25 years and is listed in *The Best Doctors in America* (Naifeh, Smith, Stec, & Madden; Woodward/White, 1997). In addition to his clinical work with children and families, Dr. Batshaw has authored several authoritative texts and published numerous articles on children with disabilities. Recognized as an international expert on inborn errors of metabolism, he has received numerous major grants from the National Institutes of Health and continues to move the field forward through his research.

Throughout his career, Dr. Batshaw has focused on providing the best care for children with disabilities by sharing his experience and passion with other medical professionals. He is currently the "Fight for Children" Chair of Academic Medicine and Chief Academic Officer at the Children's National Medical Center in Washington, D.C., and also serves as Professor and Chairman of Pediatrics at The George Washington University School of Medicine and Health Sciences in Washington, D.C. Dr. Batshaw is a Fellow of the American Academy of Pediatrics and is a member of the American Pediatric Society, the Society for Inherited Metabolic Disorders, the Society for Pediatric Research, and the Society of Developmental Pediatrics.

Before moving to Washington in 1998, Dr. Batshaw was Physician-in-Chief of Children's Seashore House, the child development and rehabilitation institute at The Children's Hospital of Philadelphia, and held the W.T. Grant Chair in Child Development at the University of Pennsylvania School of Medicine. Dr. Batshaw is a graduate of the University of Pennsylvania and of the University of Chicago School of Medicine. Following pediatric residency in his native Canada at the Hospital for Sick Children in Toronto, he completed a fellowship in developmental pediatrics at the Kennedy Krieger Institute of the Johns Hopkins Medical Institutions in Baltimore.

Dr. Batshaw's investment in the well-being of children was first sparked by his parents, both of whom were social workers; his father was involved in modernizing the juvenile justice system in Québec. Dr. Batshaw's wife, Karen, is a social worker in the field of international adoptions. His children also continue this legacy of making a difference: His daughter, Elissa, is a special education teacher; his son Michael is a social worker; and his younger son, Drew, has overcome the challenges of attention-deficit/hyperactivity disorder to graduate from Vassar College and become an Internet software engineer.

Contributors

George Acs, D.M.D., M.P.H.
Chair, Department of Dentistry
Children's National Medical Center
111 Michigan Avenue, NW
Washington, D.C. 20010

Lisa J. Bain, M.A.
Research Project Manager
Deafness and Family Communication
    Center
Department of Psychiatry
University of Pennsylvania School of
    Medicine
Philadelphia, PA 19104

Ken Bleile, Ph.D.
Professor and Department Head
Department of Communicative
    Disorders
University of Northern Iowa
238 Communication Arts Center
Cedar Falls, IA 50614

James Coplan, M.D.
Clinical Associate Professor of
    Pediatrics
Children's Seashore House of The Chil-
    dren's Hospital of Philadelphia
3405 Civic Center Boulevard
Philadelphia, PA 19104

Karen Echols, Ph.D.
Clinical Instructor, Physical Therapy
    Division
School of Health-Related Professions
University of Alabama at Birmingham
Director of Community Programs
Civitan International Research Center
1720 7th Avenue, S.
Suite 311
Birmingham, AL 35209

Andrea Edelman, M.Ed., CRC
Clinical Supervisor
Advanced Employment Readiness
    Center
Children's National Medical Center
111 Michigan Avenue, NW
Washington, D.C. 20010

Peggy S. Eicher, M.D.
Private Practice (specializing in pedi-
    atric dysphagia and feeding
    management)
4 W. Possum Hollow Road
Wallingford, PA 19086

Angelo P. Giardino, M.D., M.S.Ed.
Associate Chair, Pediatrics
The Children's Hospital of Philadelphia
3405 Civic Center Boulevard
Philadelphia, PA 19104

Penny Glass, Ph.D.
Developmental Psychologist
Children's National Medical Center
111 Michigan Avenue, NW
Washington, D.C. 20010

Mohamad S. Jaafar, M.D.
Professor and Chair of Ophthalmology
Children's National Medical Center
111 Michigan Avenue, NW
Washington, D.C. 20010

Lisa A. Kurtz, M.Ed., OTR/L, BCP
Pediatric Private Practice
16 Martin Avenue
Scarborough, ME 04074

Susan E. Levy, M.D.
Section Chief, Developmental
    Pediatrics
Children's Hospital of Philadelphia
3405 Civic Center Boulevard
Philadelphia, PA 19104

D. Michael Malone, Ph.D.
Associate Professor of Early Childhood
    Education
University of Cincinnati
One Edwards Center
Room 223 (Corry Avenue)
Cincinnati, OH 45221

Sheila Rose Mazzoli, M.Ed.
Educational Specialist and Assistive
    Technology Consultant
Montgomery County Intermediate
    Unit 23
1605B W. Main Street
Norristown, PA 19403

Gretchen A. Meyer, M.D.
Neurodevelopmental Physician
U.S. Navy
Portsmouth Naval Hospital
620 John Paul Jones Circle
Portsmouth, VA 23708

Wanda Y. Newell, Ph.D.
Education Program Director
McCormick Tribune Foundation
435 North Michigan Avenue
Suite 790
Chicago, IL 60611

Man Wai Ng, D.D.S., M.P.H.
Assistant Professor of Pediatrics
The George Washington University
    School of Medicine and Health
    Sciences
Children's National Medical Center
111 Michigan Avenue, NW
Washington, D.C. 20010

John M. Parrish, Ph.D.
Executive Director
The Erickson Foundation
701 Maiden Choice Lane
Catonsville, MD 21228

Louis Pellegrino, M.D.
Director, Division of Developmental
    Pediatrics
St. Peter's University Hospital and
    Health Systems
254 Easton Avenue
New Brunswick, NJ 08903

Craig T. Ramey, Ph.D.
Director and University Professor of
    Psychology, Pediatrics, Maternal and
    Child Health, and Neurobiology
Civitan International Research Center
University of Alabama at Birmingham
1719 6th Avenue, S.
Suite 137
Birmingham, AL 35294

Sharon Landesman Ramey, Ph.D.
Director and Professor of Psychiatry,
    Psychology, Maternal and Child
    Health, and Neurobiology
Civitan International Research Center
1719 6th Avenue, S.
Suite 137
Birmingham, AL 35294

Nancy J. Roizen, M.D.
Associate Professor of Pediatrics and
    Psychiatry
University of Chicago
Pritzker School of Medicine
5841 S. Maryland Avenue
Chicago, IL 60637

Vincent Schuyler, B.S.W., A.B.D.A.
Program Director
Adolescent Employment Readiness
    Center
Children's National Medical Center
111 Michigan Avenue, NW
Washington, D.C. 20010

Catherine Shaer, M.D.
Medical Officer
Food and Drug Administration
5 Bunker Court
Rockville, MD 20854

Bruce K. Shapiro, M.D.
Associate Professor of Pediatrics
Kennedy Krieger Institute
The Johns Hopkins Medical Institutions
707 N. Broadway
Baltimore, MD 21205

Mark A. Stein, Ph.D.
Chair, Department of Psychology
Children's National Medical Center
111 Michigan Avenue, NW
Washington, D.C. 20010

Annie Steinberg, M.D.
Assistant Professor
Departments of Psychiatry and
    Pediatrics
University of Pennsylvania School of
    Medicine
3405 Civic Center Boulevard
Philadelphia, PA 19104

Cynthia J. Tifft, M.D., Ph.D.
Chair, Division of Genetics, Endocrinol-
    ogy and Metabolism
Center for Complex Diseases
Children's National Medical Center
111 Michigan Avenue, NW
Washington, D.C. 20010

Kenneth E. Towbin, M.D.
Professor of Psychiatry & Behavioral
  Sciences and Pediatrics
The George Washington University
  School of Medicine and Health
  Sciences
Medical Director, Complex Develop-
  mental Disorders Team
Children's National Medical Center
111 Michigan Avenue, NW
Washington, D.C. 20010

**Symme W. Trachtenberg, M.S.W.,
  A.C.S.W., L.S.W.**
Director of Social Work
Children's Seashore House of The Chil-
  dren's Hospital of Philadelphia
Clinical Associate in Pediatrics and
  Social Work
University of Pennsylvania School of
  Medicine
Instructor
University of Pennsylvania School of
  Social Work
3405 Civic Center Boulevard
Philadelphia, PA 19104

Paul Wang, M.D.
Assistant Professor of Pediatrics
University of Pennsylvania School of
  Medicine
Children's Seashore House of The Chil-
  dren's Hospital of Philadelphia
3405 Civic Center Boulevard
Philadelphia, PA 19104

Steven Weinstein, M.D.
Associate Professor of Pediatrics and
  Neurology
The George Washington University
  School of Medicine and Health
  Sciences
Vice Chair, Department of Neurology
Children's National Medical Center
111 Michigan Avenue, NW
Washington, D.C. 20010

Patience H. White, M.D.
Professor of Pediatrics and Medicine
The George Washington University
  School of Medicine and Health
  Sciences
Executive Director, Adolescent Employ-
  ment Readiness Center
Children's National Medical Center
111 Michigan Avenue, NW
Washington, D.C. 20010

John Albert Wray, MB., BS., FRACP
Developmental Pediatrician
Department of Developmental
  Pediatrics
State Child Development Center of
  Princess Margaret Hospital for
  Children
Post Office Box 510
West Perth 6872, Western Australia
AUSTRALIA

Preface

All parents expect their children to be brighter, prettier, happier, and more successful than themselves. In fact, we want our children to be perfect in every way. We love them and feel responsible for them; we see them as extensions of ourselves. When we find that one of our children has a disability, we must deal with a wide range of emotions, including depression, anger, confusion, anxiety, and even embarrassment.

Some conditions, such as Down syndrome, are evident at birth, whereas other developmental disabilities, such as ADHD, may not become apparent until later in childhood. Whatever the disability, it will necessitate changes in your attitudes and expectations. It may require that you learn new skills, administer medicines, and give various types of rehabilitative and educational therapies. Initially you may feel you can't cope, but you will because your child needs you.

This book tries to answer many questions about your child's disability. It is divided into four sections. The first, Getting the Diagnosis, deals with finding out your child has a disability. This section talks about the initial feelings you may have experienced when you first learned that your child had a disability. Also discussed are steps you can take to find the right doctor to care for your child. The section helps you understand how a child develops and how to look for answers to the question "Why my child?"

The second section, Growing Up with a Disability, begins with a discussion of the prematurely born infant, the needs of some infants for early intervention services, nutrition/feeding, and dental care issues. Then, rehabilitation, medical, and behavioral therapies are explored for you. Finally, educational placements and legal rights and benefits are outlined.

The third section, Developmental Disabilities, gives practical information about the different developmental disabilities: mental retardation, Down syndrome and other genetic syndromes, spina bifida, epilepsy, cerebral palsy, hearing loss, communication disorders, eye disorders and visual impairments, autism spectrum disorders, attention-deficit/hyperactivity disorder, and learning disabilities.

Chapters in the final section, What the Future Holds, explore your options for genetic counseling, the changing health care environment, and the road to adulthood. At the end of the book is a list of suggested readings and resources (including web sites) that you may find useful. Many programs and agencies, such as specific disability organizations, have not been included because of space limitations. Any works referenced in the text are included in this list rather than in a separate reference list.

Each chapter begins with an introductory section that summarizes what is discussed. In each chapter you will find one or more vignettes about children with disabilities, and the chapters end with some answers to questions parents have frequently asked my colleagues or me. It is my belief that knowledge adds to confidence and competence. This book will primarily assure you that you can trust your own common sense and instincts. It is my hope that this book will make a difference for you and your child.

Mark L. Batshaw, M.D.

Acknowledgments

This book was the result of a great deal of effort by many wonderful people. I would like to acknowledge their contributions. First, I would like to thank all of the authors who wrote chapters in this book; one author, Dr. John Albert Wray, also suggested the title. A medical illustrator is indispensable for a work such as this, and we had one of the best, Lynn Reynolds, who created Figures 7.1, 7.2, 9.1–9.4, 15.1, 15.2, 19.1, 19.2, 20.1, 20.3–20.5, 22.1, 22.4, 26.1, and 26.3–26.7. In addition, Elaine Kasmer's classic illustrations continue to explain important concepts; five of Elaine's figures were borrowed from my textbook, *Children with Disabilities, Fourth Edition* (1997), also published by Paul H. Brookes Publishing Co.: Figures 4.1, 20.2, 22.2 and 22.3, and 26.8.

For the book to move from conception to finished product, there needs to be an effective team at the publisher. Paul H. Brookes Publishing Co. is blessed with an extremely talented staff, and I would like to acknowledge the three members who had most to do with producing this book: January Layman-Wood, Mika Wendy Sam, and Heather Shrestha. Finally, I wish to credit my associate, Margaret Rose, who organized this endeavor, keeping me and my contributors on schedule, and helped edit the manuscript.

I would also like to acknowledge the many parents, friends, and professionals who reviewed and offered comments on this manuscript. Their comments were incorporated into the final manuscript. I extend my thanks to all of these reviewers, both those who chose to remain anonymous and those who are listed here: Pasquale Accardo, Becky Adelmann, Marilee C. Allen, Susan Attermeier, Lawrence Beaser, Dorothy Bulas, George T. Capone, Elissa Batshaw Clair, Matthew D. Cohen, Barbara C. Cutler, Barbara Domingue, June Downing, Jata Ghosh, Deborah Gilbert, Karl Gumpper, Katherine J. Inge, Paul Lipkin, Sue Pratt, Patricia S. Scola, David Wargowski, Amy Whitehead, and David L. Wodrich.

When Your Child
Has a Disability

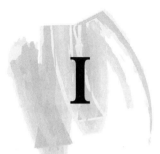

I

Getting the Diagnosis

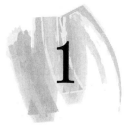

Finding Out
Your Child Has a Disability

James Coplan and Symme W. Trachtenberg

When you find out your child has a disability, it may not seem possible to return to your everyday world. This chapter discusses some of your first feelings and means of coping with them. Making contact with professionals, support groups, and other parents who share similar experiences will help you find the strength to develop and foster the health and well-being of your child. Understanding that you are not alone and that other families have gone through what you are going through is half the battle; the rest is coming up with solutions. You will end up as an expert on your child, capable of helping others. Your family can survive and emerge whole.

Marty

Sue and David had been concerned about their son Marty's development since his premature birth at 32 weeks. Marty had come home from the hospital at 2 months of age a happy, if small, baby. The early intervention therapist who came to their home noted that Marty's feet seemed stiff and tended to cross, or "scissor." At Marty's next checkup, the pediatrician diagnosed Marty as having spastic diplegia, a form of cerebral palsy (see Chapter 19) common in preterm infants. Sue and David were devastated. They cried and exchanged angry words. Sue felt guilty because she believed that her high blood pressure may have caused the early delivery. Sue and David's children responded to the tension: Marty became crankier, and 5-year-old Jody began to misbehave. David started spending more time at work to get away from the stresses at home, and Sue felt abandoned. She recognized that she needed help and spoke to the early intervention therapist, who referred her to a social worker. Sue entered into short-term counseling, and subsequently David agreed to join her. They reopened lines of communication and got some practical advice about coping with their feelings and providing behavior management for Jody. Sue and David also joined a parent support group that met monthly, and they received significant support from their extended family and their church. Most important, Marty was starting to make real progress in his early intervention program, and Sue and David derived great pleasure from every gain he made. Marty, in turn, responded to their praise and tried even harder, and Jody was brought in as a "special helper." Although Sue and David still have their moments of sadness, they are proud of their children and are glad that they have brought their family closer together.

DEALING WITH YOUR REACTIONS

When you first learned that your child had a disability, your initial response may have been shock, accompanied by a sensation of emotional numbness. This reaction is especially common when the news is delivered unexpectedly. Or, you may have had concerns about your child's development over a period of months or years. By the time your child's disability was formally diagnosed, you may not have been greatly surprised. Even under these circumstances, however, it may be difficult to hear words spoken aloud that confirm your fears. You may go through a period of denial, either before or after receiving the diagnosis. Denial is a healthy and, in some ways, necessary stage of the grieving process. On a superficial level, the reaction "It can't be" is perfectly understandable because we naturally wish bad news to be untrue. On a deeper level, denial over the short-term functions as a protective mechanism that we use to conserve our emotional energy for the critical tasks that we must accomplish, such as child rearing. This phase is normal. Problems arise, however, when denial is prolonged and you are not able to move forward on tasks necessary for your child's and your family's welfare.

When receiving bad news, people either internalize or externalize their reactions. Internalization is the process of assuming blame for misfortune. The two most common emotions experienced by people who internalize are guilt and shame. In Sue's case, it was guilt that she had high blood pressure that may have caused Marty's premature birth. Externalization refers to the process of placing responsibility for events on others. The most common feelings experienced by people who externalize are blame and anger. These two response patterns, internalization and externalization, stem from the unspoken belief that when something bad happens, "It's got to be somebody's fault."

Eventually, when we feel emotionally safe, we let our feelings show. This is usually a time of overwhelming grief. As with shock and denial, grief is a healthy emotion. Parents who are consumed by guilt, shame, blame, or anger may not be able to grieve properly. This can create significant problems in the long run. Once parents pass through the stage of acute grief, however, they come to accept the fact of their child's disability. This transition is marked by the return of some degree of optimism or at least a determination to do the best that one can. Even so, it is normal from time to time to ask yourself "*What if?*" and wonder how things might have been. It is also normal to reexperience grief at certain life cycle events, such as birthdays, school entry, and other occasions that remind you of what has been achieved and what has not.

DIFFERENCES BETWEEN PARENTS/PARTNERS

Different family members and caregivers may have different reactions to news of a child's disability. For example, the child's primary caregiver often may suspect that something is different about the child first, and, as mentioned previously, may not be that surprised to learn that the child has a disability. These differing views can cause friction between parents, especially if one is ready to hear the diagnosis but the other is still at an earlier stage in the reaction process, such as denial. Being at different stages in the grieving process is also typical because people grieve in individual ways.

Although it is no longer as true as it once was, men in our culture are still expected to be "strong" and to not show their grief. They may have more difficulty talking about their feelings. This can create a barrier for fathers in terms of working through their own grief.

Problems arise when each partner grieves privately and is unavailable to provide emotional support to the other. For example, in Sue and David's family, one parent (David) spent more and more hours at work, whereas the other (Sue) remained on the "front lines" both physically and emotionally. Mothers may be somewhat more prone to blame themselves for their child's disability, particularly if they have some questions about the pregnancy or labor and delivery.

SPECIAL CASES

The Strongly Desired or Long-Awaited Child

If you have experienced difficulty conceiving or if you have waited to have children, this wait raises the stakes emotionally. It may make it even harder than usual for you to adapt to your child's disability; alternatively, you may be more accepting than the typical parent of your child's disability.

The Unplanned Child

Rearing children requires parents to give up a tremendous degree of freedom. If you had not planned to make these sacrifices, your child's disability may make the parenting role even more difficult. You may experience feelings of rejection directed toward your child. If this is the case, it may be help-ful for you to bear in mind that many parents, even parents of wanted chil-dren, are sometimes ambivalent about their role as parents.

The Adopted Child

As with the strongly wanted biological child, the adopted child comes as a special gift. If you have adopted your child because of infertility, then you may experience a double layer of grief or anger: first, because of your inabil-ity to conceive and second, because you feel "unfairness" that your adopted child has a disability. Alternatively, you may have knowingly adopted a child who was at risk for disability because you felt you could provide much-needed love and support. If this has been the case, then sadness because of your child's disability may be compounded by a sense of personal failure—that you somehow failed to avert the bad outcome you knew was a possibil-ity when you adopted.

Blended Families

The birth of a child represents the cementing of a relationship. If you or your partner have typical children from previous relationships, it may be difficult to avoid feeling that your relationship with your present partner is somehow weakened by the birth of a child with disabilities.

TELLING THE REST OF THE FAMILY

The simple answer to the question "What do we tell the rest of the family?" of course, is "Just tell them the truth." Unfortunately, life is often not that sim-ple because different members of the family may be at very different points in the grieving process.

What Do We Tell Our Parents?

During difficult times, we tend to fall back on our accustomed relationships with our own parents. If those relationships have been supportive and based on mutual respect, then it is relatively easy to go to one's parents for comfort and support in times of distress. If the relationship with one's parents has been difficult, superficial, or distant, then sharing the news will be much harder. Sometimes grandparents are actually the first to notice a problem in the child, but they may hold their tongues until their own children are able to see and respond to the situation. If this has been the case, then getting the diagnosis out in the open may represent an opportunity for the family to come together. Sometimes, however, grandparents experience denial themselves. They, like anyone who experiences denial, may urge you "not to worry" about your child, or they may challenge the validity of your perceptions or the competency of the doctors or other professionals who have diagnosed your child's disability. Supportive grandparents should be welcomed as allies. If they are unable to fulfill this role, then they should be kept informed but prevented from intruding on your role as primary caregivers.

What Do We Tell Our Other Children?

Children, even more than adults, tend to blame themselves when they sense that an event has upset the family. Children view themselves as the center of the universe. Therefore, they magically think that they must be responsible for anything that happens in their universe. This is especially true of preschool children. The first thing you may need to do is to reassure your other children that this did not happen because of anything they thought or did. (This advice may sound strange, until you stop to ask yourself the following question: "How many times have I tried to blame *myself* for my child's disability, even though the doctors keep telling me it was not my fault?") It is also important to tell your other children that the disability is not something they will "catch." Sharing your own feelings with your other children in a way that will be understandable to them is appropriate. "Mommy and Daddy feel very sad because your brother has a problem that we can't fix," might be the explanation for a preschooler. If your other children are a little older or when your preschooler is older, simple explanations for the cause of the disability, if known, may be appropriate.

Even more important, however, is your ability to convey to your other children that their feelings are *normal*—whether these feelings consist of irrational self-blame or resentment because of the extra attention you may need to give to your child with a disability. "It's okay to feel angry. Mommy and Daddy sometimes feel like that ourselves," is often the best response, even as you remind your other children that it is *not* okay to act out these feelings of resentment in ways that can hurt other people. Saying this may be difficult for you, but it is preferable to responses such as "How can you say that about your brother? Don't you know he has a problem?" The ability to listen sympathetically to your other children in this fashion is directly linked to how well you have been able to deal with such feelings yourself. If you are still focused on your own coping, you with find it hard to give your children the emotional space they need to ventilate their own feelings.

It is also important to have one-to-one contact with each of your children on a regular basis so that they know how special they are to you. To achieve this, you will need to manage your time and work on developing a network of supportive friends, extended family, and professionals to help you out when you need it. Finally, it is important to reinforce to your children that people in a family should take care of each other. There are many good books on this subject in the children's section of larger bookstores or the public library suitable for reading with your other children. There are also sibling support groups that may be helpful.

TELLING FRIENDS AND CO-WORKERS

Some friends and co-workers may be uncomfortable listening to you speak about your child with a disability. You can set the tone for an interaction by *briefly* mentioning the disability *if needed:* "Kara's gotten to love this playground. The other kids take turns pushing her wheelchair through leaf piles, and she draws pictures in the sandbox with a long stick." Or, you may discover a co-worker with whom you have more in common than previously suspected. If you talk openly, others will usually become more comfortable and able to talk with you and be supportive. Unfortunately, however, this is not always the case. The most important things to keep in mind are your own need for ongoing contact with others who *are* able to listen sympathetically and your effort to be nonjudgmental toward friends and colleagues who may seem uncomfortable hearing about your distress.

FAMILY HEALTH

It is important that each family member get attention and affection: Mother and father individually and together should spend quality time with each child or combination of children, and you and your partner should have time together without *any* of the children. In addition, each parent needs some "quiet time" to him- or herself. This may involve a hobby, a sport or other leisure activity, or time spent at a house of worship or with friends. Even if you need to tell yourself "I'm taking this break so that when I come back, I can be a more effective parent" (rather than simply say "I've earned a rest"), by all means do so!

"Should I go back to work?" is a question frequently asked by mothers. Experience has shown that mothers who feel personally fulfilled through their job or career make more effective parents than mothers who have sacrificed their own lives out of a sense of obligation that they "must" stay home with their children. It must be recognized, however, that child care is sometimes more difficult to arrange and that caring for the child with disabilities may place extra demands on the family's time and energy. Ideally, families should make work-related decisions together and share in the responsibilities of caring for the children.

OTHER SUGGESTIONS

Here are some additional suggestions you may find helpful. Celebrate your child's successes—all of them. This recognition is most important to foster your child's social, physical, and psychological development. And surround yourself with positive people who will do the same.

Learn about your child's disability. It is best if both parents go to meetings with the doctor or other health care specialists, especially when diagnostic information is given or treatment plans are developed. If you are a single parent, try to bring a family member, friend, or other advocate with you to help support you and your child and to help you remember the information you are given. If you think of questions before the visit, write them down and take them with you to the visit. Consider using a tape recorder during the session, and ask for a copy of the report generated from the visit. Read up on the disability, attend lectures, search the web, and ask questions.

Seek help when needed, even if you never did before, but be specific about what you need. Get involved in parent support and information groups through your child's early intervention program, the medical center where your child may have been diagnosed, or through regional or national programs specific to your child's disorder.

Learn about local and national organizations that can keep you updated regarding diagnostic and therapeutic information specific to your child's problems. Publications such as *Exceptional Parent* (a general magazine for parents of children with disabilities) and reputable sites on the web, such as http://www.familyvillage.wisc.edu and http://www.pacer.org, provide useful information (see the Suggested Readings and Resources at the end of this book for more publications and organizations). Remember, however, to cross-check information you get from the web because it is not always accurate.

Learn to be an advocate for your child; get active and speak out. Advocacy may include involvement with your local school or medical center. Work with others to benefit not only your child but all children with special needs. But be kind to yourself when you discover that you are very motivated and active at one time and not at another. These ups and downs are to be expected. Listen to your body and your spirit so that you don't overwork them.

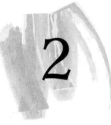

Making the Most of Doctor Visits

Susan E. Levy

In addition to a primary care physician (a pediatrician or family practitioner), your child with a disability is likely to require the care of one or more specialists (for example, a neurologist, a developmental pediatrician, an orthopedist, a neurosurgeon, or a psychiatrist). You deserve to have a primary care doctor who is interested in your child and who will direct care and provide a "medical home." This doctor should function as the care coordinator or team leader of the specialists, arranging for different types of treatment and monitoring your child's progress. Therefore, it is important to find a primary care doctor who is willing and able to spend the time that you and your child need, show sensitivity to your child's needs, and understand the treatments required for the best care for your child.

CHOOSING A DOCTOR

Many parents choose a doctor before their baby is born. Sometimes parents have developed a relationship with the doctor who cares for their older children. The birth of a child with a disability, however, presents special challenges for the doctor and marks a good time to reassess your earlier choice. You must feel assured that your child's physician has excellent clinical skills. Parents of other children with disabilities as well as organizations concerned with your child's specific disability can recommend pediatricians. You can also contact your state's chapter of the American Academy of Pediatrics, which has a list of pediatricians with particular subspecialty interests or training. Pediatricians interested in the care of children with disabilities are also likely to be members of the American Academy for Cerebral Palsy and

Developmental Medicine, the Society for Developmental Pediatrics, and/or the Society for Developmental and Behavioral Pediatrics. (See the Suggested Readings and Resources at the end of this book for contact information for these groups.) Many physicians belonging to these organizations work exclusively with children who have developmental disabilities. They often do not provide primary care but are still good resources as consultants or managers of teams of specialists who will care for your child. Many children's hospitals maintain lists of pediatricians who have an interest in children with disabilities. Compare this information with the list of pediatricians that your insurance program covers.

You'll need to assess other aspects of the physician's practice that are important to your child's care. Many knowledgeable physicians prefer not to care for children with disabilities or may be so busy that they cannot devote the time necessary to meet your child's needs. You'll also want to identify the kind of physician who best matches your family's communication styles and personalities. You may prefer a doctor with years of practice, or you may choose a recently trained pediatrician who may be closer to your age and experiences. You should find out about the doctor's availability during off-hours. Is the practice connected with a major pediatric center with subspecialist consultants that is 2 hours away, or is it associated with a community hospital that may not have all of the specific supports required by your child and family but is right around the corner?

If you already have a pediatrician for your other children, you may want to discuss with this doctor whether he or she feels comfortable taking care of your child with a disability. If the doctor feels he or she doesn't have the time or expertise to treat your child, most likely he or she will be candid and refer you to a colleague with a specific interest in children with disabilities.

A complicating factor in your selection of a doctor is the revolution going on in health care systems (see Chapter 27). HMOs (health maintenance organizations) are becoming the predominant form of health care throughout the United States because they offer a less costly alternative to the traditional fee-for-service medical care programs. A preferred provider organization (PPO) is a more costly alternative than an HMO but does offer you more freedom in choosing a physician. Because children with disabilities frequently have medical and therapy expenses that exceed the reimbursement limits of most HMOs, many middle-income families have qualified for and obtained financial support through federal programs such as Supplemental Security Income. You will need to check what limits your insurance company places on therapies and other medical services that your child may require.

Make sure you understand the limitations imposed by your insurance policy by reading the small print on the contracts *and asking* your agent when anything is unclear. You'll need to find out whether your insurance plan is accepted by the doctor or practice you would like to use or consider changing to a plan that is accepted. If you change plans, make sure that there is no clause excluding coverage for "previously existing conditions." You should also investigate which hospitals your child's doctor has a staff appointment with and whether your insurance plan gives you access to them. This information will help you make an informed choice regarding a health care provider. In some cases, you may have to balance expense against the quality of services offered. (See Chapter 27 for more on health insurance coverage.)

If you find that your child's current doctor doesn't suit your child's needs, explain your concerns to him or her. If you still feel dissatisfied or if the doctor is unresponsive or insensitive to your concerns, find someone else and don't feel guilty. It will be best for you, your child, and the doctor. If you have a managed care insurance plan, you may need to investigate limitations to changes (e.g., specified times for changes), and you will need to make sure to notify your insurance carrier of the change.

YOUR CHILD'S FIRST VISIT

How will your child's first visit differ from those of your other children? In many respects, the examination will be the same. The exact form of the exam, however, will depend on the nature of your child's problems.

To begin, the pediatrician may ask if you have any concerns. Take this opportunity to discuss problems that are troubling you regarding development, feeding, or behavior, such as "Why doesn't my son talk?" or "When will he start walking?"

The doctor will then take an extensive history of the pregnancy, the delivery, and your child's problems. The doctor will usually ask the mother whether she had spotting during the pregnancy, whether she was taking medications, and whether she has high blood pressure, diabetes, asthma, thyroid problems, or other chronic diseases. The mother may be asked if she drank, smoked, or used other drugs during the pregnancy. You may find some questions fairly personal, but they give the physician clues about the origin of your child's disability. Chapter 3 discusses some of the known associations between medications, illnesses, and disabilities. Most disabilities are not linked to diseases or to medications taken during pregnancy. Nevertheless, many mothers fear that they did something wrong during pregnancy that affected their child. Your child's first appointment is a good time to bring up any fears with your child's doctor.

The pediatrician will ask whether the labor was prolonged, whether the delivery was difficult, whether there was a premature rupture of membranes, whether a cesarean section was needed, and whether the afterbirth, or placenta, looked normal. Sometimes difficult deliveries deprive the baby of oxygen, which can result in disabilities. The doctor will ask questions about the newborn period to determine if your child appeared unaffected at birth. Were there any physical abnormalities? Information about your child's height, weight, and head size in the newborn period may indicate whether prenatal growth was typical. Low birth weight suggests that the placenta was not functioning properly and that your child did not receive adequate nourishment or oxygen before birth. Decreased head size may indicate prenatal brain damage or a brain malformation.

More questions about the newborn period might include the following: Did your baby have jaundice? Was oxygen required? Were there seizures or problems with low blood sugar? Were there infections? The doctor is looking for complications that may have caused brain damage. You may not know the answers to all of these questions, but the hospital record can fill in many blanks. You have the right to see and obtain a copy of that record. Interpretation of medical records is covered later in this chapter.

The next questions usually focus on what happened after your baby came home. Did your baby suck well after the first week? Many babies have a weak suck during the first few days of life, but infants who are overly sleepy, have a persistently weak sucking reflex, or have a weak cry may have a developmental disability. Was your child "too good"—quiet even when left alone for a prolonged period? Was muscle tone stiff, floppy, or normal? Abnormalities in tone often signal some type of brain damage.

The history taking will then move on to a listing of your child's hospitalizations, evaluations, illnesses, accidents, allergies, immunizations, and medications. Your own records and copies of records from past medical examinations can help provide this information.

Next, the doctor will take a detailed developmental history. When did your child begin to sit up, roll over, walk? When did your child coo, babble, say his or her first word? When did he or she transfer objects, self-feed? (Developmental milestones are discussed in Chapter 4.) Your baby book may help you answer these questions. But don't get flustered if you didn't write everything down or if you have trouble remembering. You aren't being graded as a parent by how many milestones you can remember. It is simply a way of determining when development became atypical. It also allows the doctor to determine if the rate of development has changed over time. Your child's doctor might ask, "Does your child appear to be better or worse than last year?" or, "How do you feel your child functions compared with other children you know who are the same age?" Parents are often surprised to find that after all of the testing is done, their initial guess at their child's developmental level usually turns out to be quite accurate.

For older children, a school history will be taken, including questions such as How long has your child been attending the present school? Is your child receiving special education services? Are you satisfied with the placement? Is your child happy at school? Have you signed off on his or her individualized education program (IEP)?

The doctor will then ask about your child's behavior. Does he or she have a short attention span? Is your child distractible, noncompliant, or hyperactive? Does he or she have sleep problems? Is your child aggressive, impulsive, fearful, or destructive? Does he or she follow directions well? Are there problems with temper tantrums, attention-seeking behavior, lying, or stealing? Does your child rock back and forth, thumb suck, tooth grind, head bang, or have other self-stimulatory or self-injurious behavior? How does your child get along with other children? Has your child received behavioral therapy or stimulant medications? With these questions, the doctor is attempting to determine the extent of behavioral problems and the steps that have been taken to treat them (see Chapter 11).

Finally, a family history will be taken to explore the possibility of genetic disorders that are more likely to occur in families. The doctor will want to know if other members of your family have similar disabilities and whether you and your spouse are related. These rather personal questions are asked to help pinpoint the nature and perhaps the cause of your child's disability. Recognition of a genetic basis for your child's disability can have implications for future pregnancies (see Chapter 26) and may also affect your child's treatment (see Chapter 16).

The Physical Examination

The physician will next perform a physical examination on your child. During the interview, the physician has likely been observing your child and forming some preliminary impressions about your child's activity level and appearance. The examination often begins with the head and ends with the toes, but the sequence varies from one physician to another. The physician or a nurse will measure your child's height, weight, and head circumference. By plotting these numbers on a chart, the physician can determine how your child's physical growth is progressing.

The physician will examine your child's eyes and may check whether your child can follow a light in all directions. Next, the doctor will use an ophthalmoscope, a magnifying lens with a light source, to look through the pupil at the back of the eye. The retina (the photographic "film" of the eye), the optic nerve, and the blood vessels in the eye can be examined to determine if there is a physical cause for any visual impairment.

Hearing may be screened by determining whether your child responds to crinkling paper or whispering or whether your child turns toward a loud noise. The physician will also examine your child's ears with an otoscope (an instrument fitted with lighting and magnifying lens systems). Scarring of the eardrum or fluid behind it may indicate a middle-ear infection. For a child with a disability, the physical exam should be followed by formal hearing and vision testing.

The pediatrician will listen to your child's heart and lungs with a stethoscope and will then feel your child's abdomen. Tenderness might indicate an intestinal problem. The doctor will judge the size of the liver and spleen because they may be enlarged in children with certain neurological disorders.

The doctor will examine your child's arms and legs to see whether they move easily and whether muscle tone is normal. By watching your child walk, by testing strength, and by moving the limbs, the doctor will answer several questions: Does your child walk or crawl typically? Are there any muscle contractures or spasticity? Are there unusual movements?

The doctor continues by testing tendon reflexes. This is done by lightly tapping against tendons at the elbow, wrist, knee, and ankle with a rubber reflex hammer. Usually the tapping causes a slight jerking of the limb; no response or a very strong jerk is abnormal. The doctor may also check for primitive reflexes that are present in newborns but usually disappear before 1 year of age, such as the rooting reflex, in which the baby turns his or her head toward an adult's hand when the adult strokes the baby on one cheek. These primitive reflexes persist after 1 year of age in children with cerebral palsy.

Medical Testing

After your child's physician has performed a physical and neurological examination, he or she may perform medical testing to further assess the disability. This section describes some of the more commonly used tests, but keep in mind that different tests are appropriate for different disabilities and that sometimes no medical tests at all are necessary. Some of the most common tests are the EEG (electroencephalogram), brain imaging such as a CT (computed tomography) or an MRI (magnetic resonance imaging) scan, chromosomal analysis, molecular analysis, and metabolic screening tests. Depending on the complexity of the test, results will take anywhere from 1 day to several months to become available. Call your child's doctor to have the test results interpreted for you. Don't just assume that the results are normal if you haven't heard anything. You will also have less anxiety once you know the test results.

The EEG, which is often called the *brain wave test,* looks for seizure activity in the brain and is not a test for mental retardation. Your child may be given a sedative before the test to induce sleep, which may bring out seizure activity. This test is described in more detail in Chapter 18.

Brain imaging studies are performed by CT or MRI scanning. The CT scan is a technique in which multiple X ray images are assembled by a computer into cross-sectional views of the brain. The MRI scan produces more precise images of the brain and uses magnetic force rather than X-rays. Both tests can show whether the brain is normal in size and assess abnormalities in brain structure. Most children with mental retardation will have either typical scans or images that show only a mild decrease in brain volume.

A chromosomal analysis is a blood test to study the number and structure of the genetic composition of your child's cells (see Chapter 26). Reasons for ordering this test include minor or major physical malformations or a strong family history of developmental delays or disorders. The chromosomal study requires about a teaspoon of blood and takes about 2–4 weeks for the results to become available.

In certain genetic disorders, such as Williams syndrome (see Chapter 16), the genetic defect may be too small to be seen in the chromosomal study but can be detected with a specific blood study for chromosomal microdeletions called *FISH* (fluorescent *in situ* hybridization analysis; see Chapter 26). Many other disorders causing developmental disabilities will likely be diagnosable in the future on the basis of specific errors or mutations in the DNA (deoxyribonucleic acid) using molecular diagnosis (specific DNA studies).

Finally, a metabolic screening test may be done on your child's blood or urine. The test detects inborn errors of metabolism in which an enzyme is defective or absent (see Chapter 16). The diseases that result—such as phenylketonuria, hypothyroidism, or maple syrup urine disease—can cause mental retardation and are treatable if detected early. The three disorders just mentioned are actually tested for as part of newborn screening testing in most states, but many other metabolic disorders are not routinely tested for in all children.

MAKING SENSE OF MEDICAL REPORTS

After all of this questioning, examining, and testing, your child's doctor will write a report. Like any other technical area, medicine has its own specialized jargon that may be difficult to understand. The following is a sample medical report for a child with a developmental delay, along with an accompanying translation that you may find helpful in interpreting what you read in your child's records. It is crucial, however, that you sit down with the doctor and go over your child's record so that you understand the important points and can ask questions. You may want to take notes as your child's doctor explains things. Most doctors are not bothered by this.

Sample Medical History

Chief Complaint: John is an 11-month-old white male referred by his pediatrician for evaluation of developmental delay.

Past Medical History: John was the 2.5 kg product of a 34-week gestation born to a 30-year-old gravida 2, para 0 mother by spontaneous vertex delivery after an 8-hour labor. The pregnancy was complicated by intermittent spotting and pre-eclampsia. Fetal activity was normal. The 5-minute Apgar score was 4.

Translation: John weighed 5 pounds and 2 ounces (2.5 kilograms × 2.2 pounds per kilogram) when he was born 6 weeks before the due date (40 weeks – 34 weeks = 6 weeks). His mother had two pregnancies (gravida 2), but this was her first live-born child (para 0); the other child was miscarried. The mother delivered normally, with the baby coming out head first from the birth canal without assistance (spontaneous vertex delivery). The mother had high blood pressure and protein in her urine during the pregnancy (preeclampsia). The fetus kicked and moved typically (normal fetal activity). At birth, however, the baby was not active and had trouble breathing. This accounts for the low Apgar score (4 out of 10), which measures activity of the newborn baby minutes after birth.

In the neonatal period the child's hospital course was complicated by RDS, and he required mechanical ventilation for 5 days. Jaundice was also present with a peak level of 12 mg/dl, which required phototherapy. At 7 days of age he developed lethargy and refused feedings. He was found to be septic with beta Streptococcus cultured from the blood and required intravenous antibiotics for 14 days. Ultrasound of his head revealed a Grade III intraventricular hemorrhage. This resolved over 2 weeks. He was discharged home at 1 month of age, feeding well and showing interest in his environment. He was noted, however, to have increased tone in his lower extremities.

Translation: In the first day of life (neonatal period), the child developed a breathing disorder common to premature infants called *respiratory distress syndrome (RDS)*. Treatment involved placing a tube down the windpipe and using a ventilator to keep the lungs expanded and filled with air (mechanical ventilation). Within days the lungs started to produce the chemical necessary to keep the lungs expanded (surfactant), and the baby could be taken off the ventilator. His liver was also immature, resulting in a buildup of the red blood cell pigment bilirubin. This turned his skin and the whites of his eyes yellow (jaundice). His bilirubin level of 12.5 milligrams per deciliter (mg/dl) was high for a premature baby, for whom a normal level is about 1–2 mg/dl. Because very high levels of bilirubin can cause brain damage, John was placed under fluorescent lights (phototherapy) to break down the bilirubin pigment. He also had a bacterial infection in his blood (sepsis) caused by the bacteria Streptococcus. Fortunately this organism was responsive to penicillin, which was given through a vein (intravenous) in his forearm.

The major concern when John was released from the hospital was that an ultrasound of his head showed some bleeding in the ventricles, or reservoirs, of the brain (intraventricular hemorrhage; see Chapter 5). This hemorrhage may have resulted from the sepsis or from lack of oxygen due to the RDS. Although repeated ultrasounds demonstrated that the blood gradually disappeared over a 2-week period, the hemorrhage placed the baby at risk for having cerebral palsy and hydrocephalus (enlarged ventricles due to an increased volume of fluid under pressure).

Developmental History: *Expressive language: John cooed at 4 months, babbled at 5 months, produced "da-da" at 7 months. Receptive language: social smile 4 months, understood "no" and played gesture games at 10 months. Gross motor skills: held head up at 3 months, sat with support at 8 months. Does not sit alone, crawl, or pull to stand. Fine motor skills: unfisted at 6 months, transferred objects at 7 months, developed a pincer grasp at 10 months. Mother feels most skills are at a 7- to 8-month level.*

Translation: John's language skills are developing typically, but there is a delay in his motor skills (see Chapters 4 and 5).

Physical Exam: Height 71 cm (10th percentile), weight 11 kg (50th percentile), head circumference 50 cm (greater than 95th percentile). John is an attractive child with an enlarged head; he seemed happy and attentive.
HEENT: No focus of infection. Anterior fontanel open. Intermittent left esotropia. Fixes and follows visually
Chest: Lungs clear
CVS: Heart sounds and rhythm normal without murmurs
Abdomen: Soft without organomegaly
Genitalia: Normal male with testes bilaterally descended
Extremities: Feet held in equinus position. Tone increased in lower extremities with clasp-knife spasticity. Achilles tendon could not be dorsiflexed to a neutral position.
CNS Examination: Cranial nerves are intact. Reflexes are 4+ in the lower extremities and 2+ in the upper extremities. Babinski sign was present bilaterally. The only persisting primitive reflex was the positive support.

Translation: When John was referred at 10 months of age, his height and weight were typical for his age (10%–50%) but his head circumference was very large, which suggested hydrocephalus. His soft spot (anterior fontanel) was soft as is normal, indicating that the brain was not under excessive pressure. There was no evidence of infection in the head, eyes, ears, nose, or throat (HEENT). The eyes were crossed (esotropia), which is common in children with cerebral palsy. Listening with the stethoscope to the chest revealed no abnormalities in the lungs.

The cardiovascular system (CVS) showed no heart murmur or other abnormality. The abdominal exam did not reveal an enlargement in the kidneys, spleen, or liver (no organomegaly). The baby's penis and testes were normal in size, and the testes were in the sac (descended). His feet, however, were held pointed downward (equinus) and the ankles (Achilles tendon) could not be flexed (dorsiflexed) to a normal walking (neutral) position. His legs were spastic with increased tone and would suddenly give way like a Boy Scout knife blade (clasped-knife). When the tendon below the kneecap was tapped lightly, the leg jerked briskly (4+ reflex). When the bottom of the foot was stroked, the big toe moved upward (Babinski sign) rather than downward as is typical at that age. All primitive reflexes should have been gone by 10 months, but in John, the positive support reflex was still present, meaning that he holds his legs stiff when an adult holds him under his arms and bounces his feet on the floor.

Developmental Testing: Cognition: Expressive and receptive language were judged to be at the 9- to 10- month level because he was able to say "ma-ma," oriented toward a bell, and exhibited understanding of gestures and "no." His problem-solving skills were also at the 9- to 10- month level, including pincer grasp. Motor: Gross motor skills, however, were delayed and felt to be around the 6-month level. He was able to roll over and sit with support.

Translation: John's cognitive (intellectual) skills were typical for his age, but his gross motor (sitting and walking) skills were delayed.

Diagnoses:

1. *Cerebral palsy—mild spastic diplegia*
2. *No significant cognitive delay*
3. *Rule out hydrocephalus*

Plans/Recommendations:

1. *Evaluation by physical therapist, occupational therapist*
2. *Referral to an early intervention program with physical therapy services*
3. *MRI scan scheduled for evaluation of suspected hydrocephalus*
4. *Return to clinic in 3 months*

Translation: All signs are consistent with a diagnosis of cerebral palsy. Because his legs are more affected than his arms, the diagnosis of spastic diplegia (spastic cerebral palsy affecting primarily the legs) was made. This is the most common form of cerebral palsy occurring in premature infants. In John's case, it probably resulted from lack of oxygen and decreased blood pressure around the time of birth, leading to a hemorrhage into his brain and damage to the part of the brain that controls leg movement.

John's intellectual abilities do not appear impaired; however, John may be at risk for further brain damage if he has developed hydrocephalus. If a CT scan confirms hydrocephalus, John will probably undergo surgery to have a drainage tube, or ventriculoperitoneal shunt, placed. This will divert the accumulating ventricular fluid into the abdominal cavity, where it can be absorbed. John will also be referred to an early intervention program (see Chapter 6). He will come back for reevaluations at 3-month intervals to make sure that he is making progress and that there are no new problems.

SUMMARY

You can best support your child by working with a medical team that will provide the expertise needed to treat his or her needs and that will give the compassion and engagement necessary to care for your entire family. This team may include a primary care physician (pediatrician or family practitioner), one or more medical specialists, and other health care professionals. You will also need to understand what is being done when your child is being examined and when tests are being performed. Learning to read your child's medical records, which you should retain copies of, will help you keep track of your child's medical progress. You should be an important member of your child's medical team, helping to make informed treatment choices. The more you know, the more you can take an active role in your child's care.

Some Questions Answered

How should I handle questions about my child's treatment?

If your child's doctor is unresponsive or doesn't have the time to answer your questions, consider getting another doctor! Doctors with busy practices may not schedule sufficient time for long explanations during a routine visit, but you should be able to make an appointment for a longer consultation during which your child's doctor can take the needed time to answer your questions.

What if I refuse to have a test done for my child?

A physician cannot perform any test on your child without your permission. In fact, for certain tests, parents have to sign a written consent form. Do not be afraid to decline a test if you are worried that your child may not benefit from it or that it carries significant risks. State your reason for refusing. Your child's doctor may be able to provide information that will allay your fears or may agree with you. In any event, you will have to make the final decision of what is best for your child.

How often should my child be examined?

How often your child goes for checkups depends on your child's medical problems. In some cases once every 6–12 months may be sufficient. In other instances, such as for a child who is having many seizures, biweekly or monthly visits may be necessary. Your child, however, should be reexamined at least once a year for the doctor to see how he or she is developing, to adjust medications, and to determine if any new therapies should be started. Generally, children are seen by the doctor less frequently as they grow older.

3

Why My Child?
Causes of Developmental Disabilities

Mark L. Batshaw

Every parent of a child with disabilities may ask at one time or another, "Why my child?" For some parents, an answer will help them understand the disorder, choose therapy, find a support group, or make decisions about having future children. But for many parents, there will be no answers or incomplete ones. In such instances, parents may expend much emotional and physical energy and money searching for a diagnosis. Sometimes the search for a cause can take precious time from the development of a treatment plan.

In general, the more severe the disability, the more likely a diagnosable cause will be found. Conversely, the majority of mild disabilities remain mysteries. This chapter discusses some of the many causes of developmental disabilities. These can originate before birth (prenatally), during birth (perinatally), or after birth (postnatally). You may discover answers to your questions while you focus on treatment.

Andrew

Andrew, a friendly and vivacious 6-year-old, had always been slow to develop, and his language was more severely affected than his other skills. He was diagnosed as having moderate mental retardation at 4 years of age and was also noted to have marked hyperactivity. His pediatrician explained to Andrew's parents that he wanted to consider genetic testing. The pediatrician also felt that Andrew had a somewhat unusual face, dissimilar from that of his parents but very similar to that of his 8-year-old brother Mitchell, who at age 3 also had been diagnosed with developmental delays. The brothers' faces were long, and their ears were large and protruding. Both boys had a heart murmur suggesting a mild problem in a heart valve. Because these brothers had similar delays and features suggestive of a specific genetic disorder, blood was obtained for a specific DNA (deoxyribonucleic acid) test for fragile X syndrome (see Chapter 16). Andrew and Mitchell were subsequently found to have fragile X syndrome. Although this knowledge did not open up any new treatment options, it did provide the family with information about long-term outcomes and encourage them to join a parent support group.

PRENATAL CAUSES OF DEVELOPMENTAL DISABILITIES

Most severe developmental disabilities have their origin before birth, either as a result of a genetic or a chromosomal disorder, exposure to damaging substances in the environment, maternal infections, or yet unknown reasons. With so many opportunities for things to go wrong, one might wonder not why so many children have developmental disabilities but why so few do. It is important to understand that although there are many causes of disabilities, each is so rare that the total number of children affected is small. About 95% of all children are born without disabilities.

Genetic and Chromosomal Disorders

Genetic disorders occur in the sperm or the egg and may affect the formation of the fetus or the production of a specific product needed for typical growth and development. The most common genetically transmitted developmental disability is Down syndrome. A second group of inherited disorders involves defects in a single gene within a chromosome (see Chapter 26). This can lead to production of less enzyme as is found in inborn errors of metabolism such as phenylketonuria, in which a toxin builds up that leads to brain damage if untreated, and in neuromuscular disorders such as muscular dystrophy, in which an important muscle protein is missing. Impaired brain development is the problem in another single-gene defect, fragile X syndrome.

Environmental Causes

Other forms of prenatal brain damage have an environmental basis. Certain substances taken in by the mother during pregnancy can harm the fetus; these are called *teratogens*. Susceptibility to the teratogen depends on the dose and timing of the exposure. If exposure occurs close to conception, it generally has an all-or-none effect; the embryo survives unaffected or dies. At the other extreme, late in the pregnancy, the teratogen may affect the size of the fetus or may precipitate premature birth but will not cause a birth defect. The most damage is likely to be done by teratogens in the first trimester, when the body organs are forming.

An extreme example of the effect of teratogens occurred in pregnant women who survived atomic bomb blasts in Hiroshima and Nagasaki. These women received massive exposure to radiation (1,000 rad or more). Those exposed shortly after conception generally had miscarriages early in their pregnancies. Those exposed around 2–4 months' gestation gave birth to babies with small heads and mental retardation. Those exposed in the third trimester tended to have babies who were born prematurely.

In contrast, medical X-rays expose a woman to very small doses of radiation; for example, a chest X-ray produces less than 0.0001 rad. Because it is unknown what amount of radiation is safe for the fetus, doctors generally avoid exposing pregnant women to medical X-rays, especially during their first trimester of pregnancy. Ultrasound and microwaves, unlike X-rays, cannot cause damage to the fetus.

Medications

A number of medications have been associated with fetal malformations. The most disastrous example occurred in the late 1950s when thalidomide was introduced in Europe to treat the nausea that can occur with pregnancy. Hundreds of infants were born with shortened limbs before the link with thalidomide was established and the drug was removed from the market.

Other medications, such as most antiepileptic drugs, have been shown to damage the fetus. Potential effects of these drugs include malformations of the baby's face, arms, legs, and spine, often with developmental delay. However, only about 10%–20% of children whose mothers take these medications are affected, and the effects appear to be more severe when the dosage is high and when medication is taken early in pregnancy. Anticancer drugs can also produce fetal malformations because they are meant to kill the most rapidly dividing cells, which are found in a pregnant woman's embryo as well as her tumor.

Vitamins generally do not cause problems during pregnancy, and multivitamins are in fact recommended for all pregnant women. However, massive doses of orally administered vitamin A contained in the acne medication Accutane (isotretinoin) and the psoriasis drug Tegison (etretinate) have resulted in face and brain malformations in infants.

Although there has been concern about other drugs, the medications just mentioned are the only ones in general use that have been shown conclusively to cause fetal malformations. Women should try, however, to take as few medications as possible during pregnancy, especially during the first trimester.

Substance Abuse

The drug most commonly associated with fetal malformations is not a prescription medication; it's alcohol. Approximately one third of women with alcoholism give birth to babies who have a spectrum of impairments called *fetal alcohol syndrome* (or its milder form, *fetal alcohol effects*), which may include mental retardation or learning and emotional disabilities, deformed limbs, a small head, and congenital heart defects. The degree of malformation depends on the amount of alcohol ingested, when it was consumed during the pregnancy, and whether drinking occurred in binges. No one has yet identified a safe drinking level; even moderate or occasional drinking may place the fetus at some risk. Until more is known, most doctors recommend that pregnant women abstain from drinking alcohol, especially during the early months of pregnancy.

Currently, there is no concrete evidence that marijuana or heroin cause fetal malformations. Cocaine and methamphetamine use during pregnancy, however, have been associated with shortened limbs and intestinal malformations, presumably because of constriction of fetal blood vessels. Heroin or methadone use by a pregnant woman may lead to a serious physical withdrawal state in the baby during the first week of life, characterized by episodes of hypoglycemia (low blood sugar) and seizures. Cigarette smoking has not been proven to cause fetal malformations but is associated with an increased occurrence of prematurity and low birth weight.

Multifactorial Conditions

In addition to purely genetic or environmental causes, sometimes interactions occur between heredity and the environment, as in cleft palate and in spina bifida (see Chapter 17). These are called *multifactorial conditions.* In spina bifida, an insufficient intake of the vitamin folic acid (an environmental factor) places certain susceptible women (a genetic factor) at an increased risk for bearing children with a birth defect of the spine. Even teratogenic effects of medications can be related to a genetic influence. The antiepileptic drug Dilantin (phenytoin) has been found to have a much greater likelihood of causing malformation in fetuses of women who have a genetically based deficiency of an enzyme that breaks down this drug.

Viral Infections

Illness in a pregnant woman, especially certain viral infections, can also affect the fetus, causing brain damage and related disabilities. Traditionally the acronym TORCH has been used to denote the most common such infections: *t*oxoplasmosis, *o*ther infections (including varicella, also known as chickenpox), *r*ubella, *c*ytomegalovirus (CMV), and *h*erpes. In the past, the most common virus causing fetal damage was rubella, or German measles. This illness causes only a low-grade fever and rash in the mother but can severely affect the fetus. Approximately one half of mothers infected with rubella during the first 3 months of pregnancy bear babies who have visual impairment, deafness, and usually mental retardation. Until 1969, when a rubella vaccine became available, epidemics occurred at 8-year intervals. Since that time, fetal rubella syndrome, which affects infants whose mothers had rubella during pregnancy, has become very rare. Women are now routinely given a blood test before they become pregnant to determine whether they have antibodies against rubella. If they do not, they are vaccinated and told to avoid becoming pregnant for 2 months. Even women who have become pregnant within several weeks of their vaccination have had unaffected babies.

Now the most commonly occurring prenatal infections are toxoplasmosis, CMV, herpes, and HIV (human immunodeficiency virus). Although there are no commonly used vaccines for these disorders, certain treatments can decrease the risk of fetal damage in some of these infections.

Toxoplasmosis is a rare illness, most commonly passed from cat to human, that can cause microcephaly (small head size), blindness, deafness, and mental retardation in 40% of children born to infected mothers. Treating the infected mother early in pregnancy with Rovamycina (spiramycin), Daraprim (pyrimethamine), sulfadiazine, and Leucovorin (folinic acid) has been shown to improve the long-term outcome for the fetus.

Chickenpox infection in the mother may also harm the fetus during the first 3 months of pregnancy, although the abnormalities are less severe and less common than they are with rubella, CMV, toxoplasmosis, or herpes. Limb or facial abnormalities and, less frequently, brain damage may result. A vaccine for chickenpox is now available but is not commonly used in adults.

CMV infections often do not cause symptoms in the mother but may cause malformations and mental retardation in the fetus. Some research suggests that 10% of all babies with microcephaly may have been affected by CMV infection of the mother during early pregnancy. Later in pregnancy, CMV infection may cause progressive hearing loss but not mental retardation in the fetus. Only a small fraction of fetuses exposed to CMV (perhaps 1 in 100) develop abnormalities. The high incidence of this infection in the general population has led to the development of a vaccine that currently is undergoing testing.

The herpes simplex virus can infect the baby before birth only if the mother develops a severe infection with a high fever and a rash. Cold sores and vaginal infections do not affect the development of the fetus. A baby born to a mother with vaginal herpes, however, is at significant risk for contracting herpes while passing through the birth canal. A generalized infection in the newborn can be life threatening and can cause mental retardation. Infants of mothers with vaginal herpes are delivered by C-section (cesarean section) to decrease their risk of infection.

The most recent concern for fetal infection is HIV, the cause of AIDS (acquired immunodeficiency syndrome). AIDS damages the body's immune system, leaving the affected individual at the mercy of infections. HIV/AIDS is primarily transmitted through unprotected sexual intercourse or through contact with HIV/AIDS-infected blood. Women who become pregnant while carrying HIV can pass it to their babies, usually around birth. Because the fetal infection begins late in gestation, it does not cause malformations but places the child at risk for developing AIDS during early childhood. The use of Zidovudine (ZDV, or AZT) therapy in combination with C-section delivery has been found to decrease the risk of mother–infant transmission. Breastfeeding is also discouraged.

Maternal Illness

Unlike the specific viral infections just mentioned, other acute viral and bacterial infections such as influenza, strep throat, and urinary tract infections do not damage the fetus. Thus, pregnant women shouldn't worry if they have a cold or fever during pregnancy and should also remember that after the first 3 months of pregnancy, malformations are unlikely to occur because the fetus's major body organs have already been formed. Research suggests, however, that in utero infections later in pregnancy may predispose the fetus to develop cerebral palsy.

In addition, certain chronic maternal illnesses place the fetus at risk. The most common of these are diabetes and seizure disorders. Fetuses of mothers with diabetes are at risk for a number of abnormalities, including spina bifida, heart problems, and malformations of the legs. Later in pregnancy there is an increased risk of toxemia (described in the next section) and premature birth. Good control of blood sugar levels appears to protect the fetus partially. At birth the infant of a mother with diabetes is likely to require treatment for hypoglycemia. With expectant mothers who have seizure disorders, the drugs used to treat the seizures rather than the seizures themselves appear to cause fetal malformations. Cessation of antiepileptic medication during the first trimester prevents malformations in infants born to these women. The risk to the fetus, however, must be balanced against the potential risk of uncontrolled seizures to the mother.

Other chronic illnesses do not cause malformations but do result in an increased risk of toxemia, prematurity, or growth retardation in the fetus. These conditions include maternal hypertension (high blood pressure) and rheumatologic disorders (rheumatoid arthritis, lupus, and so forth). As in diabetes, if the disease is managed well or is in remission, the outcome for the fetus is usually good. The drugs used to treat these diseases (other than methotrexate, used for rheumatologic disorders) are not teratogens.

PERINATAL CAUSES OF DEVELOPMENTAL DISABILITIES

Labor and delivery present a new set of potential challenges for the baby. Complications can arise during the birthing process that may deprive the baby of oxygen. This deprivation in turn can cause brain damage. Such complications include placenta previa, toxemia, premature membrane rupture, nonprogressive labor and cord prolapse, breech (backside first) delivery and twins, and prematurity.

Placenta Previa and Toxemia

Certain maternal conditions that develop later in pregnancy place the fetus at risk for brain damage; the most common of these are placenta previa and toxemia. Usually, the placenta, or afterbirth, is attached to the upper third of the uterus. In placenta previa, the placenta is implanted low in the uterus and partially covers the cervix, the entry to the womb from the vagina. When the cervix opens prior to delivery, the placenta may tear, leading to hemorrhaging. This can result in life-threatening fetal blood loss or hypoxia (insufficient oxygen transport). This requires emergency delivery, usually by C-section. Fortunately, ultrasound scanning can detect placenta previa before the onset of labor. Bed rest is usually prescribed so that the mother can carry the fetus as long as possible. Shortly before the mother's due date, an elective C-section may be performed to avoid tearing of the placenta during spontaneous vaginal delivery. Placenta previa occurs in about 1 in 200 pregnancies. The abnormality is more common in women who are older than 35 years of age or who have had multiple miscarriages or abortions. Smoking and previous C-sections also increase a woman's risk of placenta previa to some extent.

Toxemia, or pregnancy-induced high blood pressure, is most commonly found in pregnant teenagers and women older than the age of 35. Its symptoms are high blood pressure, edema (swelling), and the presence of protein in the urine. If left untreated, toxemia may lead to premature delivery, fetal brain damage, or stillbirth, which are a consequence of decreased oxygen flow to the fetus. Treatment for toxemia includes bed rest and medications, including magnesium, to control the mother's high blood pressure, but sometimes premature delivery is unavoidable. A milder form of toxemia is called *preeclampsia*.

Premature Membrane Rupture

Usually a woman's "water breaks" (the membranes surrounding the fetus tear, releasing the fluid from within the membranes) after the beginning of labor. When the membranes rupture before labor, there is a risk of infection. Thus, delivery is usually induced within 24 hours of the rupture, unless the baby has not reached full term. Delivery may be delayed in this case, but the leakage is watched closely and tested to ensure that it does not become infected. Infection necessitates immediate delivery. Otherwise, the infant may develop potentially life-threatening sepsis (a systemic blood infection) in the first weeks of life. The use of antibiotics and steroids before birth has significantly improved outcomes with premature membrane rupture by protecting the fetus from infection and stimulating the production of a surface-acting material (surfactant) that keeps the lungs expanded and reduces the fetus's risk of developing severe respiratory distress syndrome (RDS; see Chapter 5). If sepsis develops, it is treated with intravenous antibiotics; if RDS occurs, the baby often requires arterial ventilation on a respirator.

Nonprogressive Labor and Cord Prolapse

Sometimes labor does not progress because of cephalo-pelvic disproportion—the baby's head is too large or the mother's pelvis is too small to permit the baby's movement through the birth canal. If nonprogression is permitted to last a long time, the baby's oxygen supply will become depleted, placing him or her at risk for brain damage. To avoid this situation, the obstetrician will perform a C-section before the baby experiences a severe lack of oxygen.

In cord prolapse, the umbilical cord, through which the baby receives oxygen and nutrition from the mother, gets trapped between the head of the infant and the cervix and is compressed during labor contractions. This compression restricts the flow of oxygen to the baby and may lead to brain damage. Cord prolapse is another reason to perform an emergency C-section.

Breech Delivery and Twins

Breech (backside first) delivery is a problem because the baby may not move as smoothly through the birth canal as in a head-first position. Because the head has not been molded in the birth canal, it may get stuck or undergo excessive pressure during a breech delivery, thus interfering with oxygen flow to the brain. Twin or other multiple births are also risky, especially for the latter-born babies. The labor may last longer than usual, and the twins or multiples are often in breech position, complicating the delivery. Multiple births are becoming more common with the increased use of fertility drugs and in vitro fertilization. In these cases, selective abortion is sometimes considered to improve the outcome for the remaining fetuses.

Prematurity

Premature infants represent about 2% of all births. A baby born at full term has been in the womb for 40 weeks. Infants delivered before 37 weeks are considered to be premature. These infants usually weigh less than 5½ pounds, sometimes as little as 1 pound (about 500 grams). *Low birth weight* is the term used to describe infants weighing less than 2,500 grams (about 5½ pounds), and *very low birth weight* is used to describe infants weighing less than 1,500 grams (about 3½ pounds). These infants have more difficulty adapting to the environment outside the womb because their body organs are immature.

They may also suffer a number of biochemical and physical disturbances that place them at increased risk for brain damage. Among these problems are RDS and apnea (brief, periodic arrests of breathing) (see Chapter 5). Prematurity is the leading contributing factor in the development of certain forms of cerebral palsy (see Chapter 19).

ASSESSING NEWBORN NEUROLOGICAL FUNCTION: THE APGAR SCORE

At 1 and 5 minutes after birth, an Apgar score is assigned to assess a full-term baby's condition. Developed by pioneering anesthesiologist Dr. Virginia Apgar, the Apgar score gauges five characteristics: breathing rate, heart rate, skin color, muscle tone, and gagging reflex. Each is given a score of 0, 1, or 2; these scores are added to get the final score, with the maximum being 10. Scores of 6 or more at 5 minutes after birth suggest that the child has had a smooth labor and delivery; more than 97% of children with Apgar scores of 6 or higher develop typically. Although Apgar scores of 5 or below indicate some increased risk of developmental disability, more than 80% of these children also develop typically.

In fact, evidence suggests that too much blame has been assigned to labor and delivery as causes of developmental disabilities. A study by the National Institutes of Health showed that more than half of all children with difficult births actually had preexisting genetic disorders or malformations that predisposed them for birth injury. Thus, although trauma during birth may appear to have caused birth defects, the difficult birth may in fact have been the result of a problem that originated early in pregnancy.

POSTNATAL CAUSES OF DEVELOPMENTAL DISABILITIES

More than 99% of children who are born without disabilities will not subsequently develop severe developmental disabilities. Certain conditions that occur during infancy and childhood, however, may lead to brain damage. These conditions fall into four categories: metabolic disturbances, infections, traumatic brain injury, and lead poisoning.

Metabolic Disturbances

A newborn is at a greater risk for developing a severe illness than an older child is. The infant emerges from the protective environment of the womb and enters the outside world. A number of metabolic changes also must occur shortly after birth. For example, the baby's body must begin to regulate its blood sugar level. If this level drops very low, hypoglycemia develops, and the infant may have seizures. To prevent hypoglycemia in a baby at risk, extra sugar can be given from a bottle or intravenously. Although most children with hypoglycemia recover completely, severe and long-lasting hypogly-cemia can result in brain damage.

The newborn's liver also must start functioning to rid the body of toxins such as bilirubin, a yellow pigment released when the baby's fetal blood cells break down. If the baby's liver cannot metabolize all of the bilirubin that is released, the excess circulates in the baby's blood, causing the skin and whites of the eyes to take on a yellowish cast. This condition is known as jaundice. Mild jaundice is common and not dangerous. When bilirubin levels get very high, however, the toxin can accumulate in the brain, damage the nerve cells, and lead to cerebral palsy. To prevent such damage, the infant may be placed under phototherapy lights that help to break down the bilirubin into harm-less by-products.

Other metabolic disorders do not result from the usual transition from fetal life to infancy but instead represent an inborn error of metabolism. As noted at the beginning of this chapter, children can be born with a genetically inherited enzyme deficiency that places them at risk for accumulating toxins that cause brain damage. Some of these rare metabolic disorders are cata-strophic illnesses occurring in the first week of life that lead to coma and death or severe disability if unrecognized and untreated. Other disorders occur later in infancy or childhood as episodes of vomiting, lethargy, and behavioral and cognitive differences that can also cause developmental disabilities.

Infections

The newborn has an immature immune system and is therefore unable to mount an adequate defense against infection. An infant who is breast-fed is able to fight off some infections because of protection passed on through breast milk. But if this line of defense fails, bacteria and viruses that the body can easily handle in later childhood can cause a life-threatening illness. Blood poisoning (sepsis) and meningitis (infection of the spinal cord covering) are two examples of rare infections that can cause severe illness and subse-quent brain damage. Many of the metabolic and infectious problems already mentioned are an even greater threat to the premature infant than to the full-term infant.

Traumatic Brain Injury

Accidental and nonaccidental traumatic brain injury can also cause de-velopmental disabilities. These injuries range from accidents in the home (falls, drownings, poisonings), to motor vehicle accidents (passenger is not seat-belted or incorrectly seatbelted, pedestrians), to nonaccidental injury (physi-cal abuse, shaken baby syndrome, gunshot wounds, stabbings). Although these causes of disability are rare, they are also often avoidable. Providing adequate supervision and training of young children, using car seat restraints correctly (including placing children in the back seat and in safety seats), providing psychological services to families at risk for abuse, and advocating gun control legislation are some potentially effective preventive measures.

Lead Poisoning

Lead poisoning can be a major problem for families living in older homes because all paint manufactured prior to 1945 contained lead. When lead was found to be toxic to the nervous system, laws were passed prohibiting lead-based paint. However, the walls in older homes, although repainted, may have undercoats containing lead. Flaking paint and wall plaster in these homes can expose the lead and pose a serious risk for toddlers who often try to put everything into their mouths. Even minute amounts of lead can cause lead poisoning.

Mild forms of lead poisoning result in developmental delays, especially in language. Severe poisoning can lead to seizures and coma. If lead poisoning is discovered at an early stage, treatment using medications that bind to the lead and eliminate it can prevent brain damage. This treatment must be combined with a program to prevent the child from ingesting more paint containing lead: The child must be taught to avoid eating nonfood items, and the house must be made safe. With this in mind, programs have been set up in many older cities to help identify and treat affected children and to remove or encase lead paint in the homes. In some cities, funds are provided by the city or the landlord to cover these expenses and the cost of alternate housing until the lead abatement has been completed.

SUMMARY

A cause for your child's developmental disability is more likely to be found if the disability is severe. The disability may have resulted from an unavoidable problem that was present even before you knew you were expecting a baby. The physician is likely to perform tests to rule out diagnosable causes of your child's problems that were suggested by the medical history and physical examination. If no answer is found, you may be tempted to seek other opinions. Further investigations may be expensive in terms of energy and finances, and sometimes no answers are found. Researchers are uncovering new disorders and developing new tests each year, and if there is no answer regarding your child's disability at this time, there may be an answer in the future. However, having an answer is not required for starting the therapies and educational programs that form the basis for treatment of virtually all developmental disabilities. This treatment is most likely to ensure optimal outcomes for your child. The Suggested Readings and Resources at the end of this book can point you to helpful books, web sites, and support groups related to your child's disability.

Some Questions Answered

If a C-section is valuable in preventing brain damage during labor and delivery, why isn't it used more frequently?

C-sections are valuable for a number of conditions mentioned in this chapter, including cephalo-pelvic disproportion, infections, and placenta previa. However, they are used more often than necessary. Among the total number of deliveries, 50% are spontaneous vaginal births, 25% require forceps, and 25% are C-sections. Because only 10% of pregnancies are threatened by problems during labor and delivery, many C-sections are being performed for the convenience of the mother or the physician rather than out of necessity.

   C-section carries some risk to both the mother and child. The infant delivered by C-section tends to have "wet" lungs because labor contractions have not squeezed out the fluid present during fetal life. As a result, these infants may have respiratory distress during the first days of life. For the mother, the problems of C-section include risks associated with anesthesia, possible infection, and bleeding.

What medical tests might my child's pediatrician perform?

The most common medical tests are chromosomal analysis, DNA testing, blood and urine metabolic testing, and EEG (electroencephalogram) and MRI (magnetic resonance imaging) scans. Chromosomal studies look for an abnormal number of chromosomes or deletions or insertions within genetic material (chromosomes). DNA tests look for mutations in genes. Inborn errors of metabolism are tested for by examining urine and blood for accumulation of specific amino acids and organic acids. An EEG is performed to rule out a seizure disorder, and an MRI scan seeks malformations in brain development. Obviously not all of these tests are done on every child. Which tests are performed depends on the physician's differential diagnosis of the potential causes of the disability. As a result, your child may have many or few tests. Fortunately, none of these tests are painful to your child or carry a significant risk of injury.

4

How a Young Child Develops

Mark L. Batshaw

A human baby at birth may seem totally helpless but in fact is considerably more mature and requires less parental care than newborn animals of many other species do. A baby kangaroo, for example, is born while still a fetus and must spend months incubating in its mother's pouch. At the other extreme is the newly hatched turtle, which immediately goes out on its own to forage for food. Somewhere in between these two examples are human babies. Although they are totally dependent on their parents to bring them food and take care of their most basic needs, they can suck, move their limbs, see, and hear.

Humans have the longest period of "nesting" before they are able to live apart from their parents. This period of dependence varies with the abilities, experience, and education of the individual. Development of a child can be thought of as a path or a series of steps. Intelligence and motor development progress along similar paths, with simple skills preceding more complex ones. A child with developmental disabilities often follows an unusual pattern of development with certain steps missed and at a rate slower than typical. This chapter discusses the development of the central nervous system, Piaget's theory of child development, milestones of development, and developmental delay.

DEVELOPMENT OF THE CENTRAL NERVOUS SYSTEM

The brain of an infant has the same basic structure as an adult brain. It also has the same nerve cells, but these cells are immature, resembling bare saplings. Over time they will develop intricate branches, called *processes*, which make them look more like grown trees. Our ability to think arises from this network of cells and processes that intertwine and exchange information.

The growth of these processes causes the total size of the brain to double in the first year of life and triple by the second year. The typical adult brain weight of about 1 pound is reached at approximately 6 years of age.

During the first 6 months of life, not only do the nerve cell processes grow in size and complexity, but they also develop an insulating sheath called *myelin* that permits more rapid conduction of nerve impulses and the ready exchange of information between muscles, sensory organs such as the eyes, and the brain. As a result, a 6-month-old can perform more complex voluntary activities such as sitting, transferring objects from one hand to the other, and babbling.

Popular thinking previously held that newborns had poor eyesight, were unable to distinguish colors, and were incapable of learning. It has become apparent, however, that the newborn's learning capabilities were not fully appreciated. The infant can visually fix on the mother's face only minutes after birth. And newborns have color vision and show a preference for brightly colored objects. Newborns can also learn; in fact, they can learn before birth. Studies have shown that when a particular musical recording is played a number of times in the presence of the mother during the final weeks of pregnancy, her newborn baby will suck on a bottle to hear this same recording but not to hear other music. Furthermore, a newborn infant will suck to hear a recording of the mother's voice but will not do so to hear the voice of another woman. In other words, the baby has already learned preferences and has developed memory. We should not be surprised to find that newborns start out with such capacities; birth is a rather arbitrary time in human development. Development starts during fetal life, and new skills are gained throughout life.

Despite these intellectual gifts, the newborn is restricted in motor skills by involuntary primitive reflexes. Many of these reflexes are evolutionary, ancient, and protective. The infant "roots," or turns in response to a touch on the cheek in order to find the mother's nipple. This rooting response is connected to a suck reflex that allows the infant to grasp onto the nipple and draw milk from it. Other reflexes, however, may limit adaptability to the outside world. For example, when the baby's neck is jostled, his or her hands will shoot out involuntarily as if in surprise; this is called the *Moro reflex*. Imagine how difficult it would be to work or play if your hands were to shoot out whenever your neck was jostled! If a newborn baby's head is turned to one side, the arm and leg on that side extend while the limbs on the other side automatically flex; this is called the *asymmetrical tonic neck reflex*, or the *fencer's reflex* (see Figure 4.1). This action could interfere with rolling over if it were to persist beyond the first 4 months of life.

It is important to remember that both physical and neurological development proceed in an orderly fashion. Yet, that progression is more like a series of steps or rungs of a ladder than like a smooth curve; one step must be reached before going on to the next one.

Full-term infant
resting position

Asymmetrical tonic
neck reflex

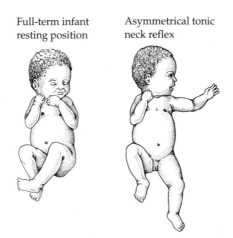

Figure 4.1.   Asymmetrical tonic neck reflex, or fencer's reflex. As the head is turned, the arm and leg on the same side as the chin extend and the other arm and leg flex.

PIAGET'S THEORY OF DEVELOPMENT

Children gain skills by a series of steps, so they may seem to rest on a plateau for some time and then suddenly hurtle to a new level. The 13-month-old baby who, after cruising around furniture for a few months, one day takes tentative independent steps toward his parents is but one example. One of the first to appreciate this pattern of development was Jean Piaget (1896–1980), a Swiss educational psychologist. Piaget's theory is useful in explaining developmental disabilities. He divided development into four stages of progressively increasing complexity of thought.

First Stage of Development: Sensorimotor

Piaget noted that prior to 18 months of age, in the period he called the *sensorimotor stage,* a child is incapable of solving problems. For instance, if the child loses something, he or she rapidly forgets it. If the child cannot see the object, he or she believes it has ceased to exist. Around 18 months, the child is able to conceptualize the problem. The child realizes the object has fallen and will search for it, knowing that it is somewhere in the immediate area even though it is out of sight. If the object is beyond reach, the child may use a stick to retrieve it. Furthermore, the child is now able to formulate a plan to attack a problem and coordinate activities to reach goals. The child, however, makes discoveries through trial and error and does not generalize successes to identical situations in the future; in other words, the child may forget what has been learned. Therefore, although a 20-month-old may finally figure out how to open a door by turning the doorknob after many attempts, the child may not remember the solution the next day but instead will follow the same trial-and-error steps used before to solve the problem.

Second Stage of Development: Preoperational

By 2 years of age the child can use language to control the environment and help solve problems. Piaget called this period the *preoperational stage of development*. The child can describe what he or she did during the day and can sing a song. The child will also ask "what" and "why" questions. Objects within the child's world can be described: A ball is round; a box is square. Thus, objects can be classified by their purpose. Opposites, such as *small* and *large* or *fast* and *slow,* are understood. The world can now be divided into subunits and understood more easily. But there are limits during this stage as well. The child is still not able to perform abstract reasoning. If water is poured from a short, wide glass into a tall, narrow one, the child says that there is more water in the narrow glass. The child also does not understand abstract concepts such as death or honesty.

Third Stage of Development: Concrete Operations

During the third stage of development, called the *period of concrete operations,* the elementary school student, 6–12 years old, learns to see complex relationships, permitting the study of academic subjects. The child is able to classify objects in sequential order according to size, weight, or time sequence. He or she can mix up panels of a cartoon and put them back in the correct order to form a story. At this stage, the child learns to solve simple arithmetic problems and to read. The child can also participate in debates, clearly stating a position although appreciating someone else's opinion. The child, however, still has difficulty dealing with hypothetical situations and abstract concepts involved in the study of science and higher mathematics.

Fourth Stage of Development: Formal Operations

According to Piaget, the final developmental period, called the *stage of formal operations,* begins at about age 12 and continues throughout one's life. Using imagination, the person is now able to project into the future and set up long-range goals. The individual is more sensitive to the needs of others and can also understand abstract concepts, isolate a problem, review it systematically, and test possible solutions. This permits the study of algebra, physics, philosophy, and other higher-level subjects. The adolescent is no longer gullible and no longer believes in fanciful stories.

The Developmental Ladder

In sum, Piaget said that intellectual development involves the addition of increasingly complex and abstract concepts at each step up the developmental ladder. Furthermore, an adult who has not progressed through all of Piaget's stages would be limited in his or her ability to function in the world. This person might be described as having mental retardation. The degree of severity of the mental retardation can be viewed in light of these developmental stages. In very general terms a person with mild mental retardation will pass through all but the final formal operations stage. Individuals with moderate mental retardation will not develop beyond the preoperational, or second, stage. And the individual with severe to profound mental retardation will generally not progress from the sensorimotor stage.

Piaget also suggested that there must be a particular level of brain maturation and development for a person to perform certain intellectual tasks. If the correct neurological organization has not been attained, no amount of practice will produce that intellectual skill. Therefore, although a child may memorize the words associated with pictures in a book, that child is not actually reading because the words do not carry contextual meaning for him or her. If the child is neurologically ready to learn a new skill, however, education will make a big difference. Without education, a child will not usually start to read or learn math independently.

Although intellectual skills require practice as well as neurological maturation, motor skills appear spontaneously when the child's nervous system has reached the proper level of development. You may have heard that children must learn to crawl before they can walk. It's not true. Traditionally, many Native American tribes routinely strapped their infants to papoose or cradle boards during the first year of life, preventing them from rolling over, sitting, or crawling. Yet, when these children were released from the boards around 1 year of age, they walked within a matter of days. They walked not because they had practiced more primitive modes of movement but because their brains had developed the proper circuitry for the skill. In sum, to move up the developmental ladder from one rung to the next, brain growth must take place.

Jennifer and Lisa

To illustrate the development of a young child, let us consider a family. Stacey and Philip have two children Lisa, age 6 years, and Jennifer, age 9 months. During her first months of life, Jennifer seemed to develop much more slowly than Lisa. At 6 months she had not rolled over, a skill Lisa had mastered by 4 months. Jennifer also didn't coo or make baby noises. She didn't smile until 4 months of age, whereas Lisa had done this at 6 weeks of age. At first Stacey and Philip thought they must have forgotten when Lisa reached these developmental levels. So they found her baby book and compared milestones. Jennifer's skills were developing but were delayed when compared with Lisa's.

Philip and Stacey were concerned but tried to put aside their fears. At Thanksgiving, however, when Jennifer was 11 months old, the extended family came together, including two cousins who were Jennifer's age. The cousins were saying a few words and walking with help, whereas Jennifer had just learned to sit and babble. Stacey and Philip decided they should see their doctor about their concerns. Their family doctor sent them to a developmental pediatrician who examined Jennifer extensively and confirmed that she had a significant developmental delay. At 12 months she was functioning at a 6-month level, or progressing at about half of the typical rate. They were told that if this continued, Jennifer would fall into the range of mild to moderate mental retardation. A 6-month follow-up appointment was scheduled, and Jennifer started in an early intervention program. An early childhood education specialist came to the family's home weekly to work with Jennifer and to give Stacey and Philip suggestions about infant stimulation activities. When reevaluated at 18 months and later at 24 months, Jennifer was making progress but was still progressing at half of the typical speed. At this time, she was diagnosed with mental retardation (see Chapter 14). At 3 years of age Jennifer began in a special education preschool program and has continued to add to her skills.

MILESTONES OF DEVELOPMENT

Developmental milestones will now be explored using Jennifer's sister Lisa as a guide. Lisa has progressed in a fairly typical fashion. It is important to understand that there is significant variation in the typical development of children. Independent sitting, for example, may emerge anywhere from 5 to 8 months, and a first word between 9 and 15 months. Also keep in mind that a mild delay in one aspect of development may not necessarily indicate a problem. A serious delay in even one area, however, may indicate a developmental disability. A delay in speech may result from a hearing or visual impairment, a delay in language and social skills may indicate autism, and a delay in motor skills may indicate cerebral palsy. Children with mental retardation have delays in all areas (language, motor, and social skills).

With this background, the different developmental milestones that Lisa passed through between birth and 6 years of age are now discussed. To help you follow the sequence of development, Tables 4.1 and 4.2 list important milestones from birth to 6 years, dividing development into four areas: gross motor skills such as running and walking, fine motor skills such as holding a block or pencil, language skills, and social-adaptive skills such as dressing. Remember that a child with a developmental delay usually follows this same sequence but does so at a slower rate.

The First 6 Months

Babies experience especially rapid development during the first 6 months life. At birth Lisa's abilities were limited to motor skills, such as moving her head from side to side and sucking, and to social skills, such as responding to sounds, looking at her mother, and crying. By 2 months Lisa demonstrated good head control (motor development) and could follow a mobile as it turned (visual development). Socially, she smiled and started to anticipate her feedings, actively kicking and gurgling at the sight of her bottle or her mother's breast. Her main communication skills were cooing and crying.

Lisa developed many new skills between 4 and 6 months. She rolled over from her back to her stomach and made swimming movements at 4 months. By 6 months she could sit briefly with support, and 1 month later she required no support at all. By 4 months her hands remained open much of the time rather than being clenched as they had been before. She developed other fine motor skills as well, including reaching, grasping, and shaking objects such as rattles. At 6 months, she could transfer objects from one hand to the other and could feed herself a cookie placed in her hand. She also helped hold her bottle. Her social skills included having a belly laugh by 4 months and enjoying a game of Peekaboo and "So Big" at 6 months. She could discriminate between her parents and other adults by 4 months, and at 6 months she could understand tones of voice and whether her parents were angry or happy. In the area of language development, she produced different sounds for different needs by 4 months; at 6 months her sounds became distinguishable as vowels and consonants, and she babbled "ba."

Six to Twelve Months

By 8 months of age, Lisa began crawling on her knees and could explore her world. She also enjoyed bouncing on her toes. At 10 months, her gross motor skills included standing with support and crawling with expertise and daring. Finally at 12 months, Lisa began cruising—walking around while holding on to furniture—and shortly thereafter walked without any support.

At 8 months her fine motor development involved exploring objects; she grabbed, twisted, smelled, tasted, and finally threw them. By 10 months Lisa could feed herself some finger foods. At 12 months she enjoyed putting objects into containers and turning pages in a book.

Lisa's social development also progressed. At 10 months she played many interactive games such as Pat-a-Cake and waving "bye-bye." At 12 months she began to take turns while playing with other children.

At 8 months Lisa babbled all of the time. Some of the sounds were "ma" and "da," although they were not specifically said to her parents Stacey and Philip. Lisa also understood the tone of voice when Stacey said "no" but did not always obey. By 10 months she said "mama" and "dada" specifically to

Table 4.1. Selected developmental milestones, birth to 2 years

Age	Gross motor	Fine motor	Language	Social-adaptive
Birth	Moves head to side, is dominated by primitive reflexes	Fixates on a face	Cries	Sleeps most of the time
1 month	Head lags	Follows 90° visually Clenches fists	Quiets to noise	Sleeps 14+ hours
2 months	Has better head control Lifts chin off mattress	Follows 180°		Smiles Anticipates feeding
3 months	Has less prominent primitive reflexes Lifts chest off bed	Follows 360° Holds hands mostly unfisted Swipes at objects	Makes cooing sounds Vocalizes more	Differentiates parents Chortles Pulls at clothing
4 months	Rolls from back to stomach Makes swimming movements	Grabs objects Holds hands at midline Shakes rattle	Produces different sounds for different needs	Has belly laughs
5 months	Rolls from stomach to back	Has raking grasp	Babbles and makes "raspberry" sounds	Frolics when played with
6 months	Rolls from stomach to back Sits briefly with support Creeps	Transfers objects between hands Holds bottle	Turns toward voice Imitates sounds Makes consonant sounds Differentiates "friendly" and "angry" voices	Searches for lost object Smiles at mirror

Age				
7 months	Bounces when standing Sits without support	Feeds self cookie Drinks from cup	Imitates noises Responds to name	Throws objects
8 months		Rings a bell	Understands "no" Says nonspecific "mama" or "dada"	
9 months	Crawls	Explores objects	Recognizes familiar words	Mouths all objects
10 months	Stands with support		Says specific "dada" or "mama"	Waves "bye-bye" Plays Pat-a-Cake
11 months	Cruises around objects	Has pincer grasp	Follows gesture command	
12 months	Takes first step	Puts objects in container Turns pages	Has two or three specific words	Takes turns
13 months	Stoops to pick up object Climbs Sits down from standing Dances to music	Points with fingers Looks for lost toy Puts cube in cup Stacks rings	Has three or four words in addition to "mama" and "dada" Looks toward named object ("Where's the ball?") Responds to name Obeys "Give it to me"	Uses trial and error to solve problems Plays responsive games Demands attention Has separation anxiety Has temper tantrums Fights sleep
14 months	Climbs stairs on hands and knees	Cooperates in dressing	Brings coat to indicate desire to go outside Names all family members	Indicates preferences in food

(continued)

Table 4.1. *(continued)*

Age	Gross motor	Fine motor	Language	Social-adaptive
14 months				Likes an audience
				Fears strangers and the dark
				Can play by self
15 months	Is in constant motion	Marks with pencil	Makes jargon	Gives kisses
		Spoon feeds	Follows one-step commands without gesture	Imitates chores
		Builds tower with blocks	Has four to six words	Negativistic
		Opens boxes	Knows one or two body parts	Indicates when wet
		Puts peg in pegboard		
		Pats textured objects		
		Pushes toy cars		
16 months	Sits on chair	Turns pages of book	Enjoys explanation of pictures in book	Hunts for missing parent
		Likes push–pull toys	Points to simple pictures	Plays in sandbox
17 months	Stands on one foot while holding on to something			Shows exploratory behavior
				Demands personal attention
				Is afraid of large animals
				Enjoys baths
				Plays Hide-and-Seek

Age				
18 months	Runs stiffly Tries to climb out of crib	Handedness is determined Scribbles Takes off clothes Puts pellet in bottle and pours it Unzips	Follow two-step commands Points to one picture in book Has 10 words—uses "no" mostly	Constantly plays with toys Uses stick to reach toy—has inventive solutions Is ready for toilet training Only puts food in mouth
19 months	Kicks ball	Builds three- or four-block tower Flushes toilet	Has 10 to 15 words Likes to be read to	Likes rocking horse Enjoys swings Pulls wagon with toys inside
20 months	Jumps	Throws ball Puts lid on box	Labels actions: "up" = pick me up Questions "what's that?"	Is possessive about toys Fears water (bath) Puts on shoes Washes hands Plays with pounding bench Engages in imaginary play—"tea party"
21 months	Walks up steps holding railing	Folds paper	Uses word combinations Uses echolalia Uses pronoun "I"	Likes bugs and other small objects

(continued)

Table 4.1. (continued)

Age	Gross motor	Fine motor	Language	Social-adaptive
22 months		Puts interlocking beads together Unwraps packages	Listens to stories Repeats nursery rhymes	Is starting to cooperate but tests limits
23 months	Walks up and down steps alone, both feet on each step Runs all of the time	Likes to fill and empty water glasses	Asks for food and drinks	"Reads" book to self Is easily frustrated
24 months	Walks backward	Matches objects Draws horizontal lines Turns on faucet	Associates names with familiar objects Has up to 50 words Distinguishes one versus many Communicates feeling using words and gestures Verbalizes toileting needs	Still doesn't share Isn't cooperative Avoids bedtime Engages in parallel play

Table 4.2. Selected developmental milestones, 2–6 years

Age (years)	Gross motor	Fine motor	Language	Social-adaptive
2–2½	Is accident prone	Turns doorknobs Has adult grip on crayon Unscrews lids Draws vertical lines Makes tower of five cubes	Utters two-word phrases Uses own name Points to and names many pictures Sings parts of songs	Is in constant motion Noncompliant—says "no" often
2½–3	Runs well Alternates feet walking up stairs	Improved hand–finger coordination Solves 6- to 12-piece puzzle Feeds self Takes off shoes and socks Draws a circle	Learns 50 words/month Makes three- or four-word sentences Gives full name Understands concept of *one* Follows three-step directions	Is bossy, moody Helps around the house Plays with others
3–3½	Stands on one foot Walks in straight line and backward Catches and kicks large ball Rides tricycle	Copies a cross Strings beads Fingerpaints and uses Play-Doh Matches colors Pours juice	Has approximately 900 words Repeats three digits Asks "How? Why?" Obeys prepositional commands (put the ball *under* the cup)	Is attached to primary caregiver Has nightmares Has improved attention Plays with dolls

(continued)

Table 4.2 *(continued)*

Age (years)	Gross motor	Fine motor	Language	Social adaptive
3–3½	Controls bowels and bladder during daytime	Undresses self Zips up	Describes actions in pictures Uses plurals and pronouns Enjoys *Sesame Street*	
3½–4	Hops Climbs jungle gym	Cuts with scissors Uses fork and spoon Puts shoes on correct feet	Makes four- or five-word sentences Likes stories and rhyming Counts to 3 Recalls events in recent past	Shares Develops playmates Has phobias Sucks thumb Begins sibling rivalry
4–5	Does forward rolls Jumps from height	Draws primitive picture of a face Copies some letters	Names nickel, dime, and penny Knows gender Enjoys jokes	Prefers children to adults Has imaginary playmates Seeks praise Likes sandbox Enjoys construction toys Dresses up as adult Washes self and brushes teeth

5–6			
Skips	Distinguishes right hand from left hand	Speaks fluently	Has Oedipal complex
Climbs, slides, swings	Draws recognizable picture of person	Knows address and birthday	Is independent
Catches ball	Copies triangle	Sings songs, tells stories	Fears death
Rides bicycle with training wheels	Copies many letters	Knows size differences	Engages in imaginative play
Dances	Prints name	Can explain what is troubling him or her	Can amuse him- or herself
	Sorts objects by size		

get her parents' attention. At 12 months, she developed a few meaningful words that only Philip and Stacey understood. Lisa began to follow simple commands accompanied by a gesture. For example, if she was holding a rattle and Stacey pointed and said "Give it to me," Lisa handed the rattle to her. As is usually the case, her understanding of language was ahead of her ability to express her own thoughts.

Twelve to Twenty–Four Months

Lisa's second year of life was spent refining the skills that she had started to gain in her first 12 months. Walking became more efficient. She no longer marched in a bow-legged fashion with her arms extended like a tightrope artist. By 13 months she could stoop to pick up objects and wiggle her body to music. By 15 months Lisa climbed stairs on her hands and knees. She started to run, could stand briefly on one foot, and could kick a beach ball at 18 months. At 20 months she could jump, and at 2 years she tentatively climbed steps and walked backward.

There were great changes in her fine motor skills during this same period. She started stacking rings at 13 months. By 15 months she would mark with a fat crayon, build block towers, open boxes, put pegs in a pegboard, and push toy cars. She also began to feed herself with a spoon and aid in dressing herself. She was clearly right-handed by 18 months and began to scribble. Improvements in her dexterity allowed Lisa to pick up a bead, place it in a bottle, and then dump it out. She was also an expert at undressing, sometimes performing this skill when her parents least expected it! At 22 months she enjoyed playing with pop-together beads and unwrapping presents. At 2 years Lisa was able to draw vertical and horizontal lines and could turn on the water faucet.

Her social skills similarly improved. At 13 months Lisa started to solve problems such as taking a lid off a box to get an object that was inside. At the same time, she developed anxieties, first of separation from her parents, then of strangers, and later of the dark. Although Lisa was able to amuse herself briefly, she preferred an audience for her antics. She gave kisses and imitated household chores, but "no" was also her favorite word. Between 15 and 18 months, her exploratory behavior increased. She could find novel solutions to problems, such as using a stick to get an object that was beyond her reach. Lisa enjoyed watching *Sesame Street*, playing in a sandbox, and engaging in Hide-and-Seek. Yet, her fears intensified, especially of large animals and, later, of baths.

The period of 18–21 months was a time of increasing independence for Lisa. She washed herself and tried to get dressed. She even showed some interest in controlling her bowels, although she did not become toilet trained until 3 years of age. Lisa's achievements included riding a rocking horse, pounding pegs into a workbench, playing on a swing, and pulling a wagon filled with toys. Imaginary games also appeared; she held tea parties and "talked" on a play telephone. She became increasingly interested in the neighborhood children, though she played tentatively and alongside rather than with them. By 2 years, she started to interact but not to share; "mine" was her most frequently used word. She was constantly testing limits to discover how far she could try her parents' patience.

Lisa's language showed perhaps the most startling changes during this second year of life. At 13 months Lisa had three or four words in addition to "mama" and "dada." By 15 months she started to use jargon, that is, to use sounds that simulate words but do not carry meaning. She knew the names of all of her family members, including Blackie, the cat. Additionally, Lisa used nonverbal communication, such as bringing Stacey her coat to indicate she wanted to go outside. At 18 months her jargon became interspersed with real words, and her vocabulary grew to 10 words. Between 18 and 21 months Lisa's vocabulary expanded to 20–30 words. She also labeled actions; for example, "up" meant "Pick me up" and "on" meant "Turn on the lights." She began to question: "What's that?" By 21 months she used the pronoun "I" and started saying a few word combinations such as "go out" and "want cookie." Lisa also echoed the last few words spoken to her by her mother. Between 21 and 24 months her vocabulary expanded to more than 50 words including a number of two-word phrases. She asked for specific foods, repeated nursery rhymes, and began to verbalize her need to go to the bathroom.

Lisa's understanding of language increased even more during this time. At 13 months Lisa turned to look at an object when Stacey said, "See the ball." She also obeyed simple commands, without an accompanying gesture. Stacey could now say, "Give it to me," without pointing, and Lisa would understand what her mother wanted. By 16 months Lisa could identify an object represented by a picture and enjoyed having Stacey read her a story about the picture. She also learned to point to her nose and to her bellybutton. At 18 months she could follow some two-step directions such as "Close the door, and then sit down." By 19 months she enjoyed having Stacey read complete stories to her. At 21 months she was ready for "touch me" books such as *Pat the Bunny*. Finally, at 2 years, Lisa distinguished the concept of *one* from *many* and other complex ideas such as *big* and *little*.

The Preschool Years: Two to Six Years

Lisa's motor skills became more coordinated and complex during the preschool years, although between 2 and 3 years she was still somewhat clumsy (see Table 4.2). This awkwardness, combined with an absence of fear and marked exploratory behavior, made her accident prone. She had many scrapes and bruises and on one occasion required five stitches. Her coordination improved between 3 and 4 years. She learned to kick a soccer ball, hop, climb a jungle gym, and ride a tricycle. Between 4 and 5 years she could do forward rolls and jump from heights. She delighted in showing off all of her skills, sometimes to the distress of Philip and Stacey. By 6 years she skipped, threw a ball, rode a bicycle, and danced.

Her fine motor skills improved along with gross motor functioning. Between 2 and 3 years Lisa learned to unscrew lids, turn doorknobs, feed herself with a fork, pour drinks, and partially dress herself. Improved eye–hand coordination allowed her to draw straight lines and circles and solve simple puzzles. Between 3 and 4 years she learned to draw a cross, finger paint, work with Play-Doh, and cut with scissors. Her dressing abilities improved, and she was able to zipper, button, and put her shoes on the correct feet. By 5 years she could draw a recognizable stick figure of a person as well as copy some letters and understand number concepts. By 6 she started to print her name and sort objects by size, color, and shape. She could also tie her shoes. She had the skills and fine motor coordination necessary for first grade.

Her social skills also improved. Between 2 and 3 years of age, Lisa had a changeable personality as is typical of this period called the "terrible twos." At times she was moody, bossy, and noncompliant. Yet, at other times she was delightful. She helped around the house and played quietly with other children. Between 3 and 4 years of age she showed an improved attention span and the ability to develop friendships with other children. By 5 years Lisa began to prefer the company of children her own age to adults, but at the same time she longed for applause from her parents. She was more able to care for herself; she could wash her hands and brush her teeth. By 6 years she was capable of imaginative and independent play.

The evolution of Lisa's language led to the expression of more and more complex ideas. Between 2 and 3 years she used short phrases and sang fragments of songs. When asked, she would tell you her name. She learned about 50 new words per month, and her understanding of language kept pace. She identified pictures in a book and followed complex three-step directions. Between 3 and 4 years, she asked her mother "How does this work?" and "Why is this?" questions, from dawn to dusk. She described actions performed in a picture, used plurals and pronouns (*we, they, he,* and so forth), and could answer questions about the recent past such as "What did you do today in nursery school?" Her sentence structure became more complex containing four to five words, and her vocabulary numbered well over 1,000 words. Lisa could also perform tasks involving prepositions, such as when instructed, "Place the block under the cup." By 5 years she enjoyed jokes and could differentiate pennies from quarters. By 6 years she had mastered more than 2,000 words. Her speech was now fluent and grammatically correct. She told stories and knew her address. When upset she could even tell her mother what was troubling her instead of just crying inconsolably.

SUMMARY

An infant is born with some cognitive abilities and much potential. The developmental sequence for each child depends on the child's capability, experience, and education. Development involves a sequence of steps leading to higher and more complex levels of understanding. Yet, until brain maturation has reached a point at which a child is capable of learning a certain skill, no amount of practice will result in the development of this skill. Intellectual skills, however, can develop from education and practice if the proper neurological circuitry is in place.

Some Questions Answered

When should I become worried about my child's development?

This is not always an easy question to answer. The difficulties of a child with severe developmental disabilities are evident in infancy. But there is a wide range of variability in children's development, and a child with a mild developmental disability may not be identified until entry into school. A slight delay only in one area may not be a cause for concern. However, a significant delay (more than 6 months) in even one developmental area should be investigated. When in doubt, have your child evaluated by a doctor—he or she may refer your child for developmental testing and, if a significant delay is found, for entrance into an early intervention program (see Chapter 6).

Certain clues can alert you to a significant developmental problem in your young child. An infant who does not awaken because of loud sounds or who is developing typically but does not utter a word by 12 months of age may have a serious hearing impairment. An infant who doesn't maintain eye contact with his parents by 2 months may have visual impairment, autism, or severe mental retardation. A child who does not roll over by 5 months or sit by 8 months or who develops an early preference for using one hand instead of the other may have cerebral palsy.

Should I believe the doctor when he says my child will grow out of it?

Many children who have mild delays in one aspect of their development will catch up over time. So, the explanation that "your child will grow out of it" may be appropriate. However, if you are still worried, if multiple areas are affected, or if your child has not "grown out of it" after 6 months or so, request a second opinion from a specialist who works with children with developmental disabilities. Depending on your child's delay, the evaluation may include formal IQ testing, a neurological examination, special education testing, physical therapy, occupational therapy, or vision, hearing, and language evaluations. This comprehensive assessment should either ease your mind that the problem is not serious or should direct you toward appropriate intervention to help your child. Don't wait long to get this second opinion because if there is a problem, early diagnosis and intervention are important.

If you have concerns, make certain that you receive answers that make sense to you. Trust your instincts as a parent; after all, you know your child best.

Who should perform the developmental evaluation for my child: a general pediatrician or a specialist?

Because your child's pediatrician or your family practitioner is the doctor who knows your child the best, start with expressing your concerns to him or her. If the physician is concerned that there is a significant developmental delay, he or she will refer you to a pediatric specialist such as a developmental pediatrician, a pediatric neurologist, or a child psychiatrist. These individuals' skills overlap a fair amount. For example, all three types of doctors have been trained to work with children who have learning disabilities, attention-deficit/hyperactivity disorder, and autism. The approach taken by each type of specialist, however, may be somewhat different. The developmental pediatrician tends to focus on the interdisciplinary care of children with different types of developmental disabilities. The child neurologist may focus more on diagnostic issues, whereas the child psychiatrist may address first the emotional and behavioral aspects of the disorder. Thus, in some cases more than one specialist may be needed. The referral that your child's pediatrician makes also depends on who is practicing in your community.

What is the difference between the terms *developmental delay, developmental disability,* and *mental retardation?*

Physicians use the term *developmental delay* to describe a young child who is slow in developing but has the potential to catch up. This contrasts with the term *mental retardation,* which implies a permanent and significant slowness in development. Mental retardation is one of the developmental disabilities described in this book. The term *developmental delay* is often used in describing a premature infant; it is rarely appropriate to be used for a child older than 2–3 years of age. Unfortunately, professionals often use the term *developmental delay* long after it has become clear that the child has mental retardation. It then becomes a way of avoiding the reality that may be painful both to the parent and to the professional.

Can you predict the rate of development of a child with cognitive impairments?

Often the rate of development can be predicted based on performance on an IQ test (see Chapter 14). A child with a typical IQ score (100) is expected to gain about 12 months of new skills each year. A child with an IQ score of 50 would be expected to gain about half that much in the same period of time. Thus, if a child with an IQ score of 50 is now 4 years old, he or she would be functioning around a 2-year-old level and would be expected to function around a 2½-year-old level when 5 years old.

How do I know the "mental age" of my child?

You can estimate your child's present level of functioning in a number of ways. If you have other children or close friends with children of a similar age, you can observe how your child compares. If you recorded your child's development in a baby book, you can compare the age at which he or she achieved specific milestones with the age your other children reached these milestones or with the typical ranges of achievement listed in Tables 4.1 and 4.2.

What can I do to increase the rate of my child's development?

As explained previously, it is not possible to change the speed at which the brain develops. There is no evidence that intelligence can be manipulated by practice. There is also no evidence that drug therapies, diets, or alternative medicine approaches have any effect on IQ scores. The teaching of skills when your child is ready to learn, however, may result in the accelerated gaining of new abilities. Thus, it is important to get your child into an early intervention program (see Chapter 6) as soon as a developmental delay has been identified.

You can help your child's development through play as well. Play is a child's work. It is through playing with objects, games, other children, and you that your child learns about the world and its relationships. Thus, having toys available that are appropriate for your child's developmental level is important. For example, your child will not be interested in playing with cars at 12 months but may become very interested when he or she is at a 2-year-old developmental level. Remember to have your child play at his or her developmental level, *not* at his or her chronological age level. Most of all, remember to enjoy playing with your child!

How much time should I spend teaching my child?

You are always teaching your child, even if you are doing it informally. When you describe the eggs or the juice to your 2-year-old at the breakfast table, you are giving information. When you take a walk and talk about the leaves on the trees, you are teaching about the world around you. If you set up a game between two children, you are educating them about sharing and taking turns. Your teaching rarely has to be formal, yet it is very important. Formal teaching can be left to your child's teacher or therapist, but the interactions you have with your child daily can stimulate and enhance his or her development in many ways.

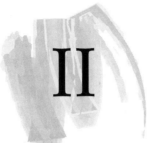

II

Growing Up
with a Disability

5

Your Baby Was
Born Prematurely

Penny Glass

A premature birth is any birth that occurs before the 37th week of pregnancy. Every year about 250,000 babies are born prematurely in the United States. Even babies born as early as 23–24 weeks can now survive. How early your baby was born is usually but not always a fairly good way of predicting the likelihood of medical or developmental complications. Most children born prematurely develop well but do have a greater risk of cognitive, physical, and behavioral difficulties than children born at term have. Rashad's and Sean's stories illustrate some of the complications faced by children who are born prematurely.

Rashad and Sean

Rashad was born at 26 weeks' gestation because her mother had toxemia (see Chapter 3). She developed respiratory distress syndrome (RDS) shortly after birth and required mechanical ventilation for more than a month. She also had a severe intestinal problem and an eye abnormality (retinopathy of prematurity). She had recurrent lung infections and poor weight gain, spending 5 months in the hospital. Despite all of this, Rashad has developed well.

Sean was born at 32 weeks' gestation following an abrupt separation of the placenta from the wall of the uterus. He was acutely ill within the first weeks of life but was allowed to go home from the hospital 6 weeks later when he was feeding well. His parents became concerned, however, when he didn't develop as well as initially expected. When evaluated at the follow-up clinic at 12 months, Sean was diagnosed with spastic diplegia, a form of cerebral palsy common in preterm infants. He responded well, however, when interacting with his parents and by 15 months said a few words. Sean had surgery to correct mild strabismus (crossed eyes). He is now a very verbal 3-year-old and is doing well in a typical preschool program. He still receives physical therapy and now walks independently.

PHYSICAL AND BEHAVIORAL TRAITS OF PREMATURE INFANTS

A number of physical characteristics distinguish your premature newborn from a full-term infant. These include a fine covering of body hair, a ruddy skin color, the absence of skin creases on the palms and feet, and the lack of ear cartilage and breast buds. Your child may lie in an extended position instead of in the more flexed posture of a full-term infant. Your baby's muscle tone also may appear loose, and he or she may seem less interested in the environment than a full-term infant is. Your baby will likely sleep most of the time. Around what would have been 32 weeks' gestation, your baby may be wakeful for brief periods, but even then, your baby may easily drift into a drowsy state. These differences lessen as your baby reaches the expected date of birth.

MEDICAL PROBLEMS OF PREMATURE INFANTS

A number of medical conditions occur mainly in preterm infants during the first months after birth. These conditions, resulting from the immaturity of their body organs, include lung disorders, ineffective breathing control, sudden infant death syndrome, brain injury, visual and hearing impairments, and gastrointestinal problems.

Lung Disorders

As with Rashad, the most common medical problem for the preterm infant is immature lung development, with RDS resulting. This condition arises from the lack of surfactant, a substance that coats the air cells (alveoli) in the lungs to keep them inflated. The decreased production of this compound allows the alveoli to collapse and makes it hard for the lungs to exchange oxygen and carbon dioxide. About one in five preemies develops RDS, and the risk increases with the degree of prematurity, ranging from 10% in infants born between 34 and 36 weeks' gestation to 60% for those born before 28 weeks. RDS was previously a fatal disease (John F. Kennedy's premature son Patrick died of this in 1963), but major medical advances since the 1970s have ensured that most children with RDS now survive.

There are a number of new approaches to prevent and treat RDS. Prenatal medication is given to a woman who is likely to deliver prematurely in an attempt to accelerate the baby's lung development. Shortly after birth, the deficient chemical, surfactant, is given to the infant through a tube in the trachea (windpipe). If RDS develops despite these efforts, life-support systems such as breathing tubes and respirators (ventilators) are used with supplemental oxygen to support the child's brain and other vital body organs. Usually the lung condition improves and the child can be taken off the ventilator and then off oxygen in a period of days to a few weeks.

There can, however, be complications with RDS. Although the mechanical ventilator and supplemental oxygen provide life support, they sometimes also damage the delicate lung tissue. This can lead to bronchopulmonary dysplasia (BPD), a chronic stiffening of the lung that interferes with oxygen exchange. BPD occurs in only a small fraction of infants with RDS. Treatment usually involves medications to decrease the causes of the stiffening, continuation of supplemental oxygen, and, in more severe cases, prolonged ventilator support.

If your infant requires prolonged mechanical ventilation, the breathing tube may be removed from the mouth and surgically inserted into the trachea through the skin at the base of the neck. The tracheostomy, or "trach tube," allows easier and safer medical care and more physical freedom for your infant. An infant with a trach tube can feed by mouth and interact socially. The trach tube is removed after the infant no longer requires a ventilator and after the risk for lung infection is sufficiently reduced.

Although most infants with BPD do not require a trach tube, they may need supplemental oxygen at home for a long time. Even after these infants no longer need supplemental oxygen, they are more vulnerable to severe respiratory infections during the first few years of life. For example, Rashad had two hospitalizations for pneumonia before she was 1 year old. By 2 years of age, a child's lungs have usually undergone a significant process of rebuilding and recovery, and the frequency of respiratory illnesses decreases. Many children who have recovered from BPD may develop a form of asthma known as reactive airway disease, which can last throughout childhood.

If your infant has BPD, he or she may experience associated developmental problems. For example, your child is likely to have muscular weakness, shortness of breath with exercise, and initial delays in motor development. This pattern generally results from your child's decreased activity and low energy reserves because his or her body is spending so much energy just to move the breathing muscles. Growth is also affected. Because lung growth is connected to overall body growth, adequate food consumption is very important to help the lungs heal. Yet, a high rate of breathing (more than 60 breaths per minute) may affect your child's ability and interest in feeding. High-calorie formula and smaller, more frequent feedings may help.

Infants with BPD cry more softly and tend to vocalize less during social play. This is thought to be the result of the competing need to control breathing. These infants' understanding of what is said, however, is usually typical.

Ineffective Control of Breathing

The immature brain does not control breathing and other muscle movement as well as the mature brain does. So, in a condition called *apnea,* a premature infant's brain may periodically and briefly "forget" to breathe. Longer episodes of apnea are accompanied by low heart rate (bradycardia). These episodes can often be prevented with stimulant medicine, such as caffeine. Episodes of apnea are very common during the first weeks after preterm birth but usually taper off as the infant approaches full-term age. Infants who continue to have episodes near the time they will be released from the hospital are likely to be sent home with an apnea monitor. If this is true for your baby, you will be trained to use the monitor and to perform CPR (cardiopulmonary resuscitation) in case your baby has prolonged apnea and bradycardia. Your child's doctor will advise you when to stop using the monitor, usually 4–5 months after what was to be your child's expected date of birth.

Sudden Infant Death Syndrome

Although sudden infant death syndrome (SIDS), also called *crib death,* occurs among full-term infants, premature infants are at an increased risk for this tragic occurrence. SIDS occurs very rarely and almost exclusively in the first 6 months of life. Research suggests that placing your premature infant to sleep on his or her back or side, rather than on the stomach, and avoiding smoking in the home cut this risk by more than half.

Brain Injury

Inadequate or absent oxygen supply to the brain, known as *hypoxia* and *anoxia,* respectively, may cause general damage to the brain in both full-term and preterm infants. Because of their immature brain development, however, premature infants have a more fragile network of blood vessels that supply the brain and are more sensitive to the physical trauma of birth, rapid shifts in blood pressure, and metabolic imbalances. Damaged vessels bleed into the ventricles, which contain ponds of fluid within the brain (intraventricular hemorrhage, or IVH), or into the surrounding brain tissue (intraparenchymal hemorrhage). If the region around the ventricles is sufficiently deprived of blood flow, an infarct (stroke) can occur and brain tissue may be lost (periventricular leukomalacia, or PVL).

Intraventricular and Intraparenchymal Hemorrhage   IVH can be diagnosed by ultrasound (see Figure 5.1) and graded according to severity. Mild bleeding (Grade I or Grade II IVH) occurs in almost half of all infants born before 32 weeks' gestation and generally has no significant developmental consequence. However, if the ventricles become engorged with blood (Grade

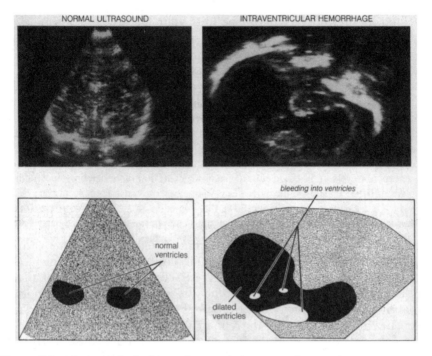

Figure 5.1.   Intraventricular hemorrhage as shown on an ultrasound.

III IVH), or particularly if the hemorrhage extends into the surrounding brain tissue (Grade IV IVH, or intraparenchymal hemorrhage), the baby's risk for developing cerebral palsy increases markedly.

In some infants, blood in the ventricles clogs the uptake of the fluid surrounding the brain and spinal cord and the ventricles enlarge significantly with fluid. This condition is called *post-hemorrhagic hydrocephalus*. If temporary, spinal taps may remove the fluid buildup or, occasionally, medications may decrease the brain pressure. If the hydrocephalus is prolonged or progressive, a neurosurgeon needs to implant a tube to drain the excess fluid (see Chapter 17).

Periventricular Leukomalacia   Approximately 5%–7% of premature infants develop PVL, the loss of brain tissue in an area that is next to the nerves that control muscle movement, especially that of the legs. The degree of tissue loss can be detected by ultrasound and more fully evaluated by CT (computed tomography) or MRI (magnetic resonance imaging) scan; the loss is designated as mild, moderate, or severe. PVL typically affects both sides of the brain, and early symptoms may not be evident until after hospital discharge. By 4 months past term, however, the infant with severe PVL is not able to maintain the head upright, has tightness in the hips and legs, has feeding problems, and/or is unable to keep a steady gaze. The full impact on development may not be determined until your child is 1–2 years of age or older. The motor impairment is usually spastic diplegia, a type of cerebral palsy in which the legs are predominantly affected (see Chapter 19). The probability that your child will have a learning disability is significantly increased, particularly with tasks that rely on visual-perceptual-motor skills. For some children with severe PVL, a form of cerebral palsy called *spastic quadriplegia* can also affect the arms as well as visual-motor and oral-motor skills. This condition persists throughout childhood and into adulthood. In more severe cases, general intellectual ability is often affected as well.

Visual Impairments

Retinopathy of Prematurity   The blood vessels on the inside back surface of the eye (the retina) are still developing during the last trimester and are susceptible to damage in the preterm infant. Retinopathy of prematurity, or ROP, consists of a disruption of retinal blood vessel development (see Chapter 22). Mild forms of ROP (Stage I or II) occur in the majority of infants born before 32 weeks' gestation, but the ROP usually regresses and normal retinal blood vessel development proceeds with minimal impact on later vision. In a minority of infants the retinopathy progresses to Stage III with an abnormal overgrowth of retinal blood vessels that could cause scarring or pulling of the retina. This is often treated with laser surgery, and infants who require laser treatment will be very nearsighted and need eyeglasses, as did Rashad, who was wearing eyeglasses by age 2. Some infants with Stage III ROP do not respond to the laser surgery and develop retinal detachment (Stage IV or V), which causes permanent visual impairment. ROP is the single most common cause of blindness in developed countries. The earlier in gestation the infant is born, the greater the risk of the disorder. Thus, all infants born prior to 32 weeks' gestation need repeated evaluations by a pediatric ophthalmologist until retinal blood vessel maturation is complete, usually around what would have been 40 weeks' gestation.

Cortical Visual Impairment   Cortical visual impairment (CVI) is a rare condition in the preterm infant that occurs most frequently in conjunction with severe PVL. The problem lies in the optic tracts, the nerves that carry visual messages from the back of the eyes to the back or occipital lobe of the brain (visual cortex), where the information is processed. Infants with CVI may initially respond to only light/dark differences and be unable to focus on a still object or follow a moving object. Usually visual function improves somewhat with time but does not become normal.

Less severe but fairly common among preterm infants and children are visual-perceptual problems. Visual perception involves the ability to discriminate, remember, and organize visual information. Visual-perceptual problems are part of many learning disabilities. (See Chapter 22 for more on visual impairments.)

Hearing Impairments

Preterm infants in general, and babies with BPD in particular, are at increased risk for hearing loss (see Chapter 20). Approximately 10% of infants discharged from neonatal intensive care units, or NICUs, may not pass their initial hearing screening, although the majority pass on follow-up. Infants who have BPD may be at increased risk for progressive hearing loss and should have follow-up testing even if they passed the initial hearing screening.

Gastrointestinal Problems

Gastroesophageal Reflux   Gastroesophageal reflux is a common problem in premature infants. It leads to abdominal discomfort, vomiting, and poor feeding and can place your child at risk for aspirating food into the lungs, causing pneumonia. This disorder results from the ineffective functioning of the muscular valve that keeps the stomach contents from backing up into the esophagus (tube to the stomach). This problem is worsened in a premature infant who requires a nasogastric (NG) feeding tube that prevents complete closure of the valve. Reflux may be lessened by placing your baby on the right side and elevating the head of the bed so he or she lies on a slope for naps and at bedtime. The reflux may also respond to thickened feeds (often using rice cereal), to frequent, small feedings (1–2 ounces at a time at 2-hour intervals), or to continuous drip tube feedings using an automated pump to regulate the flow. Many children often require medications as part of the treatment regimen (see Chapter 7). If these approaches are not successful in improving weight gain, decreasing vomiting and discomfort, and preventing aspiration, your child's doctor may suggest surgery that involves either the placement of a gastrojejunal tube (inserted through the skin of the abdomen and passed through the stomach wall and into the small intestine) or performing a Nissen fundoplication (wrapping the upper part of the stomach around the lower part of the esophagus to tighten the valve).

Necrotizing Enterocolitis   Necrotizing enterocolitis, or NEC, is a potentially life-threatening inflammation of the intestine that develops in 2%–5% of preemies in the first months after birth. Symptoms include a swollen abdomen, lethargy, and vomiting. This disorder is caused by a sudden decrease in the blood supply to the intestinal wall and may ultimately result in destruction of intestinal tissue. It may be caused by a bacterial infection, but in most cases the origin is unknown.

If NEC develops, the first treatment is to stop all feedings into the stomach and to provide or increase intravenous (IV) nutritional support. Medication may be given to treat the inflammation. Severe cases, however, require the rapid surgical removal of the damaged portion of the bowel, as was done for Rashad. Although usually life saving, in 10% of infants this surgery ends in the loss of a significant portion of the intestine, resulting in short-gut syndrome. This leads to difficulty with proper absorption of nutrients, poor growth, and chronic diarrhea. After Rashad's surgery, she experienced short-gut syndrome, and even when breast milk was gradually reintroduced to supplement the IV nutrition, she developed diarrhea. Her doctor switched her to a formula that is already partially digested. Although she was an avid feeder, Rashad was only allowed to drink small amounts at a time and would cry when the bottle was taken away. After 3 months of slow progress, Rashad's intestines healed sufficiently so that she could tolerate oral feedings and stop IV feedings.

DEVELOPMENTAL CHARACTERISTICS OF PRETERM INFANTS

Most infants born prematurely can be viewed as developing at a typical rate when their corrected or adjusted age is determined from their *expected date of birth* rather than from their actual birth date. You should use this adjusted age for monitoring your child's growth and development in the first 2 years. Preterm infants are more likely than full-term infants to have difficulty controlling the muscles of their body and paying attention. Social immaturity is also frequent during the toddler and preschool period, whereas learning disabilities are the most commonly reported finding at school age. The degree of prematurity and the type and severity of medical complications affect your child's development. Early evaluation and identification of developmental problems and, if indicated, early intervention services can attenuate the impact on your child's development (see Chapter 6).

Motor Development

Although the vast majority of preterm infants do not develop cerebral palsy, they often lack the smooth, rhythmic movement patterns of full-term infants. In the womb, the amniotic fluid and cramped uterine space provide resistance that aids in balanced muscle development. So, for the earliest born infants, muscles and joints develop in a very different environment. Your preterm baby may have spent several weeks in an isolette, which provides no resistance. As a result, your child may arch in a movement pattern that reflects muscle imbalance and makes him or her seem less cuddly. You may also notice that your infant likes to stand rather than sit when held on your lap. This is because early standing is a reflex, whereas sitting is a voluntary action. Difficulty in sitting may be a sign that your baby has increased stiffness in his or her hips or muscles in the back of the legs and may benefit from evaluation by a physical therapist. You can help by playing more while your baby is in a supported sitting position on your lap and by avoiding having your baby in a standing position. Devices such as walkers, exersaucers, and jumpers should be avoided because they encourage your baby to stand on tiptoe and walk in an abnormal pattern.

Visual-motor tasks that require the planned use of arms and hands also present more challenges for many preterm infants. Coordinating reach and grasp, scooping with a spoon, managing a standard cup, copying block constructions, and completing crayon/paper tasks can be more difficult to master. At school age, these difficulties may translate into frustration with writing tasks.

Cognitive Development

Your child's general cognitive abilities should develop at a rate typical for his or her corrected age. Fewer than 5% of premature infants are likely to function in the range of mental retardation (see Chapter 14), but this is still double the risk in full-term infants. Many preterm infants and toddlers, however, have difficulty paying attention. In childhood, the risk for learning disabilities (see Chapter 25) and/or attention-deficit/hyperactivity disorder (see Chapter 24) is in the range of 50% for infants who were born prior to 32 weeks' gestation, compared with 10%–15% for full-term infants. Subtle signs before age 4 may be harbingers of future school problems. Your infant may be more easily distracted from a task by something else in the room or by the *sound* of a voice (rather than the words being uttered). As a toddler, he or she may have difficulty listening to a story or organizing toys in pretend play. Your preschool child may have difficulty following two-step verbal directions, listening to a story in a small group, expressing feelings with words, or carrying on a conversation.

You can foster your child's cognitive development by emphasizing communication skills and social play. Early language develops around talk about common events, family names, and favorite things and through social interactions around daily routines and shared play. Talking toys, videotapes, and television do not promote your infant or toddler's language development, and how well your child watches television is not a good measure of attention span. Try to limit television/videotape time to no more than 30 minutes twice per day. Reducing distractions by having fewer toys available at a time and grouping toys that work together is a useful strategy to focus your child's attention. You can further support your child's developing intellect by encouraging efforts at listening, thinking, and problem solving. *No* evidence, however, supports the use of excessive forms of stimulation, such as toys with black-white-and-red patterns. In fact, longer attention to black-and-white patterns is a measure of *less* mature attention.

BEHAVIORAL ISSUES

The most common early behavioral difficulties that parents report are sleep disturbance, feeding difficulties, and tantrums or resistance to limit-setting. For toddlers and preschool children, the issues tend to revolve around social immaturity and activity level.

Sleep Disturbance

When you bring your preterm infant home from the hospital, it's helpful to think of him or her as a newborn and unlikely to have a good day–night, wake–sleep cycle. Your baby will likely need to be fed during the night for some time and may even need to be awakened to feed at first. Preemies frequently stretch and squirm during sleep and emit noises, seeming to be awake when they're not. Parents often report little sustained sleep beyond 2 hours at a time around the baby's due date, but as with full-term babies, the nighttime sleep period begins to lengthen around 2 months later.

You can help your baby sleep better by swaddling him or her and providing boundaries in the crib that cuddle like your arms. However, keep all covers, pillows, and soft surfaces away from your baby's face, and position him or her on the back or side rather than on the stomach. Both preterm and full-term infants at this age tend to be restless when the house is silent; a soft, steady background sound can help. Later your baby's sleep patterns will be more similar to full-term infants of the same (corrected) age.

Preterm infants are generally fussier when awake than full-term infants are. It is helpful to make sure your child is not overstimulated. He or she will be calmer if lightly swaddled when awake and will probably respond well to being held and carried. If your baby is very fussy, the pediatrician should check for medical causes of the fussiness (such as an ear infection), and you should have someone for respite or advice when you run out of coping skills.

Feeding Difficulties

The quantity of feeding receives considerable focus in the hospital, but if your baby is gaining weight adequately, the manner of feeding is often overlooked. Yet, oral feeding requires complex coordination. Feeding a premature infant is very different from feeding a full-term infant. Parents frequently say the early feeding experience is somewhat frightening because the baby may choke or even briefly stop breathing when sucking too eagerly. To avoid this, offer only small amounts of formula initially, and measure your initial success by your baby's effort and interest rather than by how much volume your infant consumes in a limited period of time. Once he or she comes home from the hospital, you may feel caught between wanting to be sensitive to your child's behavioral signals of fullness and feeling the pressure to push calories to maximize growth. It is natural for you to want your child to eat well, but pushing feeding excessively can lead to reflux, later food refusal, and picky eating that may persist beyond the time that your child needs to gain weight. Feeding problems generally respond to guidance and behavioral techniques but occasionally require medical or psychological intervention (see Chapter 7).

Acceptance of Limits

As your child moves from infancy to childhood, behavioral issues may center around your child's general acceptance of limits set by you. Parents of preemies, especially of those who have developmental problems, find it more difficult to maintain the behavior standards that they would for a full-term baby with typical development. Yet, inconsistency or avoidance of setting appropriate limits for your child can contribute to the social immaturity noted in preschoolers who were born prematurely and may impede your child's acceptance by peers (see Chapter 11).

Activity Level

Preterm children are at increased risk of being diagnosed with hyperactivity at school age (see Chapter 24). One of the early culprits may be the prolonged use of medications to prevent apnea (caffeine-related substances) and to treat reactive airway disease (Proventil or Ventolin [albuterol]). Another contributor may be the high level of physical stimulation used to encourage sustained movement in preterm babies, such as beds and seats that vibrate, bounce, swing, jump, roll, or spin in circles. You can reduce hyperactivity somewhat by limiting the number of available choices for your child, by reducing the level of sensory input and clutter in the living space, and by helping your child direct his or her energy toward creative play.

FOLLOW-UP PROGRAMS FOR INFANTS AT RISK

Many hospitals have follow-up programs for premature infants. These may involve medical and developmental specialists who evaluate and monitor your baby's development and consult with your family, your child's pediatrician, and the community early intervention program. The follow-up programs can assist you in identifying and resolving medical and developmental problems. Try to become informed about these programs before your child is discharged from the hospital; if your hospital does not have a follow-up program, ask for a referral in your county. You should also learn about early intervention programs that may be appropriate for your child (see Chapter 6).

Parenting Issues

The birth of a healthy, full-term infant is a time of celebration, when friends, family, and neighbors congregate around the baby and provide support and respite care. When your premature infant comes home, the experience may be quite different. Your child may need to be protected from contact with extended family and friends to avoid infection, and you may have little time to socialize because of the need to assume the unfamiliar and time-consuming roles of nurse and therapist. Over time, however, most families adapt, often with the help of a visiting nurse, a therapist from an early intervention program, or another parent who has had a similar experience. In addition, the extended family, especially grandparents, can be a great source of support.

In Rashad's case, her parents became adept at sharing the nursing responsibilities. Each day before work, Dad carefully measured the medication doses for the next 24 hours, marked the vials, and arranged them in sequence for his wife to give to their daughter. He mixed the formula and prepared and labeled all of the bottles for time of day. He maintained a daily log. Mom, who had taken a leave from her job, administered the medications, fed Rashad on schedule, recorded the amount consumed, and monitored her development. Initially Rashad's parents found little time to enjoy being with her, but as the medical issues began to be resolved, they felt more at ease and started to enjoy their role as parents.

SUMMARY

Medical advances since the late 1970s have markedly improved outcomes, but preterm birth does increase the risk for a number of medical and developmental complications. Close attention by your child's pediatrician, supplemented by specialists in NICU follow-up programs, can result in the early identification of developmental and behavioral problems in your child. Early intervention programs will help you encourage your child's motor and cognitive development. Although initially it may not seem easy to care for your infant, it will be incredibly rewarding to see him or her grow from being but a few pounds to becoming an active and healthy child.

Some Questions Answered

How long will my baby remain in the hospital?

The length of hospitalization depends on your baby's birth weight, gestational age, and medical complications. The discharge date is often based on when your baby can maintain a normal body temperature outside of the isolette and take in sufficient nutrients to gain weight. Stable preterm infants may be discharged home as early as 34 weeks' gestation. Most are discharged before their due date. As the date of discharge approaches, you will receive extra training to care for your infant's medical needs at home, which may include providing oxygen, operating an apnea monitor, administering medications, and using special feeding techniques.

How should I prepare our home for our baby's arrival?

In many cases, the preparation will be much like bringing home any newborn baby. It is important, however, that the house be smoke free so as not to irritate your child's already fragile respiratory system. You may also want to restrict the number of visitors to avoid exposure to infection. Keep the level of stimulation soft and gentle, and provide time for your baby and each immediate family member to get to know each other in private. It is a time for rest and recovery for the whole family.

When will my infant "catch up?"

The phrase "catch up" suggests that a premature infant needs to develop at a faster rate than if born at term. This is not a reasonable goal. Instead, a preemie whose pattern of growth and development is appropriate for his or her "corrected age" is growing and developing at a typical rate.

Does my child remember the pain experienced in the NICU?

Although a preterm infant reacts to pain by crying, like a full-term newborn he or she does not remember the experience as an older child might. Yet, it is true that even a preterm infant can be conditioned to respond by withdrawal or crying to an event such as touch, if it is repeatedly associated with a painful stimulus such as a needle stick in the heel. However, because an infant can "learn" this association, he or she can also "unlearn" it. That is, the infant can learn instead to associate touch with pleasure by its repeated association with a positive event, such as being held and fed. In fact, babies often seem less traumatized by the NICU experience than their parents are. It may be helpful for you to consider to what extent your child's behavior reflects his or her difficulty or your own difficulty in getting past the NICU experience. Professional resources are available and can help you sort this out.

6

Understanding Early Intervention

Sharon Landesman Ramey,
Karen Echols, Craig T. Ramey, and Wanda Y. Newell

Early intervention is a term that designates a systematic approach to early and continual treatment designed to meet the needs of individual children and their families. Early intervention is based on the belief that your child's lifelong development can be enhanced by the right types and amount of stimulation and preventive health care—coupled with specialized therapies, adaptive equipment, and medical interventions—*as early in life as possible.* The specific goals or hoped-for outcomes of early intervention depend on the specific needs of your child and family.

In the field of developmental disabilities, early intervention has been mandated through federal legislation. Services for children with disabilities were initially mandated under the Education for All Handicapped Children Act of 1975 (see Chapter 13). The Education of the Handicapped Act Amendments of 1986 provided additional funding for children ages 3–5 and funded the creation of a system of early intervention for children ages birth through their third birthday.

In 1986, the vision for early intervention was exciting and optimistic. Although many states had to start this activity with little experience, other states, such as Texas, Minnesota, Illinois, Maryland, and North Carolina, already had in place infant stimulation programs designed to provide early intervention for children and families. Systems for providing services to young children with hearing and visual impairments existed, and these programs were often expanded to serve a broader population of young children. Many major cities across the United States had programs for infants with disabilities, but these programs typically did not exist throughout a state before the Education of the Handicapped Act Amendments were passed in 1986. *As a parent, you now have many more choices and options to assist you in providing the best care and education for your child.*

Even though provisions exist for early intervention services nationwide, the early intervention system is complex and somewhat fragmented in many locations. The system is partially funded federally and supplemented with additional state funds. Thus, private insurance and Medicaid are often billed, and local programs must raise additional funds to make up the deficit in operating costs. Parents need to know this to understand the perspective and operation of many programs attempting to provide cutting-edge services with somewhat limited resources. This limitation, however, does not mean that the services of early intervention programs cannot fulfill the needs of children and their families. After reading this chapter, you will be better informed about your choices and how you can help your child realize his or her full potential.

SCIENTIFIC EVIDENCE FOR EFFECTIVE INTERVENTIONS

Some long-term research has provided evidence that early intervention supports and services are beneficial for many young children and their families. There is still much to be learned, however, about specific elements of programming and how best to provide services. Questions remain about which supports or services are necessary or optional, which ones are more beneficial, and what intensity of service is necessary for intervention to be effective. Parents need to look at evidence of effectiveness as well as think about their situation and the needs of their child.

Research on brain development supports the notion that good parental care, warm and loving attachments between young children and adults, and positive, age-appropriate stimulation from the time of birth benefit a child's development in positive ways. During a child's early years the brain has the greatest capacity to change and adapt with experience and stimulation. Thus, there is a strong rationale for providing very early supports to optimize your child's development. The law entitles you as a parent to be an equal partner with the professionals involved in making decisions about treatments. Because learning takes place best in a meaningful context and in an environment of love, trust, and support, a very young child usually benefits from intervention that is family focused and individualized. Although research shows that intensive programs often bring the best results for children, these may not be the best for your family because of your child's specific medical or social-emotional needs, the stress of meeting appointments, and the support needs of the others in the family may cause hardships. Group intervention may not be developmentally appropriate for a very young child or a child who is medically fragile. A balance must sometimes be achieved between the family's needs and those of the child with disabilities.

ELEMENTS OF EFFECTIVE
EARLY INTERVENTION PROGRAMS

The evidence from studies of children at risk for developmental disabilities confirms that the elements listed next are important in producing positive results for many children. Use these to guide your choices and activities.

- *The right timing:* Generally, interventions that begin earlier in development *and* continue longer benefit children the most. Specifically, intervention programs that start in the first 3 years of life and continue through school age have produced the greatest benefits.

- *Sufficient intensity:* Parents and children who participate the most consistently and support activities learned in intervention show the greatest progress. When intervention includes daily activities and stimulation, the benefits appear to be greater. Typically, many children have received only minimal early intervention supports that may not be sufficient to produce measurable benefits. Thus, parents must be ready to advocate a sufficient amount of services and supports for their children.

- *Direct engagement of the child:* Children who participate in early interventions that provide direct educational experiences show greater and more enduring benefits than do children in programs that only provide parent information and educational supports. Although home visiting and parent education are important, often additional direct services matched to a child's individual needs are necessary to promote his or her development.

- *Multiple types of supports and services:* Interventions that provide more comprehensive services to young children, including social, health, and educational services, have worked the best. Programs that focus on just one or two aspects of a child's development usually have not been as successful. Your child's needs, along with his or her strengths, should be considered when developing an individualized family service plan (IFSP).

- *Careful monitoring and responsiveness to individual needs:* Some children will make more (or less) progress from participation in early intervention programs than will other children. The reasons for these individual differences are far from clear, although undoubtedly both biomedical and behavioral factors are involved. Thus, careful monitoring of your child's progress in an early intervention program is essential, and vigorous efforts should be made to modify the supports provided to your child if results are not promising or if you see negative effects on your child or family.

- *Follow-through to maintain early benefits:* Over time, the initial positive effects of early intervention may seem to diminish. This occurs mostly when equally vigorous and high-quality supports are not continued. Parents also know that infants and young children show extremely rapid development, which may level off over time. Early intervention cannot be viewed as an inoculation that will ensure a child's continued success no matter what. Rather, positive learning experiences and needed supports must be sustained in later years. Parents must facilitate the learned activities in the child's other environments (such as with grandparents, at the zoo, or in the grocery store), or the child will learn to perform skills only in the context of environments in which the skills were taught. (Parents and children also benefit from breaks in their therapeutic schedules. Families can often use time to "regroup," but long-term therapy needs should not be ignored.)

- *Cultural appropriateness:* Interventions for children and families need to recognize and build on the family's cultural beliefs, traditions, and practices. When interventions do not respect cultural values and strengths, families are less likely to participate fully, and interventions are less likely to be effective. Please let the professionals you are working with know about beliefs and values that are important in your family.

TYPES OF EARLY INTERVENTION SERVICES

The types of early intervention services that have been funded by Part C (birth to 3 years) of the Individuals with Disabilities Education Act (IDEA) Amendments of 1997 are listed in Table 6.1. As you can see, they represent a broad range of supports. Some children may need only one or two of these services, most commonly early childhood education and family training or counseling. Other children with more significant or complex disabilities may require many of the services. In general, during your child's first 2 years of life, these services are provided in the home or child care environment, often once per week. IDEA establishes that services should be provided within the child's natural environment prior to age 3 years, which may still be the home for many families or a private preschool or child care center. Programs that group only young children with disabilities should consider including children without disabilities to provide a more inclusive environment for learning. Another provision of Part C is a seamless transition to services in the Part B school-based preschool program for children with disabilities. Early intervention staff and those serving Part B should collaborate and obtain the family's permission to assist with a smooth transition to school-based services. This process should begin when the child is 2 years of age and should be complete near the child's third birthday. The child is then covered under Part B of IDEA, which mandates its own range of services listed in Table 6.2.

HOW TO OBTAIN SERVICES

States are actually required to identify infants at risk for disability through Part C of IDEA. Most states have set up a Child Find program, often within a local health department or school district, to accomplish this. Your child's health care provider, your local public school, or the health department should be able to provide contact information. Often the health care provider

Table 6.1.   Early intervention and related services specified under Part C (birth to 3 years) of the Individuals with Disabilities Education Act (IDEA) Amendments of 1997

Services may include but are not limited to the following:

Assistive technology devices and services	Occupational therapy
Audiology	Physical therapy
Family training, counseling, and home visits	Psychological services
Health services	Service coordination services
Medical services for diagnosis or evaluation	Social work services
Nursing services	Special instruction
Nutrition services	Speech-language pathology
	Transportation and related costs
	Vision services

---

will contact the program directly for you, but a child can be referred by anyone who suspects that a child has a developmental delay or disability (parent, relative, preschool teacher, family friend). The program that you contact will need to know about your child and family and will ask questions related to your child's birth history and other details. An evaluation will be scheduled within a specified time, either at a child center or at your home, depending on the program and your preference. The teacher or therapist who evaluates your child will take a medical and developmental history from you, read any available medical records, and conduct developmental testing with your child. If a developmental delay warranting early intervention services is identified, program staff and other specialists will develop an IFSP with you to establish the goals and objective of the treatment plan. You will be asked to sign this document, and then early intervention services will begin.

SELECTING THE BEST OPTIONS FOR YOUR CHILD

Traditionally, parents relied on one or two professionals, often their child's pediatrician and a local therapist, for treatment recommendations. Yet, most pediatricians had no specialty training in developmental disabilities and often knew little about new support programs and early intervention options. Today, many more physicians are well informed, but the service delivery system is more complicated and ever-changing. To whom should you turn for up-to-date, reliable information? At least five very good sources of information can help you make choices about early intervention:

1. *University affiliated programs (UAPs) specializing in developmental disabilities* are available in every state and territory. These programs were estab-

lished by the U.S. Congress to provide information about developmental disabilities and supports to states and consumers. Many of the United States' more than 60 UAPs have developed excellent, current resource guides for families. To find the UAP nearest you, contact the American Association of University Affiliated Programs (see the Suggested Readings and Resources at the end of this book for contact information).

2. Each state has an *Interagency Coordinating Council (ICC),* an advisory group consisting of parents, professionals, policy makers, and representatives of agencies that provide or administer early intervention. The ICC in your state should be an excellent source of information about your options and legal rights (your state's UAP has contact information).

3. *Other parents,* particularly those who are active leaders in local parent organizations, often have the big picture and can provide very useful tips about how to proceed and where the best supports are in your community. There are many parent support groups that focus on particular childhood disorders and others that encompass a range of developmental disabilities. Parents in these groups can point to "weak spots" or danger areas in certain strategies or programs. Parent Training and Information (PTI) programs are funded by the Office of Special Education Programs of the U.S. Department of Education. These PTI centers provide training and information to meet the needs of parents of children with disabilities within the area served by each center. PTIs, coordinated by the Technical Assistance Alliance for Parent Centers in Minneapolis, Minnesota, can help parents to understand their children's specific needs, learn to communicate more effectively with professionals, participate in the educa-

Table 6.2.   Special education and related services specified under Part B (ages 3–5 years) of the Individuals with Disabilities Education Act (IDEA) Amendments of 1997

Services may include but are not limited to the following:

Assistive technology devices and services	Physical therapy
	Psychological services
Audiology	Recreation
Counseling services	Rehabilitation counseling services
Early identification and assessment	School health services
Medical services for diagnosis or evaluation	Social work services in schools
	Special education
Occupational therapy	Speech-language pathology
Parent counseling and training	Transportation

tional training process, and obtain information about relevant programs, services, and resources (see the Suggested Readings and Resources at the end of this book for contact information).

4. *Recent books and journal articles* concerning early intervention and your child's needs also provide useful information. Unfortunately, many public libraries do not maintain complete and recent acquisitions in this area. Instead, you are likely to obtain much better information by drawing from a combination of sources, such as on-line book services, information search services available through the Internet, or a librarian (media center expert) or skilled bookstore staff member who can help search for new publications. Many of the scientific and professional articles are written with highly specialized terms and professional jargon, and not all of these articles are directly useful to parents. Nonetheless, if you stay informed, you are likely to feel more confident about making choices. Sadly, however, parents receive secondhand information from newspaper or television accounts of "breakthroughs" that often are reported in very sketchy ways, oversimplify the findings, and obscure important qualifiers or caveats. One example is a report about nutritional supplements that might benefit children with autism, resulting in a huge parental demand for this treatment. There is not yet evidence about whether it is truly beneficial and not harmful.

5. *Professionals who are on the front line* are good sources of information. These individuals work directly with families and young children in the early intervention system. They often are aware of innovative methods and attend professional meetings where they hear news about promising new services, strategies, and supports. They also receive continuing education and have a reservoir of information from their own firsthand experience. Talking with several different professionals rather than relying on one or two usually works best. Try to visit exemplary programs or talk with professionals outside your immediate locale. This will broaden your perspective and may lead to new opportunities for programs and professionals. Be sure to inquire about how long a professional has been working in the field, where he or she received training, and how many children and families like yours the person has worked with. Asking this does not mean that it is better to get advice either from very young or older professionals; rather, it helps you to place his or her opinions in the context of his or her experience and background.

MONITORING YOUR CHILD'S PROGRESS

One of the most important things you can do is to maintain careful diaries, calendars, and folders with information about your child's progress, as well as to keep a copy of all medical records and reports. Once you have established goals for your child, be sure to watch for progress toward each of them. An important finding that appears in survey after survey is that almost all parents are very pleased or satisfied with the early intervention services they receive. This is good news but may reflect that most parents do not have a clear standard for measuring the services their child and family receive. Working with friendly and positive people is not enough—nor is simply the availability of a program for your child (even a popular program with a good reputation) adequate to ensure that your child is making optimal progress. Be vigilant while also being appreciative of those who are supporting your child's growth and development. Just as parent involvement is recognized as a vital force in children's school success, it also can make a big difference in how much children benefit from early intervention.

Tim Jr. and Angela

Sue and Tim Warren are the parents of a handsome little boy, Tim Jr., who was diagnosed with autism at the age of 18 months. Tim's father is a psychiatrist and his mother is a psychologist, and both had worked professionally with children with autism. Yet, when this became a personal experience, they were both devastated and overwhelmed—and they realized that even with all of their professional training and experience, they still had a lot to learn about how to really help their son on a daily basis. They developed an ambitious early intervention and treatment plan but found they could not locate the level of services and the trained staff they needed to carry out their plan. This led to much frustration initially. Indeed, the Warrens became parent advocates in order to help create the services they so desperately needed and to be sure that other families like theirs would have assistance. They worked with a local AmeriCorps program and also contacted the leading university-based clinics in their city to let the professionals know more about the inadequacy of early intervention services. Their son is now in elementary school in an inclusive classroom—not an easy task, but one that has many benefits for their son, their family, and the other children in the classroom. The Warrens also realize the need to better train professionals to understand the personal experience of having a child with a serious developmental disorder.

Cindy's youngest daughter, Angela, now age 3, was born with Down syndrome. Because Cindy was older than 40 when she was pregnant, she had an amniocentesis early in pregnancy. The test results indicated that her baby might be born with a disability, and Cindy was given a choice of having an elective abortion. She and her husband never considered the abortion seriously and were prepared to learn all they could about their daughter's needs. Tragically, Angela's father was killed in an automobile accident when she was only an infant. Cindy had to return to work to help support her family. Finding a high-quality child care center that would accept her daughter and making time for the many special therapy appointments and Angela's two operations have been huge challenges for Cindy. The early intervention system in the state has been exceptionally supportive and provided in-home respite care while Angela was recuperating from her operations. Cindy joined a parent support group, an idea she had rejected at first, and it has been very helpful. Angela's older brothers and sisters have gotten to know other families, and one sister and brother already plan to become health care practitioners to help children with special needs. The family considers Angela a special blessing and remembers how much joy she brought to her father. The early intervention service that meant the very most to this family was physical therapy. Because the physical therapist met with Angela twice a week, every week, for the first 2 years of her life, everyone in the family felt they had a real friend and cheerleader who helped them see that Angela was truly an individual child—and that her motor delays could be lessened if the whole family encouraged Angela to do things on her own and stay active.

SUMMARY

The early intervention system believes you are the most important team member in your child's development—the one who knows your child best and who has the greatest responsibility for your child's well-being. Many parents are overwhelmed by this responsibility at first—and by the undeniable extra burden of time and effort needed to meet their young child's needs. At the same time, research shows increasing proof that families report many unexpected benefits associated with having a child with disabilities. These include a greater appreciation for the meaning of life, a sense of greater connections to others (parents, extended family), and a true enjoyment of their child as an individual. Spiritual and religious beliefs and supports, a sense of optimism, and social support all factor into the equation for positive coping.

One of the most important lessons that parents learn—some earlier, some later—is that a great deal of what makes for effective parenting with their child with disabilities is, in fact, the same as what leads to good parenting for all children. Being responsive and attentive, encouraging independence and new learning, praising positive behavior, and preventing or eliminating negative behavior are all needed regardless of your child's exact rate or type of development. Be sure to maintain a healthy balance in your child's life, and build on his or her strengths and positive features while you also address areas of weakness. In the long run, social and emotional development are as important, or more important, in determining the quality of life for a child with disabilities as intelligence and motor abilities have been.

All children need lots of the essential ingredients in their everyday lives (encouragement, mentoring, celebration, rehearsal, protection, communication, and guidance). These essentials apply just as much to children who are at risk or who have differences in their development as they do to children who are developing typically.

Some Questions Answered

Who will provide early intervention services?

The professionals you encounter as active participants in early intervention may include pediatricians, pediatric neurologists, developmental pediatricians, physical therapists, speech-language therapists, social workers, psychologists, special education teachers, occupational therapists, audiologists, optometrists and ophthalmologists, nurses, nutritionists, and specialists who have received interdisciplinary or multidisciplinary training. To coordinate your child's and family's needs and the many professionals involved in your child's care, a case manager or service coordinator is usually assigned to help you, or you may become your family's own case manager.

How is early intervention eligibility determined by the states?

Federal legislation gives states the right to specify services by diagnoses, such as Down syndrome, cerebral palsy, or spina bifida, or by specific performance criteria. Remember that different states do not always agree about which risk conditions, such as prematurity or very low birth weight, should qualify children to receive vigorous early intervention! These decisions are somewhat influenced by politics and money; a state's cutoff point for defining a disability or a developmental delay has a direct impact on the number of children served. Thus, some toddlers with mild to moderate developmental delays are likely to be judged ineligible in many parts of the country. The 1997 amendments to IDEA encourage but do not require states to expand opportunities for some children identified as at risk and their families rather than to meet an arbitrary, strict deficit criteria.

The eligibility criteria for who is entitled to enroll in an early intervention program vary from state to state. So, many infants and toddlers who are eligible to receive services in one state may not qualify in another state, and the number and intensity of services may vary. If you move to another state, the National Information Center for Children and Youth with Disabilities (see the Suggested Readings and Resources for Chapter 1 at the end of the book for contact information) can provide assistance regarding services available in that state.

How will my child's need for early intervention be assessed?

Almost all assessment involves tests or procedures to determine a child's mental development and performance in areas such as motor development, social-emotional development, language, and cognition. The results of these assessments are critical for determining eligibility, making program decisions, and recommending action. Many programs use a play-based assessment that may appear to be informal. The assessment team, however, gains a great deal of information during this activity and often relies on information that parents provide as well.

How important is a diagnosis for obtaining early intervention services?

A criticism of medicine and other health-related disciplines is that diagnosis is often problem-centered or is focused on a child's deficits. Many parents have learned, though, that their child is much more than a diagnosis. Furthermore, professionals do not always agree on a child's diagnosis, especially if he or she has more than one sign or symptom and if the child's own behavior or health fluctuates. Professionals often check and then rule out the possibility that a child has one or more of a large number of rare conditions. This is responsible and worthwhile because detecting these conditions may lead to specific treatments or supports. At other times, however, many days, weeks, or months of assessment do not lead to any greater understanding of the nature or the cause of a child's exceptionality in development. The vast majority of children in early intervention do *not* ever have a single or a clearly confirmed diagnosis that identifies either a cause or a highly specific course of treatment.

Can professionals make predictions about my child's future?

A professional's best guess about what the future will hold for a given child is not always accurate. Today, many professionals admit to parents that they cannot, with any degree of confidence, predict what a child is likely to be able to do or what a child's later health and development will be like. So many factors determine a child's future that making predictions is very difficult. In the past, a prognosis (prediction about future health and development) given following a diagnosis often became a self-fulfilling prophecy. Each child is truly unique, and this uniqueness is in no way altered by the fact that he or she develops differently than what is considered typical. Parents of typically developing toddlers cannot predict with any certainty their children's futures. Remember also that challenges in your child's life can be healthy learning experiences, and that your support and encouragement nurture your child's well-being in the face of difficult situations.

What is an IFSP?

An individualized family service (IFSP) plan is required to be developed *before* any services can be provided. The process of developing an IFSP involves the family and professionals, who work together to identify the primary needs of the child and the family and what services and supports are best suited to meet these needs. Early intervention services consider family as the primary source for a child's learning experiences and overall well-being. The family is ultimately responsible for decision making on the behalf of the child, thus, the family should have an active voice in determining IFSP goals. Families might need support in order to assist their child with disabilities, therefore, the IFSP includes provisions for direct services for a child and his or her family.

Typically, an IFSP is used until a child's third birthday, but some preschool programs continue to use an IFSP until the child turns 5 or may use the individualized education program, or IEP, format of Part B of IDEA (see Chapter 12). The IFSP should honor parents' ideas and use language that is generally understood by all. In addition, it is vital that your family's practical situation be considered (transportation needs, work schedules, and so forth). Furthermore, it is important that you receive the information, education, training, or supports you might want to best help your child. IFSPs are required to be signed by the parents, and they have to be updated and agreed to by all major participants in your child's early intervention program. IFSPs may be changed any time parents or professionals working with the child determine that the goals need to be updated.

If your child is receiving early intervention through private means, then an IFSP may not be required because IDEA requires an IFSP only for the provision of public services. But you will want to be sure the professionals you collaborate with are seeing the big picture and allowing you to be an active participant in planning for your child's services.

What is the role of a service coordinator?

In early intervention, a service coordinator or case manager is responsible for assuring that the family is actively engaged in planning their child's and family's goals and assists in monitoring all services that are provided. This individual also makes sure that the needs of the child and family are taken into account and that there is follow-through to help the family obtain all of the recommended services. The service coordinator might even be one of your child's therapists, depending on the early intervention program.

What rights do parents or guardians have under Part C (early intervention) of IDEA legislation?

Parents or guardians of children receiving services must give written consent for any exchange of information about their child between agencies and other service providers (physicians, speech pathologists, child care workers, and so forth). Confidentiality of personal information is ensured. Furthermore, you can accept or decline any service or portion of service without jeopardizing other intervention services provided. In addition, you must receive written notice before any evaluation or change of placement or service level can be implemented. You also have the right to file a complaint regarding service.

7

Nutrition and Feeding

Peggy S. Eicher

Good nutrition is essential to foster typical growth and development, to prevent infections, and to provide the energy needed for daily activities. Yet, during early childhood many children, particularly children with disabilities, develop a feeding problem that interferes with appropriate nutrition. Your child may have different caloric needs, be unable to communicate hunger or thirst, or have difficulty self-feeding, chewing, or swallowing food. Signs of a feeding problem can be dramatic (choking or weight loss) but more commonly are subtle and/or unnoticed (increased congestion, intermittent gagging with meals, or a gradual decline in the texture, variety, or volume of food consumed). Fortunately, feeding difficulties are manageable when identified early and treated through the coordinated efforts of family members and other care providers. This chapter discusses your child's nutritional needs as well as the biology of the feeding process. This information should help you understand the influences of various medical and developmental conditions on feeding so that you are better equipped to anticipate and prevent or get treatment for a feeding problem in your child.

Esther

Esther, who has cerebral palsy, was gaining weight poorly at age 4. Although her parents were spending as much as 1 hour five times per day feeding her, Esther was not taking in enough food to stay well nourished. A feeding team evaluating Esther noted that she had a tongue thrust that tended to push food out of her mouth. She had clinical signs of gastroesophageal reflux (GER), in which stomach contents flow back up the esophagus (the tube connecting the mouth to the stomach). In addition, sitting in a parent's lap to eat did not provide Esther with enough trunk support to breathe easily or keep her head and neck upright. The team recommended that Esther's parents feed her in a special seat, thicken her liquids with cereal, and increase her food texture. Medications were also started to decrease her reflux symptoms. By the time of her follow-up visit 1 month later, Esther had gained 3 pounds, and her parents found feeding her a lot less frustrating. As her overall nutrition and growth improved, her irritability decreased, and she did much better in her preschool program.

COMMON NUTRITIONAL PROBLEMS

Good nutrition results from a balanced diet that supplies all of the essential nutrients and calories that your child needs to grow and develop. A healthy diet provides choices from each of the six major food groups: breads and cereals; fruits; vegetables; milk, yogurt, and cheese; meat, poultry, and fish; and fats, oils, and sweets. Recommended daily servings from each group include 6–11 of breads, cereal, rice, or pasta; 3–5 of vegetables; 2–4 of fruit; 2–3 each of dairy and of meat, poultry, and fish; and scant amounts of fats, oils, and sweets. For a child, these recommendations should be balanced over several days rather than for every meal.

Weight and height are important growth measurements that should be taken on a regular basis. Your child's medical care provider will plot these on a standardized growth chart that shows how your child is growing compared with a national sample of children whose growth has been measured over several years. If your child's growth follows the typical pattern of growth over time, he or she is probably getting adequate calories and nutrition. Growth that is too fast or too slow, however, is not always related to nutrition alone. Some genetic disorders, such as Down syndrome, have an atypical growth pattern, and growth charts specifically for these children are available. Some children may have a medical diagnosis, such as cerebral palsy or spina bifida, that interferes with height growth or its measurement. For these children, measurements of the skinfold thickness at the fleshy area between the shoulder and the elbow can be used to determine whether your child has too much or too little body fat. Whatever measurements are used, it is important to frequently monitor the growth of your child to optimize growth for age and quickly identify periods of undernutrition or overnutrition.

Undernutrition

The term *undernutrition* is used to describe inadequate growth or an inappropriate slowing down from your child's previously established rate of growth. This can result from inadequate caloric intake, excessive caloric expenditure, or an inability to use the calories ingested. In children with developmental disabilities, poor weight gain results primarily from inadequate caloric intake.

Atypical slowing of growth indicates the need for an evaluation to identify any difficulties your child faces in eating or digesting food.

Obesity

Certain developmental disabilities, such as Prader-Willi syndrome, Down syndrome, muscular dystrophy, and spastic cerebral palsy, predispose children to becoming overweight. Obesity itself may decrease a child's energy expenditure further by making mobility more difficult and less often attempted. It can also affect overall health, leading to elevated blood pressure and an increased risk of fractures. Yet, one of your child's most enjoyable activities may be eating. Although you will not want to take away this pleasure, you can place certain limits. One helping of food is sufficient at mealtimes, and between-meal snacks can be healthful and low in calories, such as fruits and vegetables. If you need help starting a weight control program for your child, consult a nutritionist to develop a diet and a physical therapist to plan an activity program.

Constipation

Constipation is a prolonged period (more than 3 days) without having a bowel movement or having hard stools that are difficult to pass. This is a common problem for children with disabilities. Decreased physical activity, a reduced intake of fluids and foods containing fiber, and uncoordinated bowel contractions all may contribute to the constipation. Besides making your child feel uncomfortable, constipation leads to increased abdominal pressure and slowed transit through the bowel, both of which increase the likelihood of GER. Furthermore, if your child feels full he or she will be less interested in eating.

Treatment methods for constipation vary and should be selected in consultation with your child's doctor. As much fluid as your child can tolerate should be included in his or her daily diet. Bulky and high-fiber foods, such as whole grain cereals, bran, fruits, and vegetables, can increase bowel activity. If necessary, a fiber supplement can be added. Prunes, papayas, and apricots act as mild natural laxatives. Increased exercise helps and should be encouraged when possible. When more powerful laxatives or suppositories are necessary, milk of magnesia, Malt-Supex (malt soup extract), SENOKOT (senna concentrate), mineral oil, Dulcolax (bisacodyl), or glycerin suppositories are effective (see Figure 10.5 in Chapter 10). An enema such as Fleet Enema for Children may also help the problem, but frequent use may interfere with your child's rectal muscle control and should be avoided. You may need to try a combination of approaches before your child begins to have regular bowel movements. Keep in mind that it is not necessary for your child to have a stool each day if he or she is eating and growing well. If your child is having feeding problems, however, passing a daily soft stool greatly facilitates feeding.

MECHANICS OF EATING

Your child's diet should be judged not only by the caloric and nutrient content of the food eaten but also by its texture and appeal. A high-texture diet is only appropriate for your child if she or he has the skills to flatten or grind the food, collect it, and swallow it safely. In addition, the digestive tract must be able to perform its three major functions: 1) controlled movement of food from the esophagus to the anus, 2) digestion of food, and 3) absorption of nutrients.

Although we may take swallowing for granted, it is, in fact, one of the most complex motor activities. Swallowing can be divided into a number of phases. Swallowing is controlled in the lower brain or brain stem in an area known as the "swallowing center." Branches of nerve cells from higher in the brain (the cortex) connect to the swallowing center to provide additional control over the swallowing process. Any problem affecting the swallowing center or the cortical cells connecting to it will also interfere with the coordination and function of the swallowing process. Furthermore, oral-motor skills, much like gross and fine motor skills, are greatly influenced by your child's growth and development. With brain maturation and improved voluntary control, more specific and finely graded movements can be performed.

Typically, new oral-motor skills are linked closely with the growth in oral structures. Your infant, for example, is perfectly equipped for nipple feeding, and the structure of his or her mouth makes it easy to generate suction. With growth, the jaw, mouth, and palate enlarge, allowing room for teeth, spoon feeding, and chewing. As the neck gets longer, so does the throat, requiring your child to control posture enough to maintain correct head and neck alignment to guide the bolus (mass of food ready to be swallowed) safely past the airway and into the esophagus. Any anatomical abnormality of the oral or nasal cavities, pharynx (back of the throat), or esophagus can make swallowing difficult for your child.

During suckling, the earliest pattern of taking in nutrients through the mouth, the tongue moves in and out like a wave on the wide, rhythmic motions of the jaw. Initially, it is a reflexive activity; your child will suckle whenever something enters the mouth. As your child's brain matures, the pattern is refined to become the voluntary act of sucking, in which the tongue moves up and down independent of the smaller jaw movements. Once sucking replaces suckling, usually around 5 months of age in a typically developing child, spoon feeding can be started because the food will not ride out of the mouth as the tongue moves.

The next oral-motor skill in the developmental progression is munching. Here, small pieces of food are broken off, flattened, and then collected for swallowing. Munching consists of the ability to move the tongue from side to side to deliver and later recollect the food in combination with repetitive, small jaw openings and closings. *Chewing* food and breaking it into smaller pieces does not occur until your child acquires a rotary pattern of jaw movement. This typically emerges as early as 9 months and is gradually modified with practice to the adult pattern around 3 years of age.

Because each new oral-motor skill builds on the foundation of an earlier skill, your child must have practice at each level. If medical problems, motor abnormalities, or behavioral issues limit the amount of practice your child gets with a certain skill, they can slow his or her progression to the next higher skill level and increase the risk of his or her developing a feeding problem. For example, if muscle tone or digestion issues impair your child's practice with side-to-side tongue motion, then munching will be delayed and introduction of table foods will be very difficult. In response, your child may refuse table foods, accept but gag, or become more selective. When you try harder to introduce the food, your child may refuse or gag more. If this scenario continues, a feeding problem will develop.

FEEDING PROBLEMS IN CHILDREN WITH DISABILITIES

Feeding problems can result from factors that can be categorized into three main groups: medical factors, motor factors, and learned patterns of interaction. Although one factor may cause the initial feeding disturbance, other factors may increase the complexity of the feeding problem. Such was the case for Esther, whose initial problem was GER that limited her interest in food. As time went on, her limited practice in eating slowed her oral-motor skill development. The discomfort she felt because of the GER led her to arch her back, which made it harder for her to sit down. The sections that follow describe some of the most common feeding problems in children with disabilities.

Increased Oral Losses

Losing food from the mouth before swallowing is usually a sign of oral-motor difficulty. Your child may have trouble keeping his or her lips closed, thus allowing food to escape as the tongue collects and transports it. Or, your child's mouth may stay open as a result of low tone in the facial muscles or habitual mouth breathing. Food also can be pushed out by a tongue thrust resulting from a persistent suckle pattern. Before intervening, you need to first make sure your child is not using his or her mouth for breathing. If he or she uses the mouth as an airway, it will not stay closed until your child feels comfortable breathing only through the nose. Next, try to determine if losses are less for liquids or solids and if they occur with every bite or only toward the end of the meal. If losses occur only at the end of the meal, the muscles are perhaps becoming fatigued. A speech-language pathologist or occupational therapist comfortable with oral-motor interventions can suggest exercises that will strengthen the muscles and improve endurance. If losses occur throughout the meal, try offering a smaller amount of food per bite, which allows your child to perform more controlled tongue movements. If losses increase for liquids, try thickening the fluids slightly while the therapist helps your child strengthen lip closure. If losses increase for solids, talk to your therapist about trying to place the food in the cheeks to encourage your child to move the tongue from side to side rather than in and out.

Prolonged Feeding Time

Prolonged feeding time (greater than 20–30 minutes per meal) usually results from a combination of factors. Transport of the food to the back of the mouth may be slowed because of weakened tongue movements, requiring more time between bites. Your child may slow the pace of the meal to allow more time for breathing between bites or sips or to allow the esophagus to clear if its transport is slow. If your child takes a long break in the middle of every feeding, he or she might be trying to minimize reflux symptoms by delaying eating more until he or she feels less full or until the food already swallowed is cleared from the esophagus. Prolonged feeding time can be very difficult for you and your child and signals the need for an evaluation by a feeding team.

Pocketing

Food pocketing involves holding food in the cheeks or front of the mouth. Often children who have difficulty with tongue movement have trouble bringing food to the middle of the tongue before a swallow. As a result, mashed food or chunks move toward the cheeks. If your child does not want to swallow a particular food because of its texture or taste, he or she may trap it in the cheeks or under the tongue and just behind the teeth. If pocketing occurs related to poor side-to-side tongue movement, a therapist comfortable with oral-motor intervention can provide tongue exercises for your child that will strengthen the lateral movement pattern. Pocketing to avoid swallowing can be very challenging to treat and should be evaluated fairly quickly by a therapist trained in swallowing dysfunction.

Coughing and Gagging

Coughing and gagging are normal defense mechanisms to protect against food entering the lungs. Noting when coughing and gagging occur during your child's meal may suggest which food texture is troublesome. For example, gagging on lumpy foods but not purées suggests difficulty with transporting foods with more texture. This difficulty may signal an immature oral-motor pattern or abdominal discomfort. Coughing with liquids indicates that your child is having difficulty controlling the flow of food through the throat and past the airway. If coughing or gagging occurs after a meal but not during the meal, however, reflux should be considered. Depending on the cause, treatment may include changing your child's position while feeding, altering the texture of foods, or using antireflux medication. Coughing or gagging with meals that persists over several weeks is a serious warning signal for swallowing difficulty and requires evaluation as soon as possible.

Aspiration with Meals

Aspiration is the entry of food or a foreign substance into the airway. Food can be aspirated when making its way down to the stomach or when refluxed up from the stomach. Accumulation of food in the airway causes irritation and inflammation. Depending on the amount and frequency of aspiration, this can lead to recurrent episodes of pneumonia and lung damage. Everyone aspirates small amounts of food occasionally, but protective responses such as a gag or cough help to clear it from the airway. Children with cerebral palsy who have difficulty coordinating swallowing, however, are at increased risk for recurrent aspiration. Aspiration in infants may appear as brief arrests of breathing or slowed heart rate. In older infants and children, symptoms commonly include coughing, increased congestion, or wheezing during meals. Some children aspirate without showing any protective response; this is called silent aspiration. If you suspect that your child may be aspirating, discuss the issue with your child's doctor. Very often the problem can be corrected, enabling your child to swallow safely again.

Spitting, Wet Burps, and Vomiting

It is common for infants to spit up occasionally, have wet burps, or dribble milk after feeding. Although the lower esophageal sphincter, the muscle surrounding the base of the esophagus, normally acts as a one-way valve preventing backup into the esophagus, it does not work effectively until about 12 weeks of age, when the esophagus has grown the necessary length below the diaphragm. Thus, infants who are "spitters" frequently stop spitting after 3–4 months of age. If the infant takes large volumes or has increased abdominal pressure from decreased stool production, the spitting may continue for a longer time. If the lower esophageal sphincter is uncoordinated or weakened, food and stomach acid can reflux, or flow back into the esophagus (see Figure 7.1). If your child is growing well, sleeping well, and is playful without being irritable, and advancing in oral-motor skills, the reflux is not harmful and most likely should go away by 2 years of age. Some children, however, reflux so much that it leads to a loss of needed nutrition and the possibility of aspiration. In addition, the volume and acidity of the refluxed stomach contents may cause an inflammation of the esophagus, making swallowing food uncomfortable. Repeated episodes of pneumonia, food avoidance, or back arching may indicate reflux, although these symptoms may have many other causes as well.

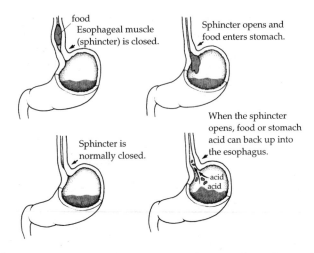

food
Esophageal muscle
(sphincter) is closed.

Sphincter opens and
food enters stomach.

Sphincter is
normally closed.

When the sphincter
opens, food or stomach
acid can back up into
the esophagus.

acid
acid

Figure 7.1.   Gastroesophageal reflux. Food typically passes down the esophagus, through the esophageal sphincter, and into the stomach. Usually, the sphincter then closes, acting as a one-way valve. If the muscle does not work properly, however, then acidic stomach contents can reflux back up into the esophagus.

Vomiting or regurgitation is also associated with other, less frequent conditions. Pyloric stenosis, in which the muscle controlling the outflow tract of the stomach is enlarged, needs to be considered in any infant with recurrent vomiting. Food intolerance, such as lactose intolerance (inability to digest the sugar contained in milk), results in bloating, vomiting, or diarrhea. In Hirschsprung disease, part of the large intestine cannot contract to push stool toward the anus, which results in backup of stool. Weak, slow, or disorganized movement through the esophagus can result in buildup of food in the esophagus or uncoordinated opening or closing of the entrance to the esophagus. Other possible causes of vomiting in newborns and young infants are inborn errors of metabolism, in which toxic products accumulate to cause nausea and vomiting.

Frequent vomiting should be discussed with your child's doctor. He or she can help you identify accompanying symptoms that suggest what the underlying cause might be and whether the vomiting could be harmful for your child. Appropriate testing may include blood tests, urinalysis, radiology studies such an upper GI (gastrointestinal) study that reveals structural abnormalities in the esophagus, stomach, and intestines, a milk scan to evaluate stomach emptying, and/or endoscopy (using a fiber optic device) to look directly at the area involved.

If reflux is diagnosed, treatment recommendations may involve changing the volume of meals and positioning your child differently after feedings. For example, your child may do better sitting up for 30–60 minutes after meals. This allows the food to move down more easily into the stomach and makes it less likely to back up into the esophagus. Over-the-counter medications such as Zantac (ranitidine) and Pepcid (famotidine) help tame reflux by decreasing stomach acid production, thus lessening the irritating potential of the refluxed material. Medications that propel the stomach contents into the intestine decrease the likelihood of reflux. Your child's physician should supervise the use of each of these medications because they have potential side effects.

Lack of Interest in Food and Refusal to Eat

Because of the coordination and muscular control required, eating is hard work for many children with disabilities. If your child also has a breathing or digestion problem, he or she may show very little interest in eating or act very hungry before mealtime but then only eat a small amount. Alternatively, your child may accept only a few favorite foods or may refuse to eat any foods at all. Although every child will try to convince a parent that only favorite foods should be served for meals, children who have a disability may be more persistent about this, especially if they have a motor or medical problem that makes them want to avoid certain foods. Keep track of what your child doesn't like to eat: Is he or she avoiding crunchy foods or meats that may be harder to chew? Is he or she avoiding certain food groups such as dairy or wheat, which may suggest food intolerance? Is he or she eating very little at meals but snacking a lot throughout the day? Is he or she filling up with liquids before the meal? Talk with your child's doctor about your child's eating patterns. He or she may recommend some simple tests to evaluate the possibility of food intolerance or may help you to formulate a trial of limiting liquids or snacks between meals. If texture seems to be the problem, a therapist skilled in oral-motor intervention can help. Food refusal and selectivity are very frustrating and can over time lead not only to serious health problems but also to ineffective parent–child interactions. A behavior therapist can be very helpful in restructuring your interactions in and out of mealtimes to make meals more effective and fun. If your child is gaining weight poorly or will only accept a few foods, complete evaluation by a feeding team is the most efficient way to identify the problem areas and develop a treatment plan.

Whom to Call and When

Because of the complexity of the feeding process, multiple specialists are frequently involved in the treatment of feeding problems. Sometimes it can be very confusing to determine whom you should go to for what problem. Basically, always start with your child's physician. Be frank about your concerns and what is happening at mealtimes. Together you will be able to list what factors may be contributing to the feeding problem and how serious the problem is to your child's health and development. In addition, your child's doctor can suggest testing for any underlying medical factors that might be contributing to the feeding problem. If there are motor problems and the feeding issue involves difficulty advancing texture or managing spoon volume, a speech-language or occupational therapist with experience in feeding should be able to help. If the feeding problem developed as a bad habit during an illness or if you think your interaction with your child in and out of mealtimes could be more effective, a behavior therapist with experience in applied behavior analysis can be helpful. A feeding team evaluation is warranted if your child has a feeding problem and is gaining weight poorly, eats only the same few foods every meal for a number of weeks, or has a persistent feeding problem for which you have already sought help from a professional. You can get information about the feeding therapy resources available in your area from local early intervention services, the United Cerebral Palsy Associations (see the Suggested Readings and Resources at the end of this book), or the university affiliated program in your state. University affiliated programs are programs linked to a university that function to provide and improve services to children with disabilities and their families (see the Suggested Readings and Resources for information on the American Association of University Affiliated Programs for Persons with Developmental Disabilities).

Tube Feeding

Sometimes, despite everyone's best efforts, a child will be unable to eat enough to grow well. In these instances supplemental feedings can be provided through tube feedings (see Figure 7.2). If your child has a temporary problem that decreases his or her ability to eat, a nasogastric (NG) tube might be used. The tube is passed through one nostril, down the esophagus, and into the stomach. If your child's problem is likely to take many months or years to improve, however, a gastrostomy tube (GT) might be a better choice. For the placement of a gastrostomy tube, a small hole is made in the abdominal and stomach walls, and a tube is inserted through the hole into the stomach. This can often be done without surgery and is called a *PEG*. If reflux is a problem, a gastrojejunal (GJ) tube may be used instead. The GJ tube is basically a combination of a gastrostomy tube and a jejunal tube, which travels through the stomach into the second section of the intestine, the jejunum, in order to prevent reflux.

A commercially prepared formula such as Pediasure or Nutren Jr. can be used with any of these tubes. The type of tube, your child's particular medical problem, and the feeding schedule determine how the tube feedings should be given. With an NG or GT tube, feedings can be given as single, large volumes of 3–8 ounces every 3–6 hours or as a continuous drip delivered at a set rate throughout the day or overnight by an electric pump. GJ tube feedings, however, must be given continuously rather than as a large volume.

The presence of a tube does not prevent your child from eating by mouth, provided there is not a concern about aspiration into the lungs. In fact, for children who have oral-motor or medical issues that make it very difficult for them to ingest enough calories for adequate nutrition, a tube can actually help

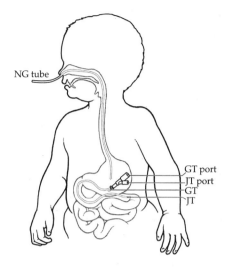

Figure 7.2.   Enteral feeding tubes bring nutrition directly into the digestive system. The nasogastric (NG) tube is placed through the nostril and into the stomach. An NG tube can be helpful when a child cannot get enough calories because of a short-term problem with oral-motor skills or swallowing. A gastrojejunal (GJ) tube is a combination of a gastrostomy tube (GT) and a jejunal tube (JT). The GJ tube has two ports. The GT port, like a GT, ends in and enables access to the stomach. The JT port, similar to a simple JT, ends in the intestine. When the stomach is not able to tolerate or digest all of the nutrition needed by the child, a GJ or a J tube can be helpful by enabling some or all of the nutrition to be given directly into the intestine.

make eating easier. Families of these children say that there is much less tension at mealtime, that the child can enjoy the food he or she eats, and that the family can look forward to mealtime as a time for positive social interaction. Of course, there are also negative aspects to having a tube: concern over whether it will be accidentally dislodged, increased difficulty finding child care, and worry about overnight feedings, to name a few.

SUMMARY

Feeding is one of the most complex activities performed by your child. Moreover, the oral-motor movements used in swallowing are learned skills. Motor function and coordination, cognitive development, medical issues, and social interactions around mealtimes all influence the learning of these skills. Fluctuation, delay, or abnormality in any of these factors can disrupt the feeding process and lead to a feeding problem. Thus, children with developmental disabilities are at increased risk for developing feeding problems.

The best way to treat feeding problems is to prevent them from occurring. Work with your child's doctor to anticipate factors that could interfere with your child's feeding success and acquisition of new skills. Then, with the help of the appropriate professional, try to minimize these factors. Because children learn how to eat, it is important to be a good teacher at mealtime. Be consistent, give clear instructions, and provide appropriate feedback throughout the meal. In addition, remember that successful eating for your child may not be the same as adequate nutrition. With the help of your child's doctor and a nutritionist, you can work out an individual nutrition plan for your child to participate in mealtimes at an optimal level as well as receive adequate calories.

Some Questions Answered

Does my child need a vitamin supplement?

If your child has a fairly typical diet or is taking formula with vitamin supplements, then no daily vitamins are needed. If your child is highly selective or drinks only juice or water, then a daily multivitamin may be helpful. (Adult multivitamins are not an acceptable substitute for children's vitamins. Adult multivitamins usually contain too much iron for a child, which can be toxic.) For all children, vitamin D is essential for adequate calcium absorption to build strong bones and teeth. A large amount of the precursor to vitamin D is stored in a person's skin and can be converted by sunlight to vitamin D. Your child may get enough vitamin D to meet his or her daily needs by going out into the sunshine.

What about trace minerals? Does my child need any of those?

According to one untested theory, many problems of people with developmental disabilities result from deficiencies in selenium, zinc, and other trace minerals, and daily supplements of the trace elements are suggested to relieve these deficiencies. There is no scientific evidence, however, to support the use of trace mineral supplements. Because excess amounts of trace minerals can be toxic, it is best to avoid giving supplements unless a specific deficiency has been identified in your child.

I suspect my child's feeding problems are caused by a food allergy. How can I find out if this is true?

Gastrointestinal food allergy continues to be a challenge for clinical diagnosis because of the variety of symptoms and lack of reliable diagnostic tests. Several types of food allergy have been described based on how quickly the symptoms begin after eating. The diagnosis of food allergy is based on a favorable response when the suspected allergen is removed from the diet and a recurrence of symptoms when the food is reintroduced. If you suspect a food allergy, speak with your child's medical care provider about your observations. It is important to maintain balanced nutrition as well as safety for your child while considering a dietary change systematically.

I've read about special diets recommended for kids with disabilities and attention problems. How do I know if they're safe for my child?

Most of these diets are based on elimination of the offending nutrient or additive, whether sugar, casein, red dye, or something else. If you are considering starting your child on one of these diets, talk to your child's medical provider about the diet and how it might affect your child's health issues. If there are no reasons to avoid a trial, you and the medical care provider (a nutritionist can also be very helpful) can formulate a dietary regimen that will provide the appropriate amount and balance of nutrients for your child. Just as important, you will be able to set up an assessment strategy to determine whether the diet is having the desired effect.

8

Dental Care for Your Child with Special Needs

George Acs and Man Wai Ng

Healthy teeth and gums are important for the overall well-being of all children and affect children's ability to chew, speak, and look attractive. Dental care is particularly important for children with disabilities because they may be more likely to have dental or periodontal disease. This chapter discusses the typical development of teeth and why children with developmental disabilities may have an increased risk for certain dental diseases and, therefore, require especially good dental care.

Luis, Janice, and Carole

Luis is a 9-year-old with cerebral palsy. His motor skills do not permit proper toothbrushing, placing him at an increased risk for developing dental caries (tooth decay). Because his tongue is always pushed toward the front of his mouth, he has an open bite and many spaces between his teeth that will require orthodontic care.

Janice is an 8-year-old with Down syndrome. The first of her permanent teeth are just coming in. But her baby teeth are very crowded, and her first permanent tooth is emerging behind a baby tooth that she has not yet lost.

Carole is a 5-year-old who had a severe head injury in a car accident at age 3 and now has mental retardation. She has also developed a seizure disorder, which is being treated with antiepileptic medication. Although Carole's parents have attempted to brush her teeth, her jaw clenching, tooth grinding, and head movements have made it very difficult, and she has had a number of cavities. This has been further complicated by overgrowth of her gums caused by the Dilantin (phenytoin) used to treat her seizures.

DENTAL DEVELOPMENT

Tooth formation begins when the human embryo is only 4–6 weeks old. A small knob of tissue begins developing for each of the 20 primary, or baby, teeth (10 in the upper and 10 in the lower jaw). As the teeth grow they develop special shapes and functions as incisors (4, used to cut food), cuspids (2, used to mash), and molars (4, used to grind). Permanent teeth begin to develop around the time of birth and harden to bone strength during early childhood. Because developing teeth are sensitive to their environment, the first few years of life can have a tremendous impact on the quality of the teeth.

Although many parents believe that the first baby tooth should emerge by the age of 6 months, there is actually a wide range in the usual ages for teeth to appear. Each child has his or her own schedule; the first baby teeth can actually come in any time between 4 and 17 months of age. What is more important is symmetry. That is, what occurs on the right side of the mouth should occur within a few months on the left, and what occurs in the upper jaw should occur in the lower jaw soon after.

A complete set of baby teeth typically takes about 2–3 years to appear. In rare instances, teeth can actually come in during the first month of life or even be present at birth; these are called *natal* or *neonatal teeth*. Although several genetic syndromes include the presence of natal teeth, the presence of such teeth alone does not always indicate an underlying disorder. These teeth do not need to be removed unless they cause significant discomfort for the mother while the infant is breast-feeding or unless they irritate the infant's mouth.

In general, when a permanent tooth emerges, a primary tooth is lost. The first permanent tooth begins to erupt (come in) around 6 years of age, and all permanent teeth, except the wisdom teeth, are in place by adolescence. These final molars, making a total of 32 permanent teeth, typically erupt between 17 and 21 years of age and may cause crowding or infection while providing little so-called wisdom. Often the emergence of both primary and permanent teeth is delayed in children with severe disabilities.

Atypical Dental Development

Disorders of number, size, shape, and calcification (mineralization) can occur as a result of disturbances at various times in tooth development. The presence of extra teeth, absence of multiple teeth, unusual shape of the teeth, inadequate mineralization (hardening), and crooked teeth that require orthodontic intervention are all more likely to occur in children with disabilities of genetic origin and place these children at increased risk for dental disease. Children with Williams syndrome (see Chapter 16) or cleft lip or palate often lack one or more teeth; children with Down syndrome (see Chapter 15) may have abnormally shaped teeth. Environmental influences can also play a role in tooth abnormalities. Nutritional deficiencies, especially of calcium and phosphorus, can result in a decrease in mineralization, which can increase the risk of tooth decay and orthodontic problems. This is particularly true if the child has physical or cognitive impairments that interfere with good dental hygiene.

ORAL DISORDERS

Tooth Decay

Tooth decay is a complex process leading to the development of cavities. It arises from bacteria that are efficient in their capability to produce cavities, a diet of carbohydrates (sugary or starchy foods, such as candy, baked goods, or pasta) for bacteria to process and turn into acids that demineralize teeth, and time for this combination to eat away at the tooth. Any break in this "chain of decay" can protect a child from developing cavities. The three most effective ways to protect the teeth are by maintaining good oral hygiene (toothbrushing, flossing, and use of fluoride), limiting sweets and carbohydrates, and eliminating the bacteria. Unfortunately, we still have not learned to prevent the growth of cavity-causing bacteria. And once present in a person's mouth, the bacteria cannot be easily eradicated. For most children, good oral hygiene combined with fewer snacks with carbohydrates can reduce the development of cavities.

About 40% of 5-year-olds and 85% of 17-year-olds have had at least one cavity. Cavities are more common in children who do not receive fluoride either from water or from prescribed supplements, such as vitamins containing fluoride. They are also more likely to occur in children with disabilities (especially mental retardation, cerebral palsy, and seizure disorders) than in typically developing children. Developmental alterations in the teeth and gums, dietary issues, reduced fluoride exposure, and inadequate oral hygiene practices all contribute to this increased risk of dental disease. It is interesting to note that children with Down syndrome tend to have a decreased risk of dental decay, because their teeth are less likely to have deep grooves and pits that provide hiding places for plaque (tartar) formation.

One form of caries that merits special attention is nursing caries, better known as *baby bottle tooth decay*. Although not all early childhood caries is due to being put to bed with a juice-filled nursing bottle, it is clear that doing so can increase a child's risk for developing rampant cavities. Because nursing caries starts on the tongue side of the top teeth, it is often hidden and therefore discovered fairly late in the process of decay. Children with malformations of the teeth, particularly if mineralization is affected, have more severe nursing caries. It is important to note that in some children who receive carbohydrate-enriched diets to encourage growth or who require long-term liquid medications containing sugar, rampant cavities may also occur. Yet, they can be prevented by cleaning your child's mouth after each feeding once primary teeth have started to erupt and by eliminating bottle feedings when putting your baby to sleep.

Periodontal Disease

Whereas dental caries affects the teeth, periodontal diseases damage the tissue supporting the teeth, the gums, and underlying bone. The connection between cavities and gum disease is that when dental plaque remains on the teeth for a long time, it becomes calcified and can cause inflammation and swelling of the gums. This can lead to periodontal or gum disease that can loosen teeth from their bony sockets.

The most common form of periodontal disease is gingivitis, which begins with inflammation and bleeding of the gums. Unfortunately, gingivitis may go unrecognized for years, leading to damage of the underlying tissues and bone. This may result in bone loss, loosening of the tooth socket, and ultimately loss of the permanent tooth. Some degree of gingivitis is present in about half of all children 6–12 years of age and in a higher percentage of children with disabilities. In addition, certain medications have the side effect of causing overgrowth of the gums, which frequently leads to periodontal disease. These include antiepileptic drugs such as Dilantin, drugs to suppress the immune system such as Sandimmune (cyclosporine), and drugs to manage high blood pressure such as Procardia (nifedipine). When the medication is stopped, the gums may recede. If treatment must continue, your child may need dental surgery to remove overgrown gum tissue.

Many developmental disabilities do not place your child at greater risk for periodontal disease. As with individuals without disabilities, however, good oral hygiene remains important. Children with certain developmental disabilities do have a higher incidence of periodontal disease. In children with Down syndrome, the combination of crowded teeth and mouth breathing leads to dry gums that bleed easily, leading to periodontal disease. Children with cerebral palsy, who may be unable to completely clear their mouths of food, are at increased risk for plaque formation, dental decay, and periodontal disease. This problem is worsened by abnormal muscle tone that interferes with routine dental care. Although children with spina bifida (see Chapter 17) do not have specific dental concerns, it is important to remember that they may require antibiotics before dental procedures if they have a ventricular shunt to treat hydrocephalus. These antibiotics prevent shunt infection from mouth bacteria. In addition, it is essential for the dentist to avoid the use of latex gloves and products as these children have a high incidence of allergy to latex.

Malocclusion

Malocclusion is a misalignment of the teeth or jaws. It can interfere with speech and chewing and can increase the risk of dental diseases. It also can affect a child's appearance, which is especially difficulty for children with self-image problems. The occurrence of malocclusion in children with certain developmental disabilities, such as Down syndrome and cerebral palsy, is about double that found in individuals without disabilities. Correcting alignment of the teeth with orthodontic treatment, such as braces, not only improves the appearance of a child's face but also decreases the risk of dental disease by making oral hygiene easier. For children with poor oral hygiene or those who have had many cavities, orthodontic braces should be postponed until it is clear that the improved oral hygiene will protect against the development of new cavities or periodontal disease. This delay is necessary because both of these problems are more likely to occur when braces are worn for extended periods of time.

HABITS AND BEHAVIORS
LEADING TO DENTAL PROBLEMS

A number of habits and behaviors can cause problems in the mouth. These include finger, thumb, and pacifier sucking, tooth grinding, mouth breathing, tongue thrusting, and involuntary chewing. Prolonged habits, typically those that extend beyond the eruption of the permanent teeth, place the child at increased risk for developing malocclusion. Fortunately, these habits can often be treated effectively using a combination of behavior management techniques (see Chapter 11) and dental appliances.

Most children who have a habit of sucking on a pacifier stop doing so by 2 years of age. Although specially designed pacifiers are available and advertised to be less likely to cause future orthodontic problems, there is no evidence to support those claims. In general, prolonged pacifier habits are less likely to affect the developing bite than prolonged thumb- or finger-sucking habits are. Although parents are often anxious to help their child stop thumb sucking, appliance therapy, such as with an orthodontic retainer, is usually not started until the child is also motivated to stop. At 7 years of age, many children can actively participate in the decision to try to stop their thumb-sucking habit, although there may be wide variation. Many of the effects of prolonged thumb sucking, such as open bite (lack of overlap of the top and bottom front teeth) may self-correct if the habit is successfully eliminated at this age.

Tooth grinding (also called *bruxism*) is quite common in young children. In most cases, it helps the child develop a comfortable bite surface on the teeth. It can occur at night, during sleep, or intermittently during the daytime. Typically, grinding occurs only intermittently and stops when permanent teeth begin to emerge. When done constantly, however, tooth grinding can become nerve-racking to parents and other caregivers. In addition, grinding wears down the teeth and may eventually change your child's bite or interfere with effective chewing. In some children with severe mental retardation, however, the grinding is excessive both in intensity and duration. Your child's dentist first must make a careful assessment of the effects on the teeth. If damage is occurring to the permanent teeth, the dentist may order a protective appliance to keep the teeth from touching.

Some children, particularly those with cerebral palsy, may have tongue thrusting habits. Because the tongue is a powerful muscle, it can move teeth. Children with very frequent tongue thrusting will often have malocclusion with an open bite and flared and spaced teeth. For children with a limited ability to control tongue thrusting, a permanent retainer may straighten the front teeth.

Occasionally, cheek and tongue chewing occur in children who have head trauma or who are in comatose states. Such involuntary chewing may result in deep bites, swelling, and ulceration of the tongue, lips, and cheeks. Although the chewing may spontaneously stop as the child's level of consciousness rises, temporary protective appliances may help prevent significant damage to the soft tissues in the child's mouth.

GOOD DENTAL CARE

You can ensure the healthiest teeth and gums possible for your child by following certain principles of dental hygiene. As a parent you play a crucial role in accomplishing this through encouraging a combination of consistent toothbrushing and flossing, fluoride supplements, and dietary regulation.

Toothbrushing

Although some children with developmental disabilities will not be able to independently brush, they can help when you guide their movements. A soft, nylon toothbrush with bristles that have rounded ends works best, but electric toothbrushes can also be used. A scrubbing motion up and down the entire surface of the front, back, and chewing surfaces of the teeth is the most effective. An adapted toothbrush with handle modifications can help the older child with cerebral palsy or other physical impairments gain independence in toothbrushing. Only a small, pea-sized amount of toothpaste with fluoride is necessary, but if foam from the paste causes problems for your child, it is fine to moisten the brush with water only. Having your child recline with his or her head tilted back may help you see the teeth better. Ideally, brushing should occur twice per day: after breakfast and before bedtime. If brushing after eating is not possible, wiping soft food debris from your child's mouth using a moist washcloth will do. You may find that brushing your child's teeth is challenging. Experimentation with different positioning may help to discover an effective and stress-free way to get through the process with an uncooperative child. You may want to consider sitting on the floor or on a chair, with your child on your lap or between your legs, facing away from you. If your child uses a wheelchair, it may be helpful to stand behind your child.

Flossing

Flossing is important because it removes debris and food particles from between the teeth, which can form the basis for dental plaque formation. Improper flossing, however, can harm the gums, so your child will need your help with this. Ask your child's dental care provider to show you and your child the best way to floss without hurting the gums. Unwaxed floss is preferred because no residue is left behind, and you may find that floss holders are helpful. Flossing once a day is sufficient and is most easily done at bedtime.

Fluoride

Water fluoridation has been the greatest boon to the prevention of tooth decay. It makes tooth enamel (the outer mineral coating) more resistant to decay and helps remineralize cavities (reharden the tooth). Some children with disabilities, however, may not drink enough water to get the needed fluoride. In this case, or in communities where water is not fluoridated, you should ask your child's dentist about fluoride supplements, either drops or vitamins. (If you do not know whether your water supply contains fluoride, your child's pediatrician or dentist can send a water sample for analysis. If supplements are required, the appropriate amount can then be prescribed.) Your child's dentist should also administer fluoride directly to the teeth at least twice each year.

Diet

It is important to consider your child's dietary needs and limitations and how they affect dental hygiene. For example, foods containing a high concentration of carbohydrates, especially if sticky, lead to plaque formation. Yet, children with chewing or swallowing problems may require low texture and high carbohydrate content. In this case toothbrushing should be done after every meal. Good choices for between-meal snacks that do not promote cavities very much include raw vegetables, unsweetened juices, milk, cheese, nuts, and popcorn; poor snack choices include caramels, sweet rolls, pretzels, and potato chips.

OBTAINING GOOD DENTAL CARE

It is important to identify a dentist in your area who can provide long-term care and guidance for you and your child. Not all dentists feel comfortable with or are good at providing care for children with disabilities. You can find an appropriate dentist through your local dental society, which maintains a list of pediatric dentists with an expressed interest in children with disabilities. It may also be helpful to contact families of children with similar disabilities who have had good experiences with a particular pediatric dentist. You can identify other families through your local school or community advocacy groups.

At a typical dental checkup, your child's teeth will be cleaned and examined, and fluoride may be applied. At some point your child's dentist may discuss whether sealants would benefit your child. Sealants are plastic coatings that are bonded to the teeth, usually the molars, to prevent decay. If cavities are found, the dentist will remove the decay and place a filling or a crown to cap the tooth. Your child's dentist will usually discuss options for care with you and your child. The need for treatment, consequences of delaying treatment, and potential physical/emotional trauma must be considered.

During the dental visit, the dentist may use behavior management techniques to help ease the examination and treatment. Many positive reinforcement techniques are available (see Chapter 11) to help the dentist provide treatment effectively and efficiently while instilling a positive attitude in the child about dental visits and tooth care. A pediatric dentist is especially trained in visual and verbal techniques such as tell-show-do and the use of verbal and nonverbal communication and is able to customize a behavioral approach to meet your child's needs. You can play an important role by providing your child's dentist with information about your child's likes and dislikes and other helpful clues. In some instances, however, the dentist will need to use devices to keep your child from moving so that your child, the dentist, and any assistants are not injured during diagnostic studies or therapy. Occasionally, a dentist may use a restraining device if your child is cooperative but experiences involuntary spasms.

Most children do not require sedation for dental examination and treatment. For some children, however, nitrous oxide (laughing gas) and oxygen inhalation sedation is an effective and safe technique for allaying a child's fear and permitting rapid examination and treatment. This sedation works quickly, can be controlled, and allows for rapid and complete recovery. It, however, requires that your child willingly breathes the sedative, which is not as effective in resistant patients. For some children, therefore, other types of sedatives or a general anesthetic are needed to ensure safe and effective treatment. If sedation or dental repair/surgery is needed, the dentist should consult with your child's primary care provider or other specialists, such as a neurologist or a cardiologist, to have a complete understanding of any unique considerations or precautions involved in treating your child. For example, if your child has a congenital heart defect or a condition that compromises the immune system, antibiotics may be recommended before a dental procedure.

SUMMARY

The dental needs of children with disabilities are varied. Although each child must be considered individually, children with disabilities as a group experience increased susceptibility to dental decay, periodontal disease, and orthodontic malocclusion. Therefore, it is important for you to promote and monitor good dental hygiene including toothbrushing habits, regular flossing, healthful diet, adequate fluoride intake, and routine dental checkups.

Some Questions Answered

At what age should my daughter have her first dental visit?

The American Academy of Pediatric Dentistry (AAPD) recommends that all children have their first dental visit around 12 months of age. Many dentists recommend a first visit even earlier, when the first tooth comes in. The AAPD has established guidelines for infant oral health that include the concept of anticipatory guidance. Starting from your child's first visit, the dentist would consider the individual needs of your child and advise about likely events during development and strategies to effectively meet the future challenges of dental growth and development.

Can I do anything to reduce the number of cavities that my child will get?

Toothbrushing, flossing, and a healthful diet can all help reduce cavities. In addition, studies have indicated that children acquire cavity-causing bacteria during the emergence of their first teeth. Parents usually inadvertently infect their child! Your breathing and handling your child allows this spread, and if you have a high bacterial count or possess bacteria that are more efficient at causing cavities, your child is at increased risk for future cavities. You can help reduce that risk by undergoing frequent dental cleanings yourself and by having all of your own cavities repaired so that you are less likely to pass your cavity-inducing bacteria to your infant.

Should my child receive sealants?

Plastic sealants can be useful in preventing cavities. They are effective when applied by the dentist to the biting surfaces of permanent molar teeth that have deep grooves or pits. This technique is particularly useful during the first 3 or 4 years after the emergence of a permanent tooth. The probability of developing a cavity on the biting surface of a permanent molar that has been erupted for 5 or more years is considerably less, so a sealant on such a tooth is not likely to be necessary. In addition, children who have evidence of tooth grinding on their permanent molars often do not require sealants because the grooves and pits in these teeth have been smoothed down.

My child falls to sleep with a bottle of formula. Will that cause nursing decay?

Some commercially available products appear not to be associated with baby bottle tooth decay, whereas others are very efficient at promoting tooth destruction. But until more information is available about why certain liquids cause cavities and others do not, children should not be allowed to fall asleep with a nursing bottle containing any liquid other than water. The same applies to children who are breast-fed. Prolonged breast feeding and falling asleep with the nipple in the mouth can promote tooth decay, as can sucking on a pacifier dipped in a sugary material. Children with gastroesophageal reflux (see Chapter 7) can also experience many cavities, even if they do not fall asleep while feeding. Because of the acid reflux, the tooth enamel will lose minerals and develop cavities.

My child is exclusively fed through a gastric tube. Are dental checkups necessary?

Even children who do not receive nutrition through the mouth are susceptible to dental disease. Good oral hygiene, dental checkups, and deep cleanings by a dentist or dental hygienist may prevent this from occurring. Periodic dental visits will also help your child get used to oral manipulation over time and prepare your child to accept dental treatment if it is required in the future.

Understanding
Rehabilitation Therapies

Lisa A. Kurtz

As a parent, you naturally want to do all you can to help your child overcome or adapt to his or her disability. Your child may benefit from a variety of therapies designed to promote development, to help cope with the demands of everyday life, and to prepare for adulthood. The most common of these include physical, occupational, and speech-language therapy. Physical therapy (PT) promotes gross motor development and helps children become mobile within their environment. Occupational therapy (OT) helps problems with fine motor and perceptual development that interfere with self-care, play, and school performance, which are the primary "occupations" of childhood. Speech-language therapy (ST) focuses on helping a child learn to communicate, including listening to, understanding, and expressing ideas through language. Table 9.1 summarizes the primary roles and functions of therapists from these three professions. Table 9.2 summarizes the qualities of an effective rehabilitation team.

Jared

When 11-month-old Jared was diagnosed with cerebral palsy, his parents enrolled him in an early intervention program, and he was evaluated by a team that included a physical therapist, an occupational therapist, and a speech-language therapist. The team agreed that it might be easiest for Jared to start with just one primary therapist who could provide therapy in the family's home while incorporating suggestions from the other team members, including Jared's parents. Marielle, the occupational therapist, devised a program of positioning suggestions, exercises, handling techniques, and play

Table 9.1. Similarities and differences among rehabilitation therapists

	Physical therapy	Occupational therapy	Speech-language therapy
Reasons to seek referral	Injury or deformity affecting lower limbs	Injury or deformity affecting upper limbs	Physical impairments affecting the mouth or throat, poor feeding
	Delay in gross motor development	Delay in fine motor or perceptual development, clumsiness	Delayed language development
	Moves differently from other children	Delayed development or frustration during daily living activities	Stuttering, poor articulation, or voice disorders
Focus of treatment			
Developmental therapy	Gross motor skills	Fine motor, perceptual, and adaptive (nonverbal cognitive) skills	Language, both expressive (speaking) and receptive (listening and understanding)
Functional skills training	Walking, transfers, and wheelchair propulsion	Activities of daily living (self-feeding, dressing, personal hygiene, play/recreation)	Functional communication, chewing and swallowing food
Exercise	Lower limbs or overall endurance	Upper limbs	Oral-motor skills
Equipment provided	Leg splints and braces, crutches, walkers, wheelchairs, adapted seats, or positioning devices	Hand splints, adapted seats or positioning devices, adapted toys or self-care devices, or switches for power wheelchairs or computers	Augmentative and alternative communication devices or adapted nipples, cups, or spoons

activities to help develop Jared's thinking and reasoning skills and to help him learn to move more easily. After familiarizing herself with the family's daily routine, Marielle taught the family ways to turn everyday activities into therapeutic experiences. Diaper changes became the ideal time to perform leg flexibility exercises and help Jared learn to reach for his toes. Although Jared had always struggled and cried during his bath, Marielle made bathtime a fun time to splash and play by recommending the use of a supportive seat that made him feel safe. Using inexpensive materials, Marielle made a special chair and tray that gave Jared the support to sit upright. Once in this position, he was better able to control his arms and reach for toys.

The speech-language therapist, Carmen, started to work with Jared when it became apparent that he was having trouble with oral-motor coordination. He was very slow to finish a meal and frequently choked or gagged on his food. Carmen taught the family how to hold Jared's jaw to give him better control during feeding, and she provided other exercises that helped him to eat more efficiently. She provided a cup that was cut out on one side to fit over his nose. In this way, Jared could drink without tipping his head back, which caused him to choke.

Shortly after his second birthday, Jared began to crawl on all fours and then pull himself up to a standing position at the sofa. At this point, Phyllis, the physical therapist, began helping Jared learn to walk. With the assistance of plastic splints to support his feet and ankles and a walker with wheels, Jared was soon able to walk around his home and other familiar environments.

WHERE TO FIND A GOOD THERAPIST

As discussed in Chapter 6, young children with disabilities are eligible for therapy free of charge through early intervention programs. Once a child with disabilities enters kindergarten, the school is responsible for providing a free and appropriate public education, which includes therapy as needed to support the child's special education program. Services available in a particular school, however, may be limited. For example, although the school might help the child learn to put on a coat to get ready for recess, the school would not be expected to teach the child to brush his or her teeth because this activity usually does not take place at school. Also, parents are not usually present during therapy at school and thus have limited opportunities to observe and practice the techniques used by the therapists. For these reasons, some parents choose to seek additional private therapy through a hospital, a rehabilitation center, a home care agency, or a private practice.

Ask the pediatrician or contact the rehabilitation department of the nearest children's hospital for suggestions about therapists in your area. Most rehabilitation departments are more than willing to offer guidance even if you do not plan to have your child attend their program. The professional associations listed in the Suggested Readings and Resources may be able to put you in touch with someone in your area who is knowledgeable about

Table 9.2.   Qualities of an effective rehabilitation therapy team

- Professionals treat parents as equal partners when making team decisions.
- All team members agree on a coordinated plan for treatment.
- Findings and recommendations are promptly communicated to everyone on the team.
- All members respect one another, even when there are differences of opinion.
- Team members regularly teach one another.
- Team members share responsibility for advocating on the behalf of the child.

pediatric therapy. You may also consider calling local colleges or universities that train therapists.

It is important that you take time to find a therapist you like and feel you can work with. Consider interviewing or visiting several therapists before making a decision, or speak to parents of other children who have attended a certain program, especially if you think your relationship with the therapist may be prolonged. Ultimately, you should choose a therapist who not only has the skills your child needs and can communicate effectively with you but who also offers convenience and affordability.

Of course, you will want to make sure your child's therapist has the appropriate training and qualifications. Although all therapists receive at least some training in how to work with children, many who choose to specialize in pediatrics obtain expertise through graduate education or through specialized training programs. Check to make sure that the therapist has knowledge of your child's particular disability or is being supervised by an experienced therapist.

PLANNING THE THERAPY PROGRAM

Good therapy is a team effort, guided by the therapist but requiring cooperation from you, your child, and other members of the team. Before the therapist can select the appropriate intervention, he or she needs to gather information about your child's current skills and the factors that promote or limit your child's abilities. This evaluation will probably include a review of previous records, an interview with you, and direct observation of your child engaging in informal play activities. Formal tests may also be used.

Once the assessment is completed, you, the therapist, and other members of your child's team should review the results and agree on a plan for therapy. Ask the therapist to explain the rationale for selecting a particular therapy approach and how long therapy may be needed. You should discuss and agree on specific goals for your child, when you hope to achieve those goals, and which therapy procedures will be used to meet those goals. In this way, you will be able to measure whether the therapy is effective by monitoring your child's progress toward those goals. If the therapist or another team member says something you do not understand, ask for a better explanation. They know that the best way to help your child is to have your full understanding and cooperation. If you disagree with something your child's therapist says, or if you are asked to do therapy procedures at home that are impractical within your lifestyle, speak up! You know your child and your family better than any professional and should never be reluctant to express your own opinions.

COMMON INTERVENTIONS USED BY THERAPISTS

Learning to Be Mobile

Exercises are used to keep your child's muscles flexible, to strengthen muscles, or to promote better endurance for activity. Passive exercises in which you manipulate your child's limbs are important if your child does not move independently, and they help to prevent joints from becoming stuck in one position, a condition known as *contractures*. The therapist will instruct you how to move your child's limbs for these exercises. It is important to pay close attention to the therapist's instructions, including how to position your child for the exercises, where to place your hands, how hard to stretch the muscles, and in exactly what direction.

Exercises for strengthening muscles require your child to move limbs actively. Often, the therapist will plan play activities that motivate your child to exercise in ways that are fun. For example, your child might be invited to play tug-of-war to strengthen the arms or encouraged to blow bubbles to strengthen the lips. The therapist will be creative in gradually increasing the amount of strength needed to perform the exercise. This is called *grading*. For example, the child who needs to build strength in the lips might start by blowing bubbles and progress to blowing on whistles or musical toys that require a larger volume of air to be pushed through the lips.

Aerobic exercises help your child to increase endurance, an important goal if he or she is inactive or overweight. Your child's therapist can show you ways to adapt exercises. For example, a child who cannot move his or her legs may learn to ride a tricycle that is operated by turning hand pedals or may practice dancing to music using only upper body movements.

Sometimes, therapists will recommend special devices to help your child achieve therapy goals. An *orthosis*, also called a *splint*, is a custom-made piece of equipment that supports a weak body part or prevents or corrects an impairment or dysfunction. Figure 9.1 illustrates two commonly prescribed splints, a resting hand splint, which helps to keep the hand open, and a molded ankle-foot orthosis (MAFO), which is made to slip into your child's shoe to support the ankle and foot during walking. Splints are most often

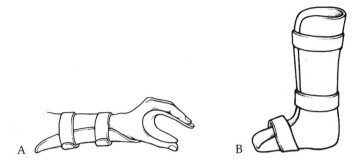

Figure 9.1.   Examples of splints: A) resting hand splint and B) molded ankle-foot orthosis (MAFO).

made of a plastic that is softened by immersion in hot water. Once softened, the plastic is cut and is molded directly onto your child's limb while the material is still warm. The process is not at all painful. Once the splint has been fitted, Velcro straps are added to hold it in place, and the therapist may line the splint with padding to make it more comfortable or to absorb moisture.

It is very important that you understand how to put the splint on, when to put it on and take it off, how to take care of the splint, and how to recognize signs that there is a problem. Ask for written instructions and a photograph or a drawing of the correct placement. Because your child is constantly growing and changing in abilities, ask your child's therapist how often he or she needs to check the splint for fit.

You may be very concerned about whether and when your child might walk. Your child's physical therapist can help you to predict your child's potential for independence as a walker, as well as his or her need for related equipment such as braces, crutches, walkers, or other aids (see Figure 9.2). It is important to make sure that the equipment properly fits your child, and that it is modified or replaced as your child grows.

Much therapy for learning to walk, called *gait training,* is required for your child to learn the movements of walking and to gain strength and balance. Not only will your child need to practice walking on different surfaces (for example, linoleum, grass, and concrete), but he or she will also need to learn to climb steps and curbs and to get around obstacles.

If a wheelchair is necessary, make sure your child receives a thorough evaluation before you make a purchase. Wheelchairs are very costly, and most insurance companies require you to wait several years before purchasing a replacement. Many models of wheelchairs are available (such as the modified stroller in Figure 9.3); usually, a team of specialists including a physical therapist, occupational therapist, wheelchair vendor, and social worker can help ensure that the wheelchair is appropriate for your child. You will want to consider how well it fits your child, how easily you and/or your child can maneuver the chair around your house or other familiar environments, how conveniently you can lift the chair into your car, and whether special features such as head supports or lap trays are needed.

Learning to Communicate

If your child is slow to develop speech or has a communication disorder, you may find yourself anticipating your child's needs, instead of waiting for your child to tell you. For example, if your child is fussy, you may offer a favorite toy instead of giving a choice. Teaching your child to communicate with others, however, is very important. As discussed in Chapter 21, communication is one of the most important activities because of its relationship to learning and to socialization. Your child's speech-language therapist will teach you ways to encourage communication during daily activities and play. Learning to speak requires your child to hear accurately, to understand or comprehend the meaning of words, and to coordinate breathing and oral movements to make speech sounds. The speech-language therapist addresses difficulties in any of these areas and will help your child develop both speech (making the correct sounds) and language (understanding and using the sounds correctly).

Some children cannot communicate effectively through speaking, including children with a profound hearing loss that has been present since birth or with severe cerebral palsy affecting the mouth. If this is the case with your child, the therapist may recommend an alternative means of communication to supplement or replace speech. Sign language is one alternative method of communication (see Chapter 20). Commonly taught to children with hearing impairments, it may also augment speech when your child has a very severe communication problem and is frustrated by his or her inability to communicate. Of course, you and other members of your immediate family will need to learn sign language along with your child.

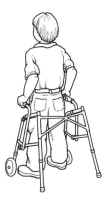

Figure 9.2.   Child using a walker.

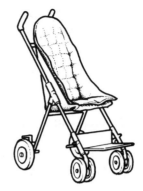

Figure 9.3. Supportive collapsible stroller.

Augmentative and alternative communication allows your child to communicate with the help of special tools and devices that substitute for or add to spoken language. These may be as simple as a board with pictures for your child to point to or as complex as computers that produce synthesized speech. Although such devices may be very expensive to purchase and maintain, your child's therapist can help you identify sources of funding through your child's school, insurance, or charitable organizations.

Learning Self-Care Skills

The degree to which your child can become independent in daily living skills will depend ultimately on the severity of his or her disability. Although your child may always require some assistance to safely and successfully bathe, eat, and dress, encourage as much self-reliance as possible. Every gain in independence will increase your child's self-esteem and provide further motivation.

Teaching self-care skills requires a great deal of patience and creativity. Families of children with disabilities often spend far more time than usual in the daily routine of getting dressed in the morning or completing a meal. It's easy to feel frustrated and to want to do too much for your child because it seems easier or faster. Remember that all children need years of practice before they get all of their clothes on properly or go through a meal without spilling. Your child's therapist can help you establish a routine that provides set times for you and your child to work on self-care skills while still allowing the time both of you need to yourselves. For example, you may find it more practical to help your child learn to use a utensil at dinnertime rather than at breakfast when you are rushing to get out of the house to work.

Feeding is usually the first self-care skill that a child learns (see Chapter 7). If your child has oral-motor problems that interfere with his or her ability to chew or swallow, you should seek advice from your child's therapist before beginning to teach self-feeding. Know what kinds of foods are safe for your child to eat, and learn what to do should your child begin to choke. Your child's therapist can also show you the best way to position your child during mealtimes and can recommend special utensils to make eating easier for your child.

Accidental spills are common and should be expected when any child first learns to self-feed. You may want to use unbreakable dishes and a plastic cloth under your child's chair to make cleanup easier. If your child takes longer than usual to finish a meal, you may wish to purchase dishes with a reservoir for hot water beneath the eating surface so that the food will stay warm for a longer time.

As you begin to teach dressing skills to your child, remember that getting dressed requires a great deal of physical movement and can be very hard for a child with poor coordination, balance difficulties, or spasticity (which causes stiffening when moving from one position to another). Get advice from your child's therapist on how to help your child relax and get into position prior to dressing so that movement is easier and on how to select clothing that is attractive, durable, and easy to get on and off. In general, slightly larger sizes, loose neckbands and cuffs, front rather than back openings, and loosely draped styles such as capes or raglan sleeves are easiest to manage. Look for clothes that wash easily because your child may perspire profusely with the effort involved in dressing and moving around. Look for clothes with reinforced seams, as your child may tend to handle clothing more roughly than usual. Try to select clothes with large or easy-to-manipulate fasteners, or, if you are handy with a sewing machine, attach Velcro fasteners behind buttons and snaps that are merely decorative.

Assistive technology consists of tools and devices that are adapted in many ingenious ways to encourage self-reliance in daily living skills. For example, children who cannot raise their arms over their head might still be able to comb their hair independently if given a lightweight comb with a very long handle. Some devices can be made at home easily, whereas others must be purchased or custom designed. Adaptations can be simple, such as enlarging the handle of a spoon so it is easier to grasp, or they can be very elaborate, such as providing computerized controls that allow your child to turn on lights or change television channels simply by looking at a target. Remember that as ingenious and helpful as some devices may be, they also can be costly and inconvenient to carry outside the home. In most cases, the fewer pieces of adaptive equipment your child needs to function independently, the easier life will be. Figure 9.4 presents an example of an assistive technology device used to help young children play with an age-appropriate toy, a jack-in-the-box.

OTHER THERAPY APPROACHES

As you begin to learn more about your child's disability, you will most certainly hear of other methods for rehabilitation. Some of these are widely

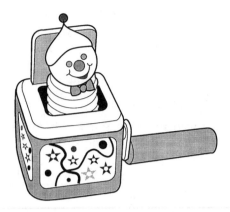

Figure 9.4.   An adapted toy. The child uses a large handle to help grasp and manipulation.

accepted and recommended, whereas others are considered more controversial. Ask your child's therapist to discuss the variety of options available for your child's rehabilitation and to recommend where to obtain any special services that may benefit your child. Table 9.3 presents some of these approaches with recommendations for how to obtain further information.

SUMMARY

This chapter has introduced some of the many rehabilitation solutions that may help your child to function as well as possible and reach his or her full developmental potential. Caring for any young child is a full-time job, as most new parents know. When your child has a disability and requires additional care and therapy, the job can seem overwhelming. As important as it is for you to provide the right therapies for your child, you must never forget your primary role as a parent. Take time to learn about your child's therapy at your own pace, and do not feel guilty if other responsibilities prevent you from doing everything your child's therapists suggest. Over time, you will find that you are increasingly comfortable with helping your child and that therapy becomes just one more part of your daily parenting routine.

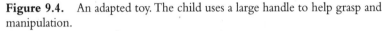

Some Questions Answered

My child has just started a therapy program. What can I do at home to help?

Your child's therapist will probably spend a portion of your child's treatment time teaching you ways to help your child. You may feel overwhelmed by

Table 9.3. Examples of therapy approaches

Type of therapy	Description	Contact for more information
Neurodevelopmental therapy (NDT)	The use of special positioning devices and therapeutic handling to help your child develop motor control. Parents are taught how to incorporate therapy techniques into their child's daily routine so that there are many opportunities for learning.	Neurodevelopmental Treatment Association 401 North Michigan Avenue Chicago, IL 60611 312-321-5151 http://www.ndta.org
Sensory integration therapy (SI)	A therapy approach that considers a child's perceptual strengths and weaknesses to create an optimal learning environment, particularly focusing on the sensations of touch, body awareness, gravity, and motion	Sensory Integration International 1602 Cabrillo Avenue Torrance, CA 90501 310-320-9986 http://home.earthlink.net~sensoryint/
Therapeutic horseback riding (hippotherapy)	The use of horseback riding and other activities using horses to achieve cognitive, physical, emotional, social, educational, and behavioral goals	North American Riding for the Handicapped Association Post Office Box 33150 Denver, CO 80233 800-369-7433 http://www.narha.org
Aquatic therapy	The use of swimming and other pool activities to promote motor skills. The reduced gravitational pull provided by an aquatic environment, often combined with use of warm water, makes movement easier for some children.	The Aquatic Exercise Association Post Office Box 497 Port Washington, WI 53074 414-284-3416

(continued)

Table 9.3. *(continued)*

Type of therapy	Description	Contact for more informatio
Therapeutic massage	The use of massage to promote a child's physical, emotional, and intellectual development and to improve parent–child bonding and attachment	American Massage Therapy Association 820 Davis Street, Suite 100 Evanston, IL 60201-4444 847-864-0123 http://www.amtamassage.org
Myofascial release	A therapeutic treatment using gentle, manual manipulation of fascia, tough connective tissue occurring throughout the body, in order to promote health and improved posture	Myofascial Release Treatment Centers 222 West Lancaster Avenue Paoli, PA 10301 800-FASCIAL http://www.vll.com/mfr/
Auditory integration training	The use of sound stimulation, provided through headphones, designed to improve the child's listening, learning, movement, organization, and self-esteem. Method is used especially with children with severe developmental disabilities, including autism.	Society for Auditory Intervention Techniques 1040 Commercial Street SE, Suite 306 Salem, OR 97302 http://www.teleport.com/~sait/

this expectation—after all, it's hard enough just doing a good job of being a parent. Speak up if you think your child's therapist expects too much (or too little) of you!

The therapist's most important job is to help you understand the goals of your child's therapy so you can find manageable ways of reinforcing them at home. For example, if your child fusses or fidgets when you teach him or her about undressing, you might motivate better cooperation by asking your child to undress for a splash in the swimming pool or to put on and take off costumes as part of pretend play. Keep sessions short, and stop if either you or your child becomes frustrated or bored. Remember that the best way to motivate your child is to give encouragement and positive reinforcement for every effort that he or she makes, whether successful or not.

How can I select toys that will help my child progress in therapy?

Many toys have educational or therapeutic value, but if your child doesn't think the toy is fun, you can be certain that he or she won't play with it for very long. Your child's therapist can suggest toys that offer the appropriate degree of developmental challenge, but also use your own ideas. If you think your child would enjoy a drum but the therapist thinks he or she cannot handle the drumsticks, the therapist might be able to modify the toy or recommend another musical instrument.

Although some companies specialize in making toys that are easier for children with disabilities to play with, many parents prefer to adapt off-the-shelf toys so the child can play with the same games that his or her peers play with. For example, puzzle pieces can be fitted with large knobs for grasping, or blocks can be made to stay together more easily using Velcro or magnets. Your child's therapist can show you where to purchase special toys and can help you to adapt regular toys.

Commonly Used Medications

John Albert Wray

A medication is a substance that is used to treat disease. There are both benefits and risks linked with medications that are commonly used in treating children with developmental disabilities. Some of these medications are used to treat illnesses such as fevers and infections that are experienced by all children. Others, such as antiepileptic and antispasticity medications, treat specific disorders associated with developmental disabilities. Although this discussion of drugs is not meant to be all-inclusive, it should give you some understanding of the types of medications that may be used and the potential side effects that your child may experience. Books with more information are included in the Suggested Readings and Resources at the end of this book.

Alphonse

Alphonse, a 1-year-old, has just been diagnosed with cerebral palsy. He was born prematurely and has had problems with irritability and gastroesophageal reflux (GER), which antireflux medication has helped. Now, his doctors are considering medication that may decrease the spasticity in his legs. His parents are trying to decide whether to have him try a new medication. What are the best questions to ask the medical team in making this decision?

GUIDELINES FOR THE USE OF MEDICATIONS

There are a number of guidelines you may wish to follow in deciding whether to use a medication and in assessing the most benefit and least risk of complications from the medication. You should apply these guidelines to nonstandard medications just as you would apply them to standard medications.

1. *Keep records of your child's medication history.* Include notes about any positive or negative reactions that your child may have had. This information can be particularly valuable if your child is receiving more than one type of medication because some medicines interact with one another. By paying close attention, you can help the doctor and pharmacist ensure that your child gets the proper medications.

2. *Use the same pharmacy (or pharmacy chain).* This step will make it easier to keep track of all of the drugs your child is receiving and to avoid adverse interactions between medications. Virtually all pharmacies now maintain computerized records of your previous orders. If you use a store with many branches, these records are centralized and permit flexibility as to which store you may choose. Most pharmacies now also give you a printout that describes potential interactions with other drugs that your child may be taking, gives written directions about administering the medication, and discusses potential side effects to watch for.

3. *Make compliance easier.* When your child must take many different medications, dosage schedules can easily get confused. Inexpensive plastic pillboxes with a compartment for each day of the week are available in most drugstores and can help reduce confusion. There are even pillboxes with alarms to remind your child when to take the medication. If your child receives chronic medication, such as antiepileptic drugs, it is important for him or her to eventually become responsible for taking the medication independently. The maturity and cognitive abilities needed to accomplish this vary in children, so there should be a gradual shift in responsibilities. The use of a pillbox as a prompt may help in this transition.

4. *Prevent poisonings.* All medicines can cause serious problems if taken in doses larger than necessary. You can minimize this risk by storing medicines in childproof containers in a locked or inaccessible cabinet, out of reach of children. Check the dosages on your child's medication to avoid overdosing, and do not increase dosage without first checking with your child's doctor. Store medicines in their original containers so that you retain dosage information and expiration dates, and do not use outdated medicines.

5. *Know why the medicine is being prescribed.* Ask questions so you know 1) what diagnoses your child's doctor has made, 2) how the medicine can help your child, and 3) what symptoms are being targeted.

6. *Know the potential side effects and interactions of a new medicine.* What are the common and less common side effects of the new medicine? What interactions may occur with the other medicines your child is taking? Should the medicine be taken before, with, or after meals?

7. *Understand how you and your child's doctor will monitor the positive and negative effects of the medicine.* Monitoring the medication is one of the most

important parts of the relationship between your family and your child's pediatrician. Before leaving the doctor's office you should have a plan (preferably written) for monitoring the medicine's effects. The written plan should also include the date of follow-up. When prescribing medicine to affect behavior, many doctors now use clinical rating scales to help monitor the drug's effects. Actual measurements of behavior are even more useful. For some medicines, it is suggested that laboratory tests be performed before the child starts the medicine and intermittently while he or she takes the medicine. The level of some medicines in the blood can be measured and is usually done at trough (just before a dose) or peak (just after a dose) times.

GENERIC VERSUS BRAND NAME MEDICATION

Generic drugs contain the same active ingredients that are found in the brand name medication, although other components of the drug, such as binders and fillers, may differ. You may be able to save a considerable amount of money by using generic rather than brand name drugs. In fact, many pharmacists encourage using generic medications, and some insurance plans and HMOs (health maintenance organizations) mandate it.

In most cases, generic substitution is safe and effective. The small variations allowable under the Food and Drug Administration (FDA) guidelines, however, may cause significant problems for certain types of drugs such as antiepileptics, in which drug levels must be kept within strict limits to control seizures with the least likelihood of side effects. Insurance companies generally permit use of brand names if specifically prescribed by your child's doctor.

If you do switch from a brand name to a generic drug or from one generic brand to another, keep track of when the change occurred and inform your child's doctor. If your child's medical problem subsequently worsens, your child's doctor can check to make sure that the medication change was not related to the change in the medical problem.

DIFFERENT SYMPTOMS, DIFFERENT DRUGS

In the following sections, you can find out more about medications grouped by their uses. Medications commonly used are discussed first: antibiotics, skin preparations and fever control, pain, and anticonstipation medications. The next section summarizes medications used for problems such as behavioral/mood control, sleep, epilepsy, GER, and spasticity. Other compounds besides medicine that your child may use are also discussed, as are vitamin and mineral supplements and immunizations. The accompanying tables list generic and brand names as well as the purpose of the drugs and some potential side effects. Table 10. 1 is a cross-referenced listing of all of the drugs mentioned in these tables. *Please remember that not every drug is listed and that*

Table 10.1.   Medications listed according to trade name

Trade name	Generic name	See usage table
Accutane	isotretinoin	10.3 Skin problems
Achromycin	tetracycline	10.2 Antibiotics
Adderall	dextroamphetamine/ampheta-mine	10.6 Hyperactivity and behavior
Advil[a]	ibuprofen	10.4 Fever
Amoxil	amoxicillin	10.2 Antibiotics
Aristocort	triamcinolone (steroid cream)	10.3 Skin problems
Atarax	hydroxyzine	10.7 Sleep problems
Ativan	lorazepam	10.6 Hyperactivity and behavior
Augmentin	amoxicillin/clavulanic acid	10.2 Antibiotics
——	baclofen	10.10 Spasticity
Bactrim	trimethoprim/sulfamethoxazole (TMP-SMZ)	10.2 Antibiotics
Bayer[a]	aspirin (acetylsalicylic acid)	10.4 Fever
Benadryl[a]	diphenhydramine	10.3 Skin problems
Biaxin	clarithromycin	10.2 Antibiotics
Botox	botulinum toxin	10.10 Spasticity
BuSpar	buspirone	10.6 Hyperactivity and behavior
Caldecort[a]	hydrocortisone (steroid cream)	10.3 Skin problems
Carbatrol	carbamazepine	10.8 Antiepileptic
Catapres	clonidine	10.6 Hyperactivity and behavior
Clearasil[a]	benzoyl peroxide 5%, 10%	10.3 Skin problems
Cleocin T	clindamycin	10.3 Skin problems
Colace[a]	docusate	10.5 Constipation
Cort-Dome[a]	hydrocortisone (steroid cream)	10.3 Skin problems
Corticotropin	ACTH	10.8 Antiepileptic
Cortizone for Kids[a]	hydrocortisone (steroid cream)	10.3 Skin problems
Cylert	pemoline	10.6 Hyperactivity and behavior
Dantrium	dantrolene	10.10 Spasticity
Depakene, Depakote	valproate	10.8 Antiepileptic
Desyrel	trazodone	10.6 Hyperactivity and behavior
Dexedrine	dextroamphetamine	10.6 Hyperactivity and behavior
Dilantin	phenytoin	10.8 Antiepileptic
Dulcolax[a]	bisacodyl	10.5 Constipation
E.E.S.	erythromycin	10.2 Antibiotics
Effexor	venlafaxine	10.6 Hyperactivity and behavior

Trade name	Generic name	See usage table
Elimite	permethrin	10.3 Skin problems
Empirin with codeine	codeine preparations	10.4 Fever
EryPed	erythromycin	10.2 Antibiotics
Felbatol	felbamate	10.8 Antiepileptic
Fulvicin	griseofulvin	10.3 Skin problems
Gabitril	tiagabine	10.8 Antiepileptic
Gantrisin	sulfisoxazole	10.2 Antibiotics
Grifulvin	griseofulvin	10.3 Skin problems
Haldol	haloperidol	10.6 Hyperactivity and behavior
Inderal	propranolol	10.6 Hyperactivity and behavior
Janimine	imipramine	10.6 Hyperactivity and behavior
Keflex, Keftab	cephalexin	10.2 Antibiotics
Keppra	levetiracetam	10.8 Antiepileptic
Kwell	lindane	10.3 Skin problems
Lamictal	lamotrigine	10.8 Antiepileptic
Lotrimin[a]	clotrimazole	10.3 Skin problems
Luminal	phenobarbital	10.8 Antiepileptic
Luvox	fluvoxamine	10.6 Hyperactivity and behavior
Maalox[a]	aluminum hydroxide and magnesium hydroxide	10.9 Gastroesophageal reflux
Malt-Supex[a]	malt soup extract	10.5 Constipation
Melatonin[a]	melatonin	10.7 Sleep problems
Mellaril	thioridazine	10.6 Hyperactivity and behavior
Metamucil[a]	psyllium	10.5 Constipation
Mycostatin[a]	nystatin	10.3 Skin problems
Mysoline	primidone	10.8 Antiepileptic
Neosporin	polymyxin B, neomycin, and bacitracin	10.3 Skin problems
Neurontin	gabapentin	10.8 Antiepileptic
Nix[a]	permethrin	10.3 Skin problems
Noctec	chloral hydrate	10.7 Sleep problems
Norpramin	desipramine	10.6 Hyperactivity and behavior
Omnipen	ampicillin	10.2 Antibiotics
Pamelor	nortriptyline	10.6 Hyperactivity and behavior

[a]Available without a prescription.

(continued)

Table 10.1.   *(continued)*

Trade name	Generic name	See usage table
Paxil	paroxetine	10.6 Hyperactivity and behavior
Pediazole	sulfisoxazole	10.2 Antibiotics
Pen-Vee K, Pentids	penicillin	10.2 Antibiotics
Phenergan	promethazine	10.7 Sleep problems
——	phenol	10.10 Spasticity
Polycillin	ampicillin	10.2 Antibiotics
Prilosec	omeprazole	10.9 Gastroesophageal reflux
Principen	ampicillin	10.2 Antibiotics
Provigan	promethazine	10.7 Sleep problems
Prozac	fluoxetine	10.6 Hyperactivity and behavior
Renacort	triamcinolone (steroid cream)	10.3 Skin problems
Retin-A	tretinoin	10.3 Skin problems
Risperdal	risperidone	10.6 Hyperactivity and behavior
Ritalin	methylphenidate	10.6 Hyperactivity and behavior
SENOKOT[a]	senna concentrate	10.5 Constipation
Septra	trimethoprim/sulfamethoxazole (TMP-SMZ)	10.2 Antibiotics
Tagamet	cimetidine	10.9 Gastroesophageal reflux
Tegopen	cloxacillin	10.2 Antibiotics
Tegretol	carbamazepine	10.8 Antiepileptic
Tenex	guanfacine	10.6 Hyperactivity and behavior
Thorazine	chlorpromazine	10.6 Hyperactivity and behavior
Tinactin[a]	tolnaftate	10.3 Skin problems
Tofranil	imipramine	10.6 Hyperactivity and behavior
Topamax	topiramate	10.8 Antiepileptic
Trileptal	oxcarbazepine	10.8 Antiepileptic
T-stat pads	erythromycin	10.3 Skin problems
Tylenol[a]	acetaminophen	10.4 Fever
Tylox	oxycodone	10.4 Fever
Valium	diazepam	10.10 Spasticity
Vistaril	hydroxyzine	10.7 Sleep problems
Wellbutrin	bupropion	10.6 Hyperactivity and behavior
Xanax	alprazolam	10.6 Hyperactivity and behavior
Xenalog	triamcinolone (steroid cream)	10.3 Skin problems
Xylocaine Viscous	lidocaine	10.3 Skin problems

Trade name	Generic name	See usage table
Zantac	ranitidine	10.9 Gastroesophageal reflux
Zarontin	ethosuximide	10.8 Antiepileptic
Zoloft	sertraline	10.6 Hyperactivity and behavior
Zyprexa	olanzapine	10.6 Hyperactivity and behavior

ᵃAvailable without a prescription.

not all potential side effects are shown; for example, virtually all medications can cause an allergic reaction, nausea, vomiting, and diarrhea in some people. Furthermore, not all of the possible drug interactions are listed. Both side effects and drug interactions should be discussed with your child's doctor or pharmacist.

ANTIBIOTICS

Antibiotics are medications used to treat bacterial and some fungal infections. They are ineffective against viruses. Common bacterial and fungal infections in all children include those of the respiratory tract, the middle ear, the urinary tract, and the skin. Because of their different modes of action, different antibiotics are effective against different microorganisms (see Table 10.2).

To determine which antibiotic will be most effective in treating a specific infection, your child's doctor may order culture and sensitivity tests. This involves swabbing your child's throat, wound, or abscess or taking a urine specimen or blood test.

For many common infections, however, your child's doctor will make a diagnosis and then begin treatment even without performing culture and sensitivity tests. This is usually the case when an ear or a sinus infection is suspected. Depending on the infection, antibiotic treatment can last from 5 days to 14 days or more. The infection may appear to clear before the antibiotic prescription has run out, often within a day or two, but the full course of treatment is important to eliminate all of the infectious organisms. The best example is strep throat, which is treated with 10 days of penicillin. Studies have shown that because people often feel better within several days, they rarely complete the full 10 days of medication; however, there is some risk of developing a bacterial infection of a heart valve with incomplete therapy. Often, the doctor may want to see your child again after the antibiotic course is finished to be sure that the infection has been cured. This is true for a middle-ear infection, in which the doctor will recheck your child's eardrum to make sure it is no longer inflamed. Although most antibiotic treatment is

Table 10.2. Common oral antibiotics

Generic name	Trade name(s)	Preparations
amoxicillin	Amoxil	C, T, L
amoxicillin/clavulanic acid	Augmentin	T, L
ampicillin	Omnipen, Polycillin, Principen	C, L
cephalexin	Keflex, Keftab	C, L
clarithromycin	Biaxin	T, L
erythromycin	EryPed, E.E.S.	C, L
penicillin	Pen-Vee K, Pentids	C, T, L
sulfisoxazole	Gantrisin, Pediazole	C, L
tetracycline	Achromycin	C, L
trimethoprim/ sulfamethoxazole (TMP-SMZ)	Bactrim, Septra	C, L

Key: C = capsules, T = tablets, L = liquid suspension or elixir.

given by mouth for a week or less, recurrent urinary tract, sinus, or middle-ear infections may lead the pediatrician to prescribe an oral antibiotic for your child for a number of months. Some rare, severe infections, such as osteomyelitis (a bone abscess), may require intravenous antibiotics for 1–2 months. In addition to taking antibiotics to help recover from an infection, your child should rest and maintain a normal intake of fluids. Your child's appetite will improve as the infection comes under control.

Skin rashes, upset stomach, and diarrhea often occur as side effects of antibiotic use. Yeast (fungal) infections in the mouth (thrush) or perineal region are also common side effects. One particular antibiotic, tetracycline, should not be given to preteenagers because it affects the development of teeth. Fortunately, other antibiotics that work just as well can be substituted; tetracycline's unique contribution is in treating acne, which occurs in adolescence when tooth staining is no longer an issue.

Some people develop allergies to medications, particularly to penicillin and some of its derivatives (for example, ampicillin and amoxicillin). An allergic reaction to penicillin can involve an itchy rash called *hives* or, rarely, severe difficulty with breathing, called *anaphylaxis*. If your child is allergic to

Commonly used to treat	Side effects
Middle-ear infections, urinary tract infections	Rash, less stomach upset than ampicillin, allergic reaction
Same as ampicillin, plus resistant bacterial infections	Same as amoxicillin
Same as amoxicillin	Same as penicillin
Penicillin-resistant infections	Upset stomach, allergic reaction
Strep throat (when allergic to penicillin)	Upset stomach, headache
Same as penicillin, skin infections	Upset stomach
Strep throat, pneumonia, rheumatic fever	Upset stomach, rash, allergic reaction
Urinary tract infections	Allergic reaction, upset stomach, lower white blood cell count
Acne, mycoplasma, pneumonia	Teeth stains in preteenagers, upset stomach, rash, kidney toxicity
Urinary tract infections, middle-ear infections	Kidney toxicity, decreased red and white blood cell count, allergic reactions

penicillin or to any other drug, make sure that the doctor knows, that your child's medical records have been flagged to indicate the nature of the reaction, and that the school nurse has been informed. Other antibiotics can be substituted safely and effectively.

SKIN PREPARATIONS

Rashes and skin problems are common in all children but are even more frequent in children who use wheelchairs or who remain in bed for very long periods of time. Rashes may be signs of viral infections such as roseola, measles, or chickenpox or can be the result of fungal or bacterial infections. They may also be of noninfectious origin, caused by an allergic reaction, sunburn, or contact with something abrasive. If caused by a virus, the rash will generally disappear when the infection clears up, although your child may need some relief of symptoms in the meantime, such as from calamine lotion on the rash or an oral antihistamine such as Benadryl (diphenhydramine). It should be noted that the combination of calamine lotion and antihistamines has little benefit over calamine lotion alone and has more side effects.

There are a number of skin preparations that may be helpful, depending on the diagnosis. Topical (rubbed on) skin medications may contain antibiotics, antifungal agents, corticosteroids (which are different from the anabolic steroids that athletes sometimes use illegally), or anesthetics and come in a variety of forms—powders, creams, ointments, and lotions (see Table 10.3). Powders increase drying and are useful in and around body fold areas, such as with diaper rash. Lotions, creams, and ointments are oil–water combinations of varying composition. Lotions are the lightest and most drying of the three, creams are somewhat heavier and oilier, and ointments are the heaviest and most penetrating. Some skin problems require treatment with oral medications in addition to or instead of these topical medications.

You can help protect your child against certain skin rashes. Having your child wear long-sleeved shirts and jeans while hiking or going into the woods can decrease the chance of exposure to poison ivy. Having your child avoid contact with foods or chemicals that have previously irritated his or her skin is helpful. Absorbent diapers, frequent diaper changes, and the use of baby powder can decrease the risk of diaper rash. Sunburn may be minimized by the "slip, slop, slap" approach: "Slip" on a long-sleeve shirt, "slop" on a sunscreen lotion, and "slap" on a hat! Sunscreen lotions now have a sun protection factor (SPF) rating. Using a lotion with at least an SPF 15 rating is recommended, although some easily burnt individuals require lotions with an SPF 20 or SPF 45 rating.

Bacterial Skin Infections

Bacterial skin infections may be treated with either topical or oral antibiotics, depending on the severity and location of the infection. Boils or other skin abscesses, in which the bacteria cannot be reached by topical medications, may require drainage of the infected area by a physician. This is usually followed by treatment with an oral antibiotic.

Acne is also a type of bacterial infection that occurs frequently among adolescents and may last for several years, with periods of improvement and worsening. It is caused by clogged sebaceous glands, or pores, that become infected. Therapy involves keeping the skin clean, removing the dirt, oil, and cell debris that can block the pores, and treating the infection. Frequent washing is important, using a nonirritating soap such as Alpha-Keri, Aveeno, Dial, Dove, Ivory, or Neutrogena. Benzoyl peroxide, the active ingredient in such products as Clearasil and Oxy-10, has been shown to be helpful in unclogging the skin pores. The topical antibiotic Cleocin T (clindamycin) also may be prescribed. Vitamin A preparations loosen cellular debris around the skin glands. There is a topical vitamin A preparation (Retin-A, or tretinoin) as well as an oral preparation (Accutane, or isotretinoin) for individuals with very severe cases. Although effective, Accutane has a number of potential side effects including causing birth defects and should not be administered to pregnant women.

Fungal Infections

Children are often troubled by fungal infections, particularly thrush, or monilia, which is caused by a yeast-like fungus called *Candida*. Other common fungal infections include athlete's foot and ringworm.

Thrush appears as a reddish rash around the genital area or as a thick white covering on the tongue or cheeks. The antifungal agent Mycostatin (nystatin) is very effective in treating this disorder. Cream and ointment preparations are used for genital infections, and a liquid preparation is used for mouth infections.

Fungi that cause ringworm and athlete's foot can be treated with another antifungal agent, Tinactin (tolnaftate). Tolnaftate is available over the counter in several formulations: cream, ointment, or powder. Your child's doctor can help you decide which formulation will be best. Ringworm can also be treated with Lotrimin (clotrimazole). If it does not completely clear up with the topical medication after 2 weeks, the oral medication Fulvicin or Grifulvin (griseofulvin) may be used.

Allergic Skin Conditions

Many skin problems are caused not by infections but by allergic reactions. Hives and certain rashes indicate an allergic response and may be treated with oral antihistamines. Another type of skin irritation, called *eczema*, can appear as a result of contact with certain types of soap, cosmetics, or other products. Eczema may also occur for unknown reasons, with inflammations appearing as itchy, scaly patches around the elbows, underarms, and neck. Steroid creams such as Caldecort (hydrocortisone) or Aristocort A (triamcinolone) can usually control the irritation. Moisturizing creams and lotions, such as Alpha-Keri, Aquaphor, Aveeno, Lubriderm, and Nivea, can be used to treat the dryness and prevent the water loss that leads to dry skin and are available without prescription.

Common scalp conditions include cradle cap in babies and dandruff among adults. Both appear as scaliness and flaking. Frequent use of a nonprescription shampoo that contains selenium sulfide (Selsun Blue), zinc pyrithione (Head and Shoulders), or salicylic acid and sulfur (Sebulex) can help treat the problem.

Insect-Related Rashes

Scabies is a skin condition caused by an infestation of the skin by mites resulting in intense itching and redness. It can occur anywhere on the body, but most often starts under the arms or in the groin region. An irritation of the scalp may be caused by infestation with lice, tiny parasites that lay their eggs in hair. Scabies and lice can both be treated using Kwell (lindane) preparations or Elimite or Nix (permethrin) preparations. Body lice and scabies are

Table 10.3.   Medications commonly used for skin problems

Generic name	Trade name(s)	Preparations
benzoyl peroxide 5%, 10%[a]	Clearasil	Cr, Lo, gel
clindamycin	Cleocin T	L, gel, O
clotrimazole[a]	Lotrimin	Cr, Lo, L
diphenhydramine	Benadryl	C, T, L, Cr
erythromycin	T-stat pads	Liquid-soaked pads
griseofulvin	Fulvicin, Grifulvin	T
hydrocortisone (steroid cream)[a]	Caldecort, Cort-Dome, Cortizone for Kids	P, Cr, O
isotretinoin	Accutane	C
lidocaine[a]	Xylocaine Viscous	Gel
lindane[a]	Kwell	Shampoo, Cr, Lo
nystatin[a]	Mycostatin	T, L, P, Cr, O
permethrin[a]	Elimite, Nix	Shampoo, Cr
polymyxin B, neomycin, and bacitracin[a]	Neosporin	Cr, O
tolnaftate[a]	Tinactin	L, P, Cr, O, aerosol
tretinoin	Retin-A	L, Cr
triamcinolone (steroid cream)	Aristocort, Renacort, Xenalog	P, Cr, O, Lo

Key: C = capsules, T = tablets, L = liquid suspension or elixir, S = suppositories, P = powder, Cr = cream, O = ointment, Lo = lotion.

[a]Available without a prescription.

Commonly used to treat	Side effects
Acne	Skin irritation, peeling
Acne (topical antibiotic)	Diarrhea, colitis, irritated eyes
Fungal infections, ringworm	Peeling skin, itching, skin irritation
Hives, allergic responses	Sedation
Acne (topical antibiotic)	Dryness, peeling skin, skin irritation
Fungal infections, ringworm	Skin rash, nausea, fatigue, confusion
Eczema, dermatitis, poison ivy	Skin irritation, dryness, rash
Severe acne	Cracked lips, conjunctivitis, muscle weakness, headache, light sensitivity, birth defects if taken during pregnancy
Cold and canker sores, sore throat	Local irritation. DO NOT USE EXCESSIVELY.
Scabies, lice	Occasionally dizziness or convulsions. Apply strictly as instructed.
Fungal infections, yeast infections (thrush)	Topically—nontoxic Orally—diarrhea
Scabies, lice	Itchiness, stinging, rash
Prevents infection of cuts	Rash
Fungal infections, athlete's foot, ringworm	Nontoxic
Severe acne	Cracked lips, conjunctivitis, muscle weakness, headache, light sensitivity, birth defects if taken during pregnancy
Same as hydrocortisone	Same as hydrocortisone

Table 10.4.   Medications commonly used for fever and pain control

Generic name	Trade name(s)	Preparations
acetaminophen[a]	Tylenol	C, T, L
aspirin (acetylsalicylic acid)[a]	Bayer	T, L, S
codeine	Empirin with codeine (with aceta-minophen)	T, S
ibuprofen[a]	Advil	C, T, L
oxycodone	Tylox (with aceta-minophen)	C

Key: C = capsules, T = tablets, L = liquid suspension or elixir, S = suppositories.
[a]Available without a prescription.

treated with cream or lotion rubbed into the affected areas. Head lice are treated with shampoo; usually one application is sufficient. This is a contagious infestation because the lice are passed on easily at child care centers or at home when children share towels, hairbrushes, and combs. Therefore, all family members should be checked for the presence of lice or nits (their eggs) on the scalp, and usually all family members receive the treatment.

Painful Skin Conditions

Some skin conditions are painful. Anesthetic solutions, such as Xylocaine Viscous (lidocaine), can be applied to the mouth and are effective in deadening the pain associated with canker sores, severe sore throats, cold sores, or throat infections. Anesthetic ointments or sprays are also available for sunburn (Bactine, Solarcaine).

Skin Sores

Skin sores, also called *bedsores* or *decubitus ulcers*, occur when the skin and underlying tissue break down as a result of pressure, poor nutrition, and/or inactivity. Children who use wheelchairs, such as children with severe forms of cerebral palsy, muscular dystrophy, or spina bifida, are particularly susceptible. The best approach to treatment is prevention—maintaining good nutrition and hygiene of the skin, using foam or sheepskin to relieve pressure points, and frequently changing positions to reduce prolonged pressure to specific areas—usually bony protuberances such as the hips or the backbone.

Commonly used to treat	Side effects
Fever, pain	Liver toxicity with severe overdose
Fever, pain, inflammation	Upset stomach, allergic reactions, dizziness, prolonged bleeding time, Reye syndrome
Pain	Dizziness, nausea
Fever, pain, inflammation	Blurred vision, stomach ulcers, abnormal kidney function
Pain	Dizziness, nausea

If your child develops skin sores, a doctor's opinion is necessary. Your child should be treated immediately to prevent the development of deep infections.

FEVER CONTROL AND PAIN MEDICATIONS

In children, fevers are most frequently associated with viral illnesses such as the flu, measles, or chickenpox, although bacterial infections such as strep throat can also cause fever. There are two good reasons to treat high fevers. First, very high fevers, above 102 °F (38.5 °C), are quite uncomfortable. Second, high fevers occurring in children younger than 4 years can be associated with convulsions. Most fevers, however, do not reach a level that requires intervention; some evidence even suggests that fever may aid the body in fighting off certain infections.

If your child's fever does exceed 102 °F, some treatment may be required. You can give your child a sponge bath in lukewarm water and use light covers in bed. Alcohol rubs should not be used because the alcohol can be absorbed through the skin and cause intoxication. If high fevers continue for more than a day or if your child is difficult to rouse, you should consult your child's doctor as there may be an infection that requires antibiotics.

Aspirin and acetaminophen (such as Tylenol) are the most commonly used medications to treat fevers (see Table 10.4). Even these drugs, however, have possible serious side effects. Aspirin has been associated with an increased risk of Reye syndrome, a rare, virus-related illness of childhood that causes inflammation of the liver and brain. Aspirin should, therefore, not be used by children with viral illnesses, particularly flu or chickenpox.

Table 10.5.   Medications and dietary supplements commonly used to treat constipation

Generic name	Trade name(s)	Preparations
bisacodyl[a]	Dulcolax	T, S
docusate[a]	Colace	C, L
senna concentrate[a]	SENOKOT	T, L, granules
malt soup extract[a]	Malt-Supex	T, L, P
psyllium[a]	Metamucil	P

Key: C = capsules, T = tablets, L = liquid suspension or elixir, S = suppositories, P = powder.

[a]Available without a prescription.

Aspirin may be given safely to children for other conditions, such as to control pain or inflammation, but when in doubt, acetaminophen is a safer choice.

Acetaminophen has similar effects as aspirin in treating fever and pain but does not reduce inflammation. It is now the most commonly used anti-fever agent. It has few side effects and is usually easier on the stomach than aspirin. It is not associated with an increased risk for Reye syndrome. A toxic overdose of acetaminophen (10–100 times the normal dose), however, can lead to severe liver damage.

Ibuprofen (such as Advil) is also frequently used for relief from pain and fever. Children's strength ibuprofen is now available without a prescription. In the rare instance that a more powerful pain medication is needed, such as after surgery, codeine or its related compound oxycodone is often used, sometimes in combination with acetaminophen (Empirin with codeine, and Tylox respectively).

Acute pain, such as from a fall or sports injury, can also be relieved by resting and elevating an injured limb and by applying an ice or cold pack. Ice can be placed in a plastic bag, then wrapped in a cloth and applied to the injured area for 5–10 minutes. Commercially made cold packs can also be used. After a 10-minute break, the pack can be reapplied. This treatment is most effective *immediately* after an injury.

ANTICONSTIPATION MEDICATIONS

Constipation can be a major problem for any child. Decreased physical activity, a reduced intake of fluids, and uncoordinated bowel contractions all contribute to the problem. Treatment methods other than the use of medicines are discussed in Chapter 7. These methods revolve around increasing fluid and fiber intake, increasing physical activity, and promoting regular toileting.

Commonly used as	Side effects
Laxative (review with physician)	Uncommon, abdominal cramps
Stool softener (review with physician)	Nausea, rash
Laxative (review with physician)	Uncommon, abdominal cramps
Laxative (review with physician)	Uncommon, abdominal cramps
Fiber supplement, bulk forming	Abdominal cramps

Laxatives, stool softeners, and fiber products are commonly used to combat constipation (see Table 10.5).

BEHAVIORAL AND MOOD CONTROL MEDICATIONS

In many cases, behavior management techniques (see Chapter 11) are effective in addressing behavior challenges in children. Sometimes, however, medication is needed. The most common reasons for using behavior medication in children are to control hyperactivity and aggression and/or to prevent self-injury. All of the behavior medications work by altering the chemical environment of the brain (see Table 10.6). They can have important interactions with other medications, and some can cause problems if stopped abruptly. So, you should seek the advice of a doctor before your child starts or stops any of these medications. The doctor may ask you and your child's teacher to fill out a behavior checklist and rating scales, which will give objective evidence of the drug's effectiveness. If your child uses the medication on a long-term basis, the doctor may also suggest a "drug holiday" once per year to make sure that the drug is still needed.

Attention-deficit/hyperactivity disorder (ADHD) is often treated with stimulant medication such as Ritalin (methylphenidate), Dexedrine (dextroamphetamine), Adderall (dextroamphetamine and levo-amphetamine), or Cylert (pemoline) (see Chapter 24). Catapres (clonidine)—used originally to control high blood pressure in adults—and its newer cousin, Tenex (guanfacine), may also be used to control hyperactivity, although they are less useful in improving attention span. Clonidine may also be useful in controlling aggression and tics, particularly if your child has other neurological problems. The most common side effect is sleepiness, which often dissipates if the medication is increased slowly. This side effect can actually be a help to a child with hyperactivity and sleep problems if the medicine is given at bedtime.

Table 10.6.   Medications commonly used for hyperactivity and behavior problems

Generic name	Trade name(s)	Preparations
alprazolam	Xanax	T
bupropion	Wellbutrin	T
buspirone	BuSpar	T
chlorpromazine	Thorazine	C, T, L, S, injection
clonidine	Catapres	T
desipramine	Norpramin	T
dextroamphetamine	Dexedrine DextroStat	T, spansule (regular, sustained release)
dextroamphetamine/ levo-amphetamine	Adderall	T, spansule (regular, sustained release)
fluoxetine	Prozac	C, L
fluvoxamine	Luvox	T
guanfacine	Tenex	T
haloperidol	Haldol	T, L
imipramine	Janimine, Tofranil	C, T
lorazepam	Ativan	T, injection
methylphenidate	Ritalin	T (regular, sustained release)

Key: C = capsules, T = tablets, L = liquid suspension or elixir, S = suppositories.

Commonly used to treat	Side effects
Anxiety	Respiratory depression, drowsiness, drooling, swallowing difficulties
Depression, attention-deficit/hyperactivity disorder (ADHD) with depression	Nervousness, tremor, headache, palpitations, abdominal cramps, nausea, weakness, dizziness
Aggressive behavior, anxiety	Drowsiness, dizziness, headache
Hyperactivity, aggressive behavior	Weight gain, drowsiness, decreased attention, movement disorder (may be permanent), low blood pressure, lower seizure threshold, liver toxicity
Aggressive behavior, tics, hyperactivity	Rash, dry mouth, sedation, dizziness, headache, constipation. DO NOT ABRUPTLY STOP MEDICATION because of risk of rebound high blood pressure.
Depression, ADHD	Same as nortriptyline
Hyperactivity, poor attention span	Same as methylphenidate
Hyperactivity, poor attention span	Same as methylphenidate
Depression, obsessive-compulsive disorder, behavior on autism spectrum	Skin rash, insomnia, weight loss, nausea, headache, weakness, stomach upset, excessive sweating
Same as fluoxetine	Same as fluoxetine
Same as clonidine	Same as clonidine but less sedating
Same as chlorpromazine	Same as chlorpromazine
Bed-wetting, depression, hyperactivity, poor attention span	Drowsiness, rapid heart rate, dry mouth, skin rash
Anxiety, seizures, aggression	Respiratory depression, drowsiness, drooling, swallowing difficulties
Hyperactivity, poor attention span	Loss of appetite, upset stomach, headache, irritability, suppression of weight gain, increased heart rate, insomnia, moodiness

(continued)

Table 10.6.   *(continued)*

Generic name	Trade name(s)	Preparations
nortriptyline	Pamelor	C, L
olanzapine	Zyprexa	T
paroxetine	Paxil	T
pemoline	Cylert	T (long acting)
propranolol	Inderal	C, T
risperidone	Risperdal	T
sertraline	Zoloft	C, T
thioridazine	Mellaril	T, L
trazodone	Desyrel	T
venlafaxine	Effexor	T

Key: C = capsules, T = tablets, L = liquid suspension or elixir, S = suppositories.

Sleepiness is less of a problem with guanfacine. After long-term therapy, the medication should be gradually discontinued to prevent rebound hypertension following sudden withdrawal.

Another medication used to lower high blood pressure, Inderal (propranolol), has been used to treat aggression and rage behaviors (as well as migraines). It is generally safe, although it may worsen symptoms of asthma, and children with Down syndrome may need lower than normal doses as the drug seems to accumulate in their blood. Antiepileptic medications (see Table 10.8) such as Tegretol (carbamazepine) and Depakene/Depakote (valproic acid/valproate) have also been used with some success in treating behavior problems.

Certain drugs used in psychiatry have also found use in treating behavior disorders in children with developmental disabilities. These include antipsychotic, antidepressant, and antianxiety medication.

Antipsychotic medications include the drugs Haldol (haloperidol), Thorazine (chlorpromazine), and Mellaril (thioridazine) as well as the more

Commonly used to treat	Side effects
Depression, ADHD with depression	Low blood pressure, tinnitus, gastroesophageal discomfort, dry mouth, blurred vision. Very rarely, sudden death from cardiac arrhythmia has been reported.
Aggressive behavior	Same as risperidone
Depression	Same as fluoxetine
Hyperactivity, poor attention span	Liver dysfunction, headache, irritability
Aggression, rage reactions, migraines	Dizziness, stomach upset, fatigue
Aggressive behavior	Drowsiness, movement disorder (less frequent than with chlorpromazine), constipation, weight gain, nasal stuffiness
Same as fluoxetine	Same as fluoxetine
Same as chlorpromazine	Same as chlorpromazine
Depression	Rash, dry mouth, blurred vision, constipation, dizziness, drowsiness, weight loss
Depression	Drowsiness, insomnia, nausea, headache, dizziness

recently developed atypical neuroleptics such as Risperdal (risperidone), Zyprexa (olanzapine), and BuSpar (buspirone). Antipsychotic medications have more serious side effects than the stimulants discussed previously. Although controlling hyperactivity and aggressive behavior, antipsychotic medication may decrease attention, increase seizure activity in children with epilepsy, and in rare instances cause liver damage. With prolonged use, they carry a significant risk of producing disorders of movement (tremors and odd postures). This is much less likely to occur with the newer forms of these drugs. These drugs, however, should be reserved for children with the most severe behavior problems that do not respond to other therapies.

Tricyclic antidepressant medications such as Tofranil (imipramine) and Norpramin (desipramine) can be useful in the treatment of ADHD, tic disorders, obsessive-compulsive disorders, and depression. There have been rare reports, however, of life-threatening cardiac arrhythmias (irregular heart rhythms), so an EKG (electrocardiogram) should be obtained before starting your child on a tricyclic antidepressant and at intervals during its use.

Table 10.7.   Medications commonly used for sleep problems

Generic name	Trade name(s)	Preparations
chloral hydrate	Noctec	C, L, S
diphenhydramine[a]	Benadryl	C, T, L
hydroxyzine	Atarax, Vistaril	C, T, L
melatonin[a]	Melatonin	T
promethazine	Phenergan, Provigan	T, L, S

Key: C = capsules, T = tablets, L = liquid suspension or elixir, S = suppositories.
[a]Available without a prescription.

Pamelor (nortriptyline), Tofranil (imipramine), and Norpramin (desipramine) are the most commonly used of this class of medication. They begin to improve mood within about 1–3 weeks. Prozac-like antidepressants, also called selective serotonin reuptake inhibitors (SSRIs), have gained in popularity. These drugs, including Prozac (fluoxetine), Zoloft (sertraline), Paxil (paroxetine), and Luvox (fluvoxamine), are more specific in their actions than the tricyclic antidepressants are and have fewer side effects. SSRIs have found use in stabilizing mood disorders and have some positive effects in children with behaviors in the autism spectrum (see Chapter 23).

Finally, antianxiety drugs related to Valium (diazepam) such as Xanax (alprazolam) have been used to treat behavior disorders in which anxiety seems to precede aggressive or disruptive behavior. After long-term treatment is completed, the medication is tapered off slowly to prevent withdrawal reactions. SSRIs may also benefit children with anxiety disorders.

SLEEP MEDICATIONS

Many children have trouble falling asleep or staying asleep at night. Treatment differs depending on the underlying problem. You should always discuss your child's sleep problems with the doctor because some important medical disorders, such as GER and airway obstruction, may be contributing to the problem. Behavior management approaches should be tried first. It is important to develop a nighttime routine. This might include a bedtime story, quiet games, or another calming activity. The room should be darkened (with a night-light if your child fears darkness), and household noise should be kept to a minimum. If your child has difficulty either falling asleep or staying asleep, try gradually lengthening the time you take to respond to requests for attention.

Commonly used for	Side effects
Sedation	Upset stomach, habit-forming
Antihistamine, sedation, treatment of allergic reactions	Dry mouth, dizziness, upset stomach, thicker secretions
Antihistamine, antianxiety, sedation	Dry mouth, tremor
Sedation	Studies not complete about long-term effects and side effects
Antihistamine, sedation, treatment of allergic reactions	Low or high blood pressure, lower seizure threshold

If your child has a persistent problem falling asleep, a mild sedative may be helpful (see Table 10.7). The most commonly used sedative is chloral hydrate. Once your child gets used to a typical sleep pattern, usually in 2–3 weeks, the medication can be gradually withdrawn, and there will be a lasting improvement in sleep. Chloral hydrate is not addictive over a short period of time and in the dosage used to treat sleeplessness. Other sleep medications include antihistamines such as Benadryl (diphenhydramine), Atarax (hydroxyzine), and Phenergan (promethazine) and antianxiety agents such as diazepam (see Table 10.10). Melatonin, a nonprescription hormone involved in the sleep–wake cycle, may be particularly helpful for sleeping problems in children with visual impairment; it has also been used to induce sleep in children with severe mental retardation. The long-term effects of melatonin, however, are not known, and there is considerable variation in concentration among the brands available. In general, sedatives should not be continued for longer than 6–8 weeks without discussing the situation with your child's doctor.

Unfortunately no drug is useful in correcting problems with early-morning waking. If your child is rising early, that is, between 5 A.M. and 6 A.M., you may want to move bedtime to later in the evening. Having your child avoid afternoon naps after the toddler period is also helpful in establishing a typical sleep–wake cycle.

ANTIEPILEPTIC DRUGS

Seizures are the result of uncontrolled stimulation of nerve cells in the brain (see Chapter 18 for more on seizure disorders). Antiepileptic drugs work by a variety of mechanisms to make seizures less likely to occur or to decrease their intensity and spread. Different medications are prescribed for different

Table 10.8. Antiepileptic medications

Generic name	Trade name(s)	Preparations
ACTH	Corticotrophin	Injection
carbamazepine	Carbatrol, Tegretol	T, L, sprinkles
clonazepam	Klonopin	T
ethosuximide	Zarontin	C, L
felbamate	Felbatol	T, L
gabapentin	Neurontin	C
lamotrigine	Lamictal	T
levetiracetam	Keppra	T
oxcarbazepine	Trileptal	T
phenobarbital	Luminal	T, L (contains 14% alcohol)
phenytoin	Dilantin	C, T, L
primidone	Mysoline	T, L
tiagabine	Gabatril	T
topiramate	Topamax	T, sprinkles
valproic acid/valproate	Depakene, Depakote	T, C, L, sprinkles

Key: C = capsules, T = tablets, L = liquid suspension or elixir.

types of seizures (see Table 10.8). Some of these drugs can be used for multiple types of seizures. Antiepileptic medications can have significant interactions with other medications and cause problems if they are stopped abruptly. You should seek the advice of the doctor before your child stops any of these medications.

Your child's doctor will start with one antiepileptic drug and increase the dose gradually until either seizures are controlled or side effects appear. A

Seizures or other disorders commonly treated	Side effects
Infantile spasms	Infection, high blood pressure, irritability, drowsiness
Grand mal, partial, behavior problems	Drowsiness, dizziness, rash, low red and white blood cell count
Minor motor, infantile spasms, partial, grand mal, behavior problems	Drowsiness, drooling, swallowing problems, dizziness, personality changes
Absence	Liver toxicity, sedation, unsteady walk, stomach upset, sleep disturbance
Grand mal, partial, absence	Severe anemia, liver damage, insomnia, weight loss
Partial, pain	Fatigue, unsteady walk, sleepiness
Partial, grand mal, absence, minor motor, behavior problems	Stomach upset, fatigue, rash, unsteady walk, headache
Partial	Drowsiness, infection, dizziness
Partial, generalized	Dizziness, drowsiness
Grand mal, partial, minor motor	Hyperactivity, rash, irritability, sleepiness
Grand mal, partial	Rash, dizziness, gum swelling, excessive hair growth
Grand mal, partial	Same as phenobarbital
Partial	*Increased* seizures, sedation
Grand mal, partial, minor motor	Cognitive impairment, kidney stones, weight loss
Grand mal, minor motor, partial, petit mal, infantile spasms, behavior problems	Liver damage, hair loss, weight gain, polycystic ovaries

small proportion of children will require a combination of two drugs; it is rare that more than two antiepileptic drugs are required to achieve seizure control. Once your child's condition has stabilized, drug levels in the blood are tested about twice per year to ensure that they are in a proper range. Drug levels are tested more frequently when the medication dosage is being changed. Blood tests to detect potential side effects also may be taken; these may include liver function tests and blood cell counts.

Table 10.9.   Medications commonly used for gastroesophageal reflux

Generic name	Trade name(s)	Preparations
aluminum hydroxide and magnesium hydroxide[a]	Maalox	L
cimetidine	Tagamet	T, L
omeprazole	Prilosec	C
ranitidine	Zantac	T, L

Key: C = capsules, T = tablets, L = liquid suspension or elixir.

[a]Available without a prescription

ANTIREFLUX MEDICATION

Children with cerebral palsy or other movement disorders are apt to have problems with food refluxing, or backing up, from their stomach into their esophagus (see Chapter 7). This can occur because the muscular valve that separates the stomach and the esophagus (the tube connecting the mouth to the stomach) doesn't work properly. The acidic stomach contents can then flow backward from the stomach into the esophagus, causing inflammation. Treatment consists of having your child eat in a good sitting posture, giving smaller and more frequent meals, and using medications that help to empty the stomach or decrease stomach acidity (such as Tagamet [cimetidine], Zantac [ranitidine] and Prilosec [omeprazole]) (see Table 10.9). Occasionally surgery is necessary to tighten the junction between the stomach and esophagus. Sometimes children with severe feeding disturbances who are not receiving adequate calories for growth may require feeding through a special tube inserted into the stomach.

ANTISPASTICITY MEDICATIONS

Antispasticity medications are used to decrease muscle tone in children with spastic cerebral palsy (see Chapter 19). Unfortunately, the medications currently available have a high incidence of side effects (see Table 10.10). Essentially, many of the oral medications affect the muscle tone of the entire body and can also cause sedation. If they are going to work well, however, they should become effective within the first week of therapy. Withdrawal of the medication should be gradual as physical dependency can develop. The medication must be evaluated to determine if the benefits outweigh the side effects. A physical medicine specialist, neurologist, or physical or occupational therapist should measure your child's muscle tone and motor abilities before and during treatment. The specialist will determine whether the treatment makes it easier for your child to roll over, sit, stand, or use the toilet.

Commonly used to treat	Side effects
Stomach acidity (review with physician)	Constipation, diarrhea
Ulcers, stomach acidity	Diarrhea, rash, dizziness
Ulcers, stomach acidity	Headache, diarrhea, blood disorders
Ulcers, stomach acidity	Sedation, rash, constipation

Some antispasticity medications affect the brain control of muscle tone, such as the oral medications diazepam, Ativan (lorazepam), and Klonopin (clonazepam) (see Table 10.8 for the latter) or Lioresal (baclofen), which can be given orally or by infusion into the spinal canal by a special pump. Other antispasticity medications decrease the ability of the muscle to contract, as in the case of Dantrium (dantrolene), which can be given orally, and Botox (botulinum toxin) or phenol, which can be given by injection into certain muscle groups.

VITAMINS AND MINERALS

Supplemental vitamins and minerals are not usually necessary for children in developed countries. Although a normal diet contains sufficient amounts of vitamins, however, an unbalanced or inadequate diet may be vitamin deficient. It is recommended that all children who live in areas where drinking water is deficient in fluoride receive a fluoride supplement (see Chapter 8). In addition, children who are not ambulatory, who use a wheelchair, or who are taking the antiepileptic drug Dilantin (phenytoin) may need supplemental vitamin D. Calcium supplements may also be helpful for children who do not walk or who are susceptible to serious bone fractures; discuss supplementation with your child's doctor. Complete formulas, such as those used for tube feeding (such as Complete B, Isocal, Pediasure, and Sustacal), already have sufficient quantities of vitamins and minerals added, so additional vitamin supplements are not needed if your child receives one of these formulas.

Supplemental vitamins and minerals may also be prescribed in certain other situations: Iron supplements such as Fer-in-sol are usually recommended after infancy if your child has iron-deficiency anemia. Because of the risk of iron poisoning, children should not receive adult multivitamins containing iron supplements. Other vitamin deficiencies may appear as a skin condition

Table 10.10.   Medications commonly used for spasticity

Generic name	Trade name(s)	Preparations
baclofen	——	T (see text for special intraspinal preparation)
botulinum toxin	Botox	Injection
dantrolene	Dantrium	T
diazepam	Valium	T, L
lorazepam	Ativan	T, L
phenol	——	Injection

Key: C = capsules, T = tablets, L = liquid suspension or elixir.

or hair loss. If you have questions about whether your child needs vitamin or mineral supplements, you should ask your child's pediatrician.

ALTERNATIVE MEDICATIONS AND TREATMENTS

Alternative medication, also called nonstandard or nonconventional therapy, includes a number of approaches to treatment that are not within the mainstream of medicine. There is a long and checkered history for these approaches, which have not been tested scientifically nor approved through the normal process of the FDA. In the 19th and early 20th centuries, these were called *patent medicines* and included "Carter's Little Liver Pills for everything that ails you" and even Coca-Cola (which then contained small amounts of coca, or cocaine, and was used as a "pick me up"). Most have proven to be without value and have faded rapidly into history; some have been found to be dangerous, such as Laetrile, which was touted to treat cancer but actually accelerated death in some instances. Still, some therapies, such as acupuncture, have been part of different cultures for centuries and may well have benefits that are just beginning to be recognized in Western culture.

The common factor in the use of these alternative medications has been a search for approaches to disorders for which traditional medicine did not have effective treatments or cures. As this is the case for many developmental disabilities, you are likely to learn of alternative treatments from friends or family, in books, and on the Internet. Discuss these approaches with your child's physician before trying them because there could be negative interactions with your child's current treatment. Your child's doctor can also share

Commonly used to treat	Side effects
Spasticity	Drowsiness, dizziness, low blood pressure, stomach upset
Spasticity	Needs careful dosing as can paralyze muscles
Spasticity	Liver damage, weakness, diarrhea, drowsiness
High muscle tone, seizures, anxiety	Respiratory depression, drowsiness, drooling, swallowing difficulties
Same as diazepam	Same as diazepam
Spasticity	Pain at site of injection

experiences in using these treatments or help you evaluate articles and statements made about these approaches.

Practitioners in alternative medicine refer to some of their medications as "nutrients." The human body is extraordinarily complex, and the actions and interactions of all substances are rarely simple. These interactions may be confusing to your family and your child's physician. Such nutrients and any other alternative medication, including high-dose vitamin supplements, should always be included in your child's medication history. Because of the complex actions of nutrients and drugs, the section Guidelines for the Use of Medications at the beginning of this chapter should apply to nutrients and other nonstandard medication just as it applies to standard medications.

Alternative medications are not subject to the same rigorous control as conventional medications are. Many alternative medications are self-prescribed, whereas others are prescribed by practitioners of alternative medicine. Before considering the use of alternative medications for your child, you should consider your health practitioner's training. If an alternative medication or new and controversial therapy is perceived as useful, usually conventional medical science will perform studies to test its true utility. In fact, an office at the National Institutes of Health (NIH) now provides funding for studies of alternative medicine. Of course, this delay in scientific testing can be frustrating but is the best way of distinguishing a real effect of a medication from an apparent but unrelated effect. The extraordinary number of alternative medications and therapies and the conflicting reports of their usefulness are confusing for families. This makes the relationship that your family has with your child's primary caregiver even more important.

IMMUNIZATIONS

Vaccinations are used to protect children from catching infectious diseases. They offer protection by stimulating the child's natural defense system, the immune system, to prepare it to attack infectious organisms that the child may come in contact with. During infancy, all children should receive vaccinations against the following diseases: hepatitis B; diphtheria, pertussis, and tetanus (these three vaccinations are usually given together as a DPT or DTaP vaccine); polio; measles, mumps, and rubella or German measles (these three are given together as the MMR vaccine); Hemophilus influenzae type b to protect against Hemophilus meningitis; pneumococcal pneumonia; and varicella (chickenpox). The suggested immunization schedule is summarized in Figure 10.1. There are an increasing number of vaccinations and combinations, and changes to the immunization recommendations are inevitable. Most of these vaccinations protect your child for life. The tetanus vaccine, however, should be repeated every 10 years, and a second MMR shot is required during the teenage years.

In general, children with disabilities should receive the same immunizations as typically developing children, with one exception. The pertussis (whooping cough) vaccine should not be given to children who have progressive neurological conditions or uncontrolled seizures. These children should receive separate diphtheria and tetanus immunizations instead of the combined vaccine. Some children with severe disabilities, especially those

Age→ Vaccine↓	Birth	1 mo	2 mos	4 mos	6 mos	12 mos	15 mos	18 mos	24 mos	4–6 yrs	11–12 yrs	14–16 yrs
Hepatitis B	Hep B	Hep B		Hep B		Hep B					(Hep B)	
Diphtheria, tetanus, pertussis			DTaP	DTaP	DTaP		DTaP			DTaP	Td	
H. influenzae type b			Hib	Hib	Hib	Hib						
Polio			IPV	IPV	IPV					IPV		
Measles, mumps, rubella						MMR				MMR	(MMR)	
Varicella						Var					(Var)	
Hepatitis A										Hep A—in selected areas		

Figure 10.1. Recommended childhood immunization schedule. Bars show range of recommended ages for immunization. Ovals show vaccines to be given if previous doses were missed or given before the recommended minimum age.

who are bedridden or who are susceptible to pneumonia, may benefit from vaccines for flu (trivalent influenza). For children younger than 9 years old who have not received the flu vaccine before, the vaccination requires two shots at 1-month intervals; for older children, just one shot is recommended. They must be given each fall, as the vaccine changes from year to year depending on the specific viral strain that is circulating.

Vaccines generally have few side effects. Some children become irritable, develop a low-grade fever after 24–48 hours, or have pain or swelling at the site of the injection. Acetaminophen can be given for the fever, and cold compresses may relieve pain at the injection site. Some vaccines contain an inactivated live virus. Live vaccines are generally not given to children who have a fever or who have a weakened immune system. The older version of the pertussis vaccine was very rarely associated with serious side effects, including high fevers, seizures, screaming spells, allergic reactions, and brain damage. The newer acellular pertussis vaccine, however, will safely protect your child from whooping cough, which although rare can be very serious (but, again, should not be given if your child experiences progressive neurological conditions or uncontrolled seizures). The acellular vaccine is less likely to have significant side effects. Children who are allergic to eggs may be unable to tolerate certain vaccines that have been produced in eggs, including the vaccines for measles, mumps, and influenza.

WHAT TO KEEP IN THE HOME MEDICINE CABINET

Every home needs a well-organized medicine cabinet. Ideally, you should be able to lock your cabinet. Keep items for coughs and colds, cuts and rashes, and poisonings. The most frequently used items that you will not want to run out of include a range of different sizes of sterile dressings (Band-Aids), antiseptic skin ointment for abrasions and cuts, gauze pads, medical bandages, calamine lotion and cotton balls, burn cream, acetaminophen, an antihistamine, and steroid ointment. Some useful instruments include tweezers and scissors. A bottle of ipecac syrup, a medicine used to induce vomiting in the event of poisoning, should also be included. It is also wise to keep a standard first-aid chart with step-by-step guidelines on hand for emergency situations. Your medicine cabinet could also contain a small emergency kit that you can take in your backpack or car.

Children can be poisoned by ingesting products ranging from their own medications to houseplants (see Table 10.11). United States law requires that labels on containers of hazardous substances include the generic name of the toxic chemical and first-aid instruction in the event of accidental ingestion. *Before taking any action after a poisoning, you should call the poison control center in your city or region.* The number should be listed in the front of your telephone directory. *Different types of poisonings require different action.* For example, it is dangerous to induce vomiting after poisonings from kerosene or

Table 10.11.   Toxic and nontoxic products

PRODUCTS THAT ARE USUALLY NONTOXIC

Antacids	Crayons	Modeling clay
Antibiotics	Deodorants	Newspapers
Ball-point pen inks	Hair products	Pencils
Bath soaps	Hand creams	Shampoos
Chalk	Latex paint	Toilet water
Cigarettes	Laxatives	Toothpaste
Colognes	Matches	Water-based glues
Contraceptive pills	Mercury from a	and pastes
Cosmetics	thermometer	

PRODUCTS THAT ARE TOXIC

Moderately toxic	*Very toxic*	*Extremely toxic*
Antifreeze	Ammonia	Herbicides
Bleach (sodium	Dishwasher granules	Insecticides
hypochlorite)	Drain cleaners	Strychnine
Epoxy glues	Lead paints	
Mothballs	Petroleum products	
Nail polish remover		
Stain remover		

COMMON DRUG INTOXICANTS

Amphetamines	Aspirin	Dilantin (phenytoin)
(stimulants)	Sleeping pills	Iron preparations
Antihistamines	Digitalis	Antidepressants

PLANTS THAT ARE TOXIC

Asparagus fern	Oleander	Some types of
Daffodils	Poinsettia	mushrooms
Dieffenbachia	Rhubarb leaves	Yew
Holly		Yarrow

gasoline, and it is dangerous to induce vomiting if your child is unconscious. Manual methods of inducing vomiting, such as sticking a finger down the throat, rarely work and can be dangerous.

SUMMARY

Medications should be used only if necessary and only when there is a clear plan of which symptom is being treated, which side effects may occur, and how the problem will be followed up. When used appropriately, medications can decrease the impact of your child's disability and improve the quality of life.

Some Questions Answered

I'm concerned because my 3-year-old daughter who has cerebral palsy and epilepsy refuses to take her antiepileptic medication. What can I do?

Refusal to take antiepileptic medication is a very serious problem. Try to make taking the medication part of your child's routine. Try some simple rewards to induce her to take the medicine. Some medicines can be crushed and given in a sweetener or can be diluted with orange juice. Other medicines are available in other forms that may be easier for your child to take. Check with your pharmacist and your child's doctor about these other formulations.

My 6-year-old son, who has ADHD, has just started taking Ritalin, and he is not going to sleep right away. Should I do anything about that?

Sleep problems among children taking this kind of medication are quite common. Sometimes the sleep problem improves after a few weeks. You should discuss this possible side effect and any other concerns you have with your child's doctor. The problem could be unrelated to the medication, so you will want to keep the pediatrician informed—he or she may have other suggestions for helping your son's sleeping problem.

Encouraging
Appropriate Child Behavior

John M. Parrish

Effective parenting is based on an understanding of your child and his or her current developmental level and needs. You will need to assist your child to develop new skills while providing love and other supports. To enhance as well as understand your child's development, you can learn key ways to encourage your child's appropriate behavior.

Each of us has our own views about what amounts to a behavior problem. Some of us are upset by a child's slightest whimper, whereas others can tune out a tag team match! In this chapter, a behavior is considered to be a problem when it occurs too often or too seldom or is inappropriate to the child's developmental level or for the situation at hand. Some problematic behaviors and challenging skill deficits that are common among children with disabilities include

- Aggression
- Attention problems
- Disruptive behaviors
- Feeding problems
- Impulsivity
- Dressing difficulties
- Toileting difficulties
- Noncompliance with parental requests and teacher recommendations
- Self-injurious behavior

- Self-stimulatory behavior (such as hand flapping or body rocking)
- Social skills deficits
- Tantrums

When behavior puts your child or others in danger of injury, it's definitely time to get help. When faced with a less severe behavior problem, you may wait, hoping it will get better. In many instances, however, difficult behaviors only worsen. When in doubt, it is wise to ask for assistance *before* your child's behavior becomes unmanageable.

HOW TO FIND HELP

Friends and relatives are often quick to offer advice about your child's behavior problems. At times it may seem to you that everyone is an authority when it comes to managing your child's problem behavior! If common-sense approaches have not worked, however, and you feel concerned about your child's behavior, you may wish to seek the help of an expert in child behavior management. Be sure that the professional has experience dealing with the behavior problems of children with disabilities and relies on well-documented, scientifically sound procedures. Ask the behavior specialist to outline how he or she would approach the particular problem behaviors. A competent specialist will be able to offer you *practical* advice on what to do and what not to do.

To locate a skilled behavior specialist, also called a *behavior analyst* or a *behavior therapist,* begin by asking your child's pediatrician for recommendations. If you live near a child development center that serves children with disabilities, you may be able to find a qualified specialist there. In addition, you can contact the psychology or special education department of your local school district, hospital, or university for services or for referral to a qualified professional.

If you cannot find someone in your area who specializes in caring for children with disabilities, consider finding a nearby professional who is willing to consult with a specialist from some distance away. Ask the local therapist to help you identify an expert. Alternatively, you may choose to travel to arrange an evaluation by a specialist and then ask the specialist to assist you in designing a community-based program for your child that you can put in place with the help of a professional closer to home. The therapist you select will expect you to be an active participant in your child's evaluation and ongoing care. You will be asked to keep appointments, make a good-faith effort to follow recommendations, and perhaps keep records of your child's behavior as a means to evaluate progress. Avoid therapists who claim that they can solve every problem or who say they will work just with your child, not with you or your child's teachers. Professional organizations that may be able to recommend skilled therapists are listed in the Suggested Readings and Resources.

THE BEHAVIOR MANAGEMENT PROGRAM: GETTING STARTED

At your initial visit, the therapist will work with you to understand your child's overall developmental progress, current strengths, and physical and emotional health. While taking into consideration your child's special needs, the therapist will identify and define your child's behavior problems, including the occasions that elicit misbehavior. This assessment may include interviews, rating scales or questionnaires, and direct observations of your child during interactions with you and others. The therapist will ask about your general concerns and for specific examples that illustrate those concerns. For instance, if you say your child is "mean," "stubborn," or "lazy," the therapist will want to know what your child does that warrants those labels: Does he or she hit other children? Does he or she argue or talk back a lot? Does he or she fail to complete chores at home?

Once your child's problem behaviors have been identified in terms of what he or she says and/or does that is of specific concern to you, the therapist will discuss the behaviors with you in greater detail. You will be asked to estimate each problem behavior's frequency, duration, and intensity and to describe the circumstances under which each behavior is most likely to occur. For example, if your child has frequent outbursts of anger, the therapist will want to know what triggers them. Do they start when you ask your child to stop some favored activity or to complete a chore? Or, does withholding a treat or privilege from your child set off a tantrum?

The therapist will also want to know how you react to your child's misbehavior. Whether your child continues to misbehave depends, in large part, on your actions. For instance, if you give in to your child's demands when tantrums occur, the tantrums are likely to continue or even intensify. Similarly, if you allow your child to avoid completing a chore because he or she is having a tantrum, the tantrums are likely to recur the next time the child is asked to complete a chore.

In addition to asking you about what typically happens before and after the challenging behavior, the therapist is likely to arrange situations during which your child's misbehavior can be observed firsthand. Toward the end of the assessment, the therapist will ask you which behaviors require the most attention and what strategies, successful or not, you have already tried. After completing the evaluation, the therapist will describe and discuss recommended interventions. If several different behaviors require attention, the order in which they are addressed will depend on the severity of each problem, the degree of effort required on your part to manage the particular behavior, and most important, your preference about where to begin. The therapist will want a commitment from you to participate actively in a short-term program.

Behaviors that can be managed easily or those that are potentially dangerous are usually targeted first. Intervention for behaviors that are not dangerous but are more difficult to alter, such as self-stimulatory behavior or persistent screaming, is often delayed until you have experienced some early successes with more manageable behaviors.

POSITIVE REINFORCEMENT: EMPHASIZING
WHAT YOUR CHILD ENJOYS AND DOES WELL

Before tackling your child's problem behaviors, the therapist may advise you to make simple changes to your child's everyday living situation or routines that can relieve stress and make a difference in how your child behaves. For example, you may want to purchase fun toys and games or useful adaptive communication devices and other equipment that are developmentally appropriate for your child. The therapist may also work on strengthening your child's appropriate behaviors. This is done through a method termed *positive reinforcement.* Positive reinforcement involves offering a preferred object or activity to your child in response to your child's desired behavior, in order to increase the frequency of that behavior in the future. Appropriate reinforcers include providing words of praise or concrete rewards, such as special foods or activities. Social activities, such as playing a game with a parent, can be highly motivating. The list of reinforcers is nearly endless and will vary from child to child and from time to time.

You may want to ask your child to suggest what he or she would prefer as a reward. With a child who is younger or who has a cognitive disability, you may adopt an indirect approach by permitting your child to do what comes naturally. If your child chooses repeatedly to lie down on the couch, watch television, listen to music, twirl string, suck his or her fingers, eat a cookie, or make noises, that activity could be used to reinforce appropriate behavior. You should not assume that what you like or what you think your child should like will work.

Some parents of children with disabilities believe that their children have no preferences. This is almost always not the case. Even children with multiple and severe disabilities have likes and dislikes. With such children, reinforcers may be more difficult to detect, but they exist nonetheless. You can identify them with the help of the therapist.

Once you have identified your child's preferences, you must determine which ones would be appropriate reinforcers. First, you should be able to deliver the reinforcer immediately after the behavior has occurred, rather than after some time. In this way, your child can learn to recognize which behaviors result in reinforcement and which do not. Second, the reinforcer should be provided only when appropriate behavior occurs and should not be available at other times. Third, reinforcers should be provided frequently and in small amounts. It is better to give verbal approval several times per day than to offer the child a movie ticket at the end of a week of good behavior. Fourth, offer a variety of reinforcers in small quantities so that your child does not lose interest too quickly. As an alternative, you may want to use reinforcers such as points or tokens that can be redeemed at a later date for a variety of special treats.

Finally, the reinforcers should be compatible with the goals of your child's management program. An overweight child should not be given high-calorie snacks as a reinforcer, nor should a withdrawn child be permitted to spend long periods of time alone in a room as a reward. The reinforcers should be inexpensive, readily available to you but not to your child, easily dispensable, interesting, novel, and should not cause side effects. Once reinforcers have been identified, you need to provide them consistently. When interacting with your child, be certain to notice when he or she is being good so that you can reinforce that behavior.

PLANNED IGNORING: WHEN IT'S
BETTER TO LOOK THE OTHER WAY

Children frequently act up in order to get attention. You will be more successful in encouraging your child's good behavior when you minimize the attention given to your child's misbehavior. For example, if you give your child attention during a whining episode, you may be increasing the likelihood of whining in the future. Similarly, when you scold your child for interrupting your conversation or making loud noises, you may be reinforcing that behavior. If your child receives attention for misbehavior, poor conduct may persist or even increase.

In such situations, planned ignoring can be effective in decreasing problem behavior. Planned ignoring involves withholding attention and other positive reinforcers following the occurrence of a problem behavior. It should not be used to address dangerous or destructive behaviors, such as self-injury, aggression, or property damage. Consistent ignoring of your child's nagging, whining, or crying will usually result in a decrease in these bothersome acts. Planned ignoring, however, typically does not work immediately. At first, you may see an increase in the rate, duration, and intensity of the behavior before you see a reduction.

For planned ignoring to be effective, you must use it consistently over an extended period of time and be willing to endure flare-ups in your child's behavior. For example, consider if your child pleads for a cookie before supper. You may have responded to the pleas by asking your child to wait. Ultimately, you may have given in to the persistent requests and crying. Using planned ignoring, you will remind your child once that the cookie will be available after supper is eaten. Then, if your child continues to beg for a cookie, you will go about your business without further talk about the cookie. The first few times such a procedure is implemented, your child probably will ask for the cookie over and over again. With consistent ignoring from you, over time the begging and crying will gradually decrease. If, however, you occasionally give in to the crying and produce a cookie, you have taught your child that begging and crying for a long enough period will result in a cookie. Planned ignoring must be followed to completion to be effective in teaching a new behavior.

Although easy to understand, this procedure is hard to follow. You may find it difficult to ignore annoying behavior. Instead, you may find yourself issuing a string of "no," "don't," and "stop" commands. Unfortunately, by providing this attention, negative though it is, you could be unintentionally reinforcing your child's problem behaviors. So, the next time your child gets on your nerves with some frustrating behavior, try to ignore it! As many parents do, you can learn to ignore consistently your child's minor disruptive behavior. And, if you persist in withholding your negative attention, you will find that your child's behavior will improve greatly over time.

DIFFERENTIAL REINFORCEMENT: BEING MINDFUL OF WHAT YOU REINFORCE

Your child may exhibit some behaviors that you want to change and others that you want to reinforce. In this case, positive reinforcement and planned ignoring can be combined to form a procedure known as differential reinforcement. For example, you would be providing differential reinforcement if you were to ignore your child's tantrums but praise cooperative play. In many situations, differential reinforcement is a better solution than planned ignoring alone because it teaches a youngster when behavior is appropriate and when it is not.

SHAPING: HELPING YOUR CHILD LEARN NEW SKILLS

Sometimes you may want to teach your child a behavior that is not currently part of his or her repertoire. Given that the behavior does not occur, you have no opportunity to reinforce it. In these cases, you may use a procedure called *shaping*. Shaping involves reinforcing the behaviors displayed by your child that most closely resemble the behavior you wish your child to learn. Multiple opportunities for your child to acquire and practice new skills should be arranged. Whenever your child behaves in a manner that approximates the desired skill, you should reward these efforts.

Consider teaching your child to shoot a basketball. You would first teach skills such as how to stop dribbling, how to grip the basketball when shooting, how to position the body for a shot, how to pinpoint the basket, and how to deliver a shot in proper form. Each time your child's performance approximated a needed skill, you would reinforce the efforts. Once such basic mechanics have been taught, you would have your child practice shooting from a very short distance until several baskets in a row were scored.

Then you would direct your child to move back a few steps and so on until he or she was able to shoot accurately from greater and greater distances.

Shaping is most often used to help children learn new daily living skills, such as how to dress, eat with utensils, use the toilet, select clothing, cross the street, and use public transportation. For detailed information about how to teach your child specific daily living skills, please refer to the very useful book *Steps to Independence: Teaching Everyday Skills to Children with Special Needs, Third Edition,* by Baker and Brightman (see the Suggested Readings and Resources at the end of this book for more information).

INSTRUCTION AND IMITATION: SHOWING YOUR CHILD WHAT TO DO

Besides shaping, two other methods are commonly used to teach new behaviors. One is termed *instructional training;* the other is called *imitation training*. Instructional training is used to teach new behaviors to children who can follow verbal directions. You describe what you want your child to do, then you acknowledge and praise your child when he or she attempts to follow your instructions. If your child lacks the language skills needed for instructional training, you may teach behaviors using imitation. Here, you demonstrate how to do the task or behavior and then have your child copy what you just demonstrated. Again, praise your child for any attempt made to imitate what you did. Instructional and imitation training can also be combined.

Shala

Shala's parents decided that it was time for her to learn to brush her teeth. They gave verbal instructions and reinforced them with demonstrations of how to brush teeth. They began by having her look directly at them as they issued the request. This got her attention. Next, they would make a simple and specific request in a matter-of-fact but firm voice: "Shala, go into the bathroom and brush your teeth." The therapist had told them that children are not likely to follow through with requests that are expressed in either an angry or apologetic manner. Also, the therapist warned them to avoid putting the request in the form of a question such as "Do you want to . . . ?" because the child then has the option of saying "no" to the request. After giving the instruction, Shala's parents silently counted from 1,001 to 1,010, giving Shala approximately 10 seconds to begin her trip to the bathroom. The therapist had told Shala's parents that they should not reason with her during this time but should just wait. The waiting was perhaps the most difficult part of the process.

Her parents were told to express their approval if Shala headed toward the bathroom. They were to ignore whining or tantrums. When Shala hadn't moved by the count of 1,010, they repeated the request exactly as they had stated it the first time. This time, however, they also pointed in the direction of the bathroom. After 10 seconds, if Shala still had not headed toward the bathroom, her mother or father was instructed to guide her gently there, ignoring any protests. Fortunately, this was not necessary.

Once Shala was in the bathroom, her mother reminded her to brush her teeth. However, given that Shala did not know how to perform the task, her mother taught her by breaking down the task of toothbrushing into small steps. These steps included finding the toothbrush and toothpaste, wetting the toothbrush, putting on the toothpaste, holding the toothbrush at a 45-degree angle to the teeth, brushing the top teeth in a circular fashion, and so forth.

To teach a skill such as toothbrushing, you can either begin with the first step or with the last step. Beginning with the first step is called *forward chaining;* beginning with the last step is called *backward chaining.* In forward chaining the first step in the task is learned, then the second step is learned, and then the two steps are combined. This chaining is continued until all steps have been learned and practiced together. With backward chaining, you start by helping your child with every step except for the last one. The next time, you give your child an opportunity to complete this final step independently before you offer any feedback or assistance. If your child needs help, you give it repeatedly until he or she learns this step. The next time, you help with every step except the last two. When those two steps are mastered, you help with all but the last three steps, and so forth. An advantage of backward chaining is that with each trial, the child successfully completes the task. This repeated success may boost your child's self-confidence and prevent frustration.

NEGATIVE REINFORCEMENT

So far, this chapter has focused on the use of positive reinforcement and planned ignoring in combination with instructional and imitation training to enable your child to develop new skills. Another group of procedures, however, can be used to increase appropriate behaviors. These procedures rely on negative reinforcement and are often confused with punishment. Negative reinforcement of a particular behavior occurs when that behavior results in the ending of an unpleasant situation. Many outcomes of negative reinforcement occur in our daily lives. We move inside to escape the cold, we stop at a red traffic light to avoid an accident, we wear sunglasses to reduce glare, and we take off a shoe to remove a pebble.

Negative reinforcement, too, is likely to be at work between your child and you. Indeed, it is possible that your child's misbehavior is being supported by negative reinforcement. For example, if your child refuses to eat spinach, and you throw out the spinach in response to whining, you are negatively reinforcing the inappropriate behavior by removing the unwanted food. In this way you are encouraging your child through negative reinforcement to continue to refuse to eat spinach.

When your child's problem behavior is sustained by negative reinforcement, the solution is to not allow the inappropriate behavior to result in avoidance of or escape from the task at hand. For instance, rather than giving in and throwing out the spinach, the effective parent ignores the child's complaints and refusal to eat and structures the situation so that the child completes the task at hand (eating spinach) before being permitted to engage in a preferred activity (such as eating dessert, going outside, or watching television).

Negative reinforcement can also be used to promote appropriate behaviors. Consider a child who is such a fussy eater that he or she is becoming underweight. The child's parents and therapists have previously tried varying the content, texture, and temperature of the food. They have tried encouraging the child to eat, but nothing works. A feeding specialist has been consulted and has ruled out a biological explanation for the problem. At this point a therapist may become involved and help the parents to use both negative and positive reinforcement to get the child to accept food.

During the learning sessions conducted at mealtime, the therapist presents the child with a spoon laden with food and says, "Take a bite." If the child accepts and swallows the food, the therapist immediately gives words of praise, hugs, and offers a brief opportunity to play with a toy. In this way positive reinforcement is contingent on food acceptance. If the child refuses to accept the food immediately, the therapist waits 3 seconds before gently supporting the child's jaw so that he or she safely accepts the food. The child quickly learns that the physical guidance can be avoided by accepting the presented bites. This "avoidance learning" is a direct result of the process of negative reinforcement.

PUNISHMENT

Positive and negative reinforcement, if successfully applied, both result in an increase of a desired behavior over time. In contrast, punishment of a behavior leads to a decrease in that behavior in the future. For example, you may punish your child for running across a busy street by scolding him or her. Punishment can also involve withdrawal of a privilege, such as taking away television time because your child was aggressive, not permitting play outside because your child did not complete a homework assignment, or removing a favorite toy because your child had a tantrum. Although punishment is a given in our imperfect world and no dogma or doctrine prohibiting its occurrence has proved enforceable, professionals often refrain from recommending the use of punishment because it can result in unwanted side effects, such as frustration, resentment, and counteraggression on the part of the punished person, and overreliance on coercive tactics on the part of the punisher. These contribute over time to problematic relationships. In contrast, positive reinforcement strategies promote appropriate behavior while being less disruptive to the child's and family's routine. You should use positive reinforcement strategies consistently before you use any punishment. Typically, punishment will reduce inappropriate behaviors only temporarily. Over time, punishment may teach your child what not to do but seldom teaches your child what to do instead of misbehavior. On a daily basis, it is better to focus on what you want your child to do and to use instructional and imitation training to teach your child how to do it.

Nevertheless, in some cases, punishment procedures may be necessary if attempts at positive reinforcement have failed and if the behavior is severe. Time-out is one strategy that can work, for example, when private statements of mild disapproval ("I'm unhappy that you didn't sit down at the table when I asked you the first time") make little difference to your child. Using this method, you remove your child briefly from sources of positive reinforcement. Time-out usually involves guiding your child to calm down briefly in a quiet area where there is nothing for your child to do. During time-out, objects and activities your child enjoys must be kept beyond reach or, preferably, out of sight altogether. Effective use of time-out depends on several factors. When used, you should give time-out consistently and preferably in response to only one or two severe problem behaviors targeted for change. The duration of time-out should be short, usually 1–3 minutes; longer time-outs can be counterproductive because the child may be able to delay or escape from doing the requested task. Finally, time-out is most effective when it is used infrequently. When time-out is over, redirect your child's attention to the task at hand or to the next play opportunity. Do not harp on the previous incident that resulted in a time-out.

If, under the guidance of a therapist, you decide to use a punishment procedure, use the following guidelines:

1. Be sure that you can deliver the indicated brief, mild punishment to your child safely and consistently. The punishment is not likely to be effective if your child can ignore verbal reprimands, play with a favorite toy during time-out, or get out of losing a privilege.

2. Apply the punishment confidently and not in graded steps. A firm but matter-of-fact "no" is better than an apologetic request to stop followed by loud reprimands when your child does not obey. Avoid lectures, nagging, scolding, threatening or sarcastic remarks, extended time-outs, excessive fines, or any physical aggression that may frighten or hurt your child.

3. In the beginning, apply punishment immediately each time the targeted inappropriate behavior occurs. As the child's behavior improves, there will be less and less of a need to use punishment.

4. Eliminate any positive or negative reinforcement that is responsible for the problem behavior. When your child misbehaves during a work activ-

ity, ensure that the task is completed. Then, simply state the cause or reason for the punishment, describe the consequence (such as loss of a privilege), and enforce it.

5. Be careful that the delivery of punishment is not associated with the later delivery of reinforcement. For example, you may be overwhelmed with guilt for removing a privilege from your child. As a result you may shower your child with affection and reassurances of your love afterward. Expressing your love in the context of apologizing for having disciplined your child may send a confusing message.

6. Avoid prolonged or extensive use of punishment; it often loses its effect if it is used too long or too frequently.

Barry

Barry is a 9-year-old with mild mental retardation and a seizure disorder. When he took his antiepileptic medication, he remained seizure-free, but he resisted taking the medication and consequently had multiple seizures that interfere with his life at home and school. His mother had been unsuccessful in getting him to take his medication and sought the help of a behavior therapist.

The therapist first determined the percentage of doses Barry accepted. She then checked whether Barry had the necessary skills to swallow his medication without difficulty. In fact, Barry did have trouble swallowing pills, so the therapist taught him how to take the medication through instruction and demonstration. Initially, she gave Barry very small capsules. Then, she presented larger and larger capsules until Barry was able to swallow capsules of the size originally prescribed. During this shaping procedure, she acknowledged any successful swallows and allowed Barry to select and enjoy a special privilege, such as watching a favorite videotape for 30 minutes. At the same time, if Barry resisted accepting the medication by turning his head, using his hands to block the capsule, or whining, the therapist ignored these nondangerous behaviors. Rather than back away when these problem behaviors occurred or scold Barry for his misbehavior, the therapist calmly continued giving the medicine, thereby not permitting these behaviors to be reinforced negatively. If Barry attempted to avoid taking the capsule by showing aggressive behavior toward the trainer, he was given a brief timeout, followed immediately by continuation of the capsule administration. If he threw presented capsules on the floor, he was instructed to pick them up and throw them away, and then he lost a privilege, such as listening to music. As Barry's difficult behaviors subsided, he was given an opportunity to practice taking the capsules himself with minimal guidance. Throughout this training sequence, the therapist kept records of Barry's performance to refine his behavior management program and to determine when training was no longer necessary. In addition, the frequency of seizures was monitored to document that Barry's increased acceptance of medication resulted in improved seizure control.

PARENT EDUCATION AND TRAINING

Behavior management for your child is most effective if it is designed by you in collaboration with a therapist and is then carried out by you. Therefore, therapists often seek to help you manage your child's behavior problems, rather than manage these concerns for you. Such help may range from telephone consultations to intensive clinic- or home-based parent training programs. Less structured forms of parent training include the use of "how-to" books on behavior management, magazine articles on positive approaches to parenting, and lectures and workshops.

Parent training begins with the therapist's describing what causes your child's problem behaviors and the supports and services needed to change these behaviors. Basic principles are illustrated using examples drawn from your daily life. Next, you will get specific procedures to try at home. The therapist demonstrates these recommended strategies either by working directly with your child while you watch, by role playing, or by showing a videotape of what to do. Following this, you will have an opportunity to rehearse the demonstrated skills so that you can practice and improve your newly learned strategies while the trainer provides you with supportive advice.

To help you try these skills at home, the therapist often shares a written list of "do's" and "don'ts." You may be asked to observe and record the occurrence of targeted appropriate and inappropriate behaviors. After you have practiced for 1–3 weeks, the therapist will review your child's progress with your child and you. On the basis of your written records and your verbal description of your child's behavior, the therapist will work with you to make adjustments to the management program until it works well.

Once your goals have been reached, you no longer need to attend regularly scheduled appointments. Instead, the therapist likely will remain in contact with you via occasional appointments and telephone contacts to troubleshoot with you. If your child's behavior takes a turn for the worse, it may become necessary to resume regular clinic visits. Otherwise, you can occasionally call the therapist to talk about your child's progress.

SUMMARY

If you are concerned with your child's behavior, do not despair. Simply act now! Through reading or receiving some professional consultation from your child's pediatrician or a behavior therapist, you can quickly learn how to provide your child with the love and discipline that he or she needs to learn how to behave appropriately.

Some Questions Answered

Do all children with disabilities have behavior problems?

Many children with disabilities do not have behavior problems. Because they sometimes lack some social skills, however, children with disabilities are at an increased risk to develop behavior problems compared with children without disabilities.

When my child misbehaves, is it best to be tolerant because he has a disability? And will he grow out of the misbehavior?

A child with a disability requires effective instruction (including discipline) as much as a child who is developing typically. Although you may adjust your overall expectations of your child given the disabilities, it is nonetheless quite important to teach your child how to behave appropriately. It is true that some problem behaviors improve spontaneously; however, many worsen if left alone. Once a behavior is in your child's repertoire, it is very likely to persist unless you do something about it.

As a parent, I should know how to manage my child's behavior. Isn't asking for help admitting that I have failed as a parent?

Parenting any child is challenging. Just as is true with any other skill, effective parenting skills must be learned. Sometimes, you can learn them best under the guidance of a professional. If your child has behavior problems, you may need to do more than read a book on your own. Don't be afraid to get help. Many factors combine to determine how your child behaves. The important message to remember is this: You may or may not be a part of the problem, but for sure, you can be a big part of the solution.

Your Child's Educational Rights

Sheila Rose Mazzoli

Educational programming for your child offers an opportunity to work with various professionals to help your child reach his or her full potential and realize the goals you have for him or her. Yet, sorting out who is responsible, what services are available, and how they will be provided can be confusing. To make matters worse, educators tend to use many specialized terms such as *inclusion* and acronyms such as LD and IEP. Therefore, you need to ask as many questions as necessary to be sure you have a full understanding of what is being discussed.

Inclusion is the placement of a child with special needs in a general classroom environment with supports. LD stands for *learning disability*. The most important acronym to be familiar with is IEP, which stands for *individualized education program*. This is a report designed to provide a description of the intended education program, related services, goals and objectives, and specially designed instruction for your child. The IEP must assess the ability of the general education curriculum to meet your child's needs and what modifications may be required. The focus is on accomplishing this in the least restrictive environment (LRE), that is, the one that offers your child the greatest access to the general education curriculum. The IEP ensures that the particular school program developed for your child complies with the federal mandate (described in the next section).

Special education services are governed by federal, state, and local laws that are designed to foster collaboration between your family and your school in the design and development of your child's program. These laws also offer protections and rights to you and your child. Making sense of the process and paperwork involved, however, can be daunting for both families and educators, and the best results are attained by your keeping open and ongoing communication with your child's school.

THE LAW

Public Law 94-142, the Education for All Handicapped Children Act (later named the Individual with Disabilities Act [IDEA] of 1990), has been in effect since 1975, covering children 3 years of age and older. This law brought an end to the exclusion of students with disabilities from local schools and ensured that they receive a free and appropriate public education. It requires that each child being considered for special education programming be evaluated in the areas of concern by a qualified examiner. It also requires that written parental permission be obtained before this evaluation. If special education services are deemed necessary, the parent(s) must be involved in the development, approval, and revision of the program. IDEA requires that an IEP be designed to meet the special needs of your child and that this program be documented in writing. The law further requires that programs and services be provided to your child in the least restrictive environment. Programs that are as similar to what other students would attend are considered less restrictive than segregated classes or programs in other buildings or locations. Finally, the law established due process procedures to resolve disagreements between you and the school regarding programming and placement.

As a result of this law, a diverse group of programs is available to your child. To comply with the law, the U.S. Department of Education has established procedures by which your child is evaluated and by which an appropriate program of special education and related services is developed and implemented. Unlike programs in general education, which are based on curricular goals for all students, programs in special education are designed to address the specific needs of your child.

Every state develops its own regulations consistent with federal requirements but may also enact additional regulations. Likewise, local school districts must follow federal and state regulations but may develop other related policies and procedures. In some cases, state regulations are more stringent than federal regulations. For example, federal regulations mandate that reevaluation occur at least every 3 years, whereas some states require reevaluation every 2 years. In all cases, whichever regulation offers the most protection to your child must be followed.

On June 4, 1997, the federal government amended and reauthorized IDEA as Public Law 105-17. In evaluating the history and impact of IDEA, Congress obtained testimony from many individuals and organizations involved over the 20-year course of its implementation. Some people expressed concerns that too many children in special education were dropping out of school and that too many minority children and children with limited English proficiency were being placed inappropriately in special education classes. There was also evidence that too much emphasis was being placed on paperwork that was irrelevant to education. Finally, some individuals voiced concerns that children receiving special education services were not reaching their potential due to the use of a parallel curriculum that lowered expectations rather than the use of the general education curriculum. On the basis of this testimony and study, Congress concluded that IDEA needed to be strengthened and improved. They summarized the objectives of the amendments to IDEA as follows:

1. To strengthen the role of parents

2. To ensure access to the general curriculum

3. To facilitate interactions with students without disabilities

4. To focus on teaching and learning while decreasing unnecessary paperwork

5. To be responsive to the growing needs of an increasingly diverse society

6. To ensure that schools are safe and conducive to learning

7. To encourage parents and educators to work out differences using non-adversarial means

Jill, Erin, and Sam

Jill was born 6 weeks early and had many complications in her first week of life. She was subsequently diagnosed with mild spastic cerebral palsy and was provided a home-based early intervention program, with weekly visits from a physical therapist. When Jill was 3 years of age, she began attending a special preschool program 3 days per week; then at age 4, she started going to the program 5 days per week.

When Jill turned 5, her parents felt it was important for her to be included in a general education classroom. Jill underwent psychoeducational testing at the local school, and the results suggested that she could function with assistance in a general education class. An IEP was developed for Jill that included physical therapy three times per week. Jill's parents were pleased with this plan and approved it. Jill then attended a general kindergarten class that had a paraeducator (teacher's assistant). By the end of the school year, however, it was clear that Jill's development in preacademic skills (learning the alphabet, writing her name, knowing number concepts), fine motor coordination (pencil skills), and social interactions was delayed. Jill's kindergarten teacher and parents felt that she would benefit from another year in kindergarten. So, she remained there for the next school year, with occupational therapy added to her physical therapy to improve her fine motor skills. These therapy sessions were provided in the classroom (and thus are called *pull-in services*).

Erin was born with Down syndrome. Following early intervention and special preschool programs, she was placed in a special education classroom in kindergarten and stayed there through elementary school. As academic demands increased toward the end of the fifth grade, however, the difference between Erin's skills and those of her classmates in the special education classroom widened. As a result Erin was placed in a Life Skills classroom for her middle-school years, where she received instruction in basic or functional reading and math, community living skills, communication, and prevocational skills. Erin is currently in a Life Skills program at her local high school. She continues to receive instruction in fundamental academics, communication, social skills, and vocational skills but leaves the high school after lunch each day to go to a worksite at a nearby industrial complex. She works in the mailroom with a job coach, who also supervises another student working in the copy center. The job coach assists Erin with necessary skills, helps her hone her interpersonal skills, and serves as a liaison between Erin's employer and school. She has already established relationships with support agencies through the individualized transition plan (ITP) component of the IEP meetings that began when Erin was 14. Not only has the team been looking into employment for Erin, but they have also begun to look into supervised living arrangements and Erin's use of public transportation in her daily life.

In kindergarten, Sam's mild behavior problems were attributed to his being "all boy." His first-grade teacher noticed, however, that Sam struggled more than the other children with writing. His verbal expression was far more creative and rich than what he was able to produce on paper. The more he focused on trying to produce a neat paper, the more the quality of his writing content deteriorated. The instructional support teacher suggested matching Sam with another student who would help him organize ideas in a logical sequence. Sam received sentence starters and other aids to help organize his thoughts and received think sheets to help improve his writing content. Despite some improvement in his handwriting, Sam was struggling again as writing demands increased in the third grade. He was evaluated by a multidisciplinary team that included a reading specialist, a psychologist, an occupational therapist, and his general education teacher. The evaluation results indicated that Sam had a learning disability, and his IEP team decided that with additional supports and services, Sam should remain in his current placement in his current school. He will receive both direct services and consultation from an occupational therapist, and he will use a portable word processor for longer class assignments. He will also receive support in the classroom from an itinerant teacher to work on study skills and organization.

SPECIAL EDUCATION AS A PROCESS

The identification, evaluation, and provision of special education services make up a process that takes place during a specified time period. A referral for special education consideration is made if a child with a designated disability is thought to be in need of special assistance or if a student in a general education program is having difficulty that has not been resolved through modification of materials and the curriculum and is suspected of having a disability. A referral must be made in writing and can be made by a parent, a general or special education teacher, a counselor, or an administrator. Parents are asked for written permission for their child to be evaluated by a team of specialists and are given a copy of their rights. Known as the *procedural safeguards notice,* this lengthy document spells out the procedures and regulations that educators and specialists must follow when a child is thought to have special educational needs. Topics in the procedural safeguards notice include the following:

- When notice must be given to parents
- What must be included in the notification
- When prior parental consent must be obtained
- What happens when a parent refuses consent
- Right to an independent evaluation
- Dispute resolution systems, including mediation, prehearing conferences, and impartial due process hearings
- Parental claims for tuition reimbursement
- Rights regarding discipline and suspension
- Surrogate parents
- Rights pertaining to education records
- Complaint procedures
- Applicable laws and regulations

Once a referral is made, the school district has a limited time to complete the evaluation, prepare the evaluation report, and deliver it to you.

The Multidisciplinary Evaluation

The purpose of the multidisciplinary evaluation is to gather information to enable your child to make progress in an educational program. A well-done evaluation will guide the instruction for your child, evaluate progress, provide data and recommendations regarding eligibility for specific programs, and make recommendations regardless of whether he or she is found to need special education services. The evaluation team includes a psychologist and other specialists in areas of concern (for example, a speech-language pathologist, a physical therapist, or an occupational therapist). The two main questions that the evaluation should address are 1) Does my child have a disability? and 2) Does he or she need special education and related services?

Only when a child with a disability needs specially designed instruction does he or she become eligible to receive special education programs and services. For example, if the evaluation team determines that your child's academic difficulties come from a lack of instruction in reading or math or from limited English proficiency, your child will not be identified as having a disability. The evaluation should also consider special factors, such as hearing or visual impairments, behaviors that impede your child's or others' learning, communication needs, and use of assistive technology devices and services.

The evaluation team may use a variety of assessment tools, strategies, and sources of information, including your input. The evaluation must be sufficiently detailed to allow the team to determine whether your child has a disability and, if so, which areas should be addressed in his or her IEP. The information gathered might include academic performance, learning problems, social and adaptive behaviors, physical abilities, results from instructional evaluations and vocational/technical assessments, interests, preferences, and aptitudes. From all of the information gathered, the team must identify your child's strengths and needs as well as the degree of need for special services. Once the report is generated, all team members must sign it to designate their agreement with the report. If individual team members disagree with the information in the report, they must attach comments to it. This report and all the comments form the basis for the IEP meeting.

The IEP Meeting

The IEP meeting is required to develop the IEP for your child. Your input in this meeting is critical to ensure that your priorities are included in the plan. You will be invited in writing to attend the meeting, which should be held at a mutually convenient time and place. One of the greatest challenges in the process is scheduling the meeting at a time that does not interfere with instruction or the parents' work schedules and that allows all participants to attend.

The law requires not only that a parent should attend the meeting but also that a special education teacher and a representative from the local education agency (school district) should attend. This individual is typically a principal or supervisor who is knowledgeable about the curriculum and is authorized to commit resources. New to IDEA is the requirement that a general education teacher attend the IEP meeting if it is thought that your child may participate in general education instruction. The educational agency can invite anyone else who may contribute to the IEP. You are also allowed to invite people to the IEP meeting. Often it is a good idea to invite a friend or service provider who can help advocate for your child's rights. This might include individuals who provide private services to your child (such as a physical therapist or a speech-language therapist) so that there can be consistency in approaches. All materials should be provided to you in your native language, and the school district should provide interpreter services, if needed. When appropriate, your child should also attend the meeting.

You can think of the meeting as an opportunity to discuss evaluations of your child, to share information that may not come through in assessments, to hear what others think is important to occur in your child's education program, and to plan with other team members the programs and services that can accomplish the goals. The meeting is best begun positively with discussion of outcomes that your child and your family desire and your child's strengths to meet those outcomes. Needs are often determined by the discrepancies between your family's desired outcomes and the skills that your child possesses to reach these outcomes. Also discussed are your child's educational accomplishments. This information will come from assessments and observations done as part of the comprehensive evaluation, as well as from your child's current teachers and service providers. It is important for you to share any information that may affect your child's daily performance, such as unusual sleep patterns, seizure activity, medications and their side effects, or behavioral issues.

The result of this discussion is the listing of your child's educational strengths and needs. From these needs, the goals and objectives of the education program are developed. Many students have needs in multiple areas. If this is the case with your child, it is helpful to come to the meeting prepared with your own thoughts about educational priorities. The school day is less than one half of your child's day. Some skills, such as dressing and bathing, can be better addressed in the home, where they naturally occur. Other skills, such as toileting and eating, require a coordinated, consistent effort during your child's day and should therefore be included as part of the educational plan. In addition, it is important that you look at long-term and life goals as you draw up the priorities for the year.

IEP meetings are most effective when all participants have studied the evaluation reports, prioritized what they feel is most important, and prepared a list of questions to be answered. Teachers will often come to the meeting with a draft IEP containing their ideas and plans. Likewise, you need to come prepared so that the meeting can be most effective and efficient.

Following the discussion of strengths and needs, the team needs to consider the ways in which your child can participate in the general education program. It is important to have the input of your child's general education teacher regarding expectations for typical students as well as the usual pace and modes of instruction. On the basis of your child's strengths and needs, participation and accommodations are considered.

An IEP meeting can be reconvened if more information is needed or if time constraints interfere. Even though the plan that is being developed generally covers 1 year, an IEP can be written for a shorter period of time. This may be the case when there have been major changes in your child's program or when there are concerns about adjustment and functioning in a new environment. You have the right to request an IEP meeting whenever you feel it is needed. Frequently, if you share your concerns directly with the school, modifications can be made without the need for a formalized IEP meeting. But if you are concerned about your child's goals, services, or placement and have been unable to resolve these concerns directly with the educational staff, you should request another IEP meeting.

Developing the IEP

Although there is no federally mandated format for the IEP, some states have suggested an outline that ensures that all legally mandated components are included. Typically the IEP begins with a front page containing your child's name, address, and birth date. Often there is a signature page to keep track of who attended the meeting. This list may be helpful to you when trying to remember who participated in the meeting, especially because many of the professionals may be new to you. You are asked to sign this sheet as well to record your attendance. Your signature on this page in no way signifies consent as to what is being discussed and planned for your child.

The first required element of the meeting is a review of the special considerations that must be addressed before developing an IEP. These considerations are in the form of questions and include the following:

1. Is the student blind or visually impaired?

2. Is the student deaf or hearing impaired?

3. Does the student exhibit behaviors that impede his or her learning or that of others?

4. Does the student have limited English proficiency?

5. Does the student have communication needs?

6. Does the student require assistive technology devices and services?

If the answers to any of these questions is yes, then the team must address the issue in the student's IEP.

These questions are followed by the heart of the IEP, the educational plan for the next year based on your child's present skills and performance. It may include reports from your child's teachers and therapists, formal psychoeducational evaluations, information from the school nurse, and input from you, your child's physician, and private therapists/tutors you may have consulted. These reports are compiled into a comprehensive report that allows your child's areas of strength and need to be identified. Because the focus is for all students to participate in the general education curriculum as much as possible, a statement must be included in the IEP that explains the extent that the student will be removed from the general education classroom and why this is necessary.

The next step is to develop a plan that will address your child's strengths and needs. The law requires that beginning when the student is age 14, he or she must have an ITP. The ITP focuses on a course of study (such as courses for college preparation or a vocational education program) that prepares the student for the transition from the public education system by age 21. Once your child is within 3 years of high school graduation, a graduation plan needs to be developed that describes what requirements your child will need to meet in order to graduate, either by passing course requirements or by meeting IEP goals and objectives (see Chapter 28). When a transition plan is required, the IEP team also needs to discuss postschool outcomes in community living, employment, and postsecondary education/training. From these decisions, the team addresses the activities and instruction that will help your child achieve the postschool outcomes. The law also requires that in preparation for transition planning the IEP identify appropriate community resources for achieving this plan (such as a community college) and invite their participation as active members of the team. There is also a requirement to monitor the fulfillment of community agencies' commitments made as part of the planning process.

The next section of the IEP contains a description of the measurable goals to be accomplished over the course of the school year. These should tie directly into your child's needs. The goals and objectives should be written in a way that clearly explains what will be learned, how success will be measured, and the schedule for evaluation of success.

The next section deals with what program modifications might be needed for your child to be successful and what specially designed instruction he or she requires. This might include allowing your child to take tests without time limits, to use a computer and other assistive technology, or to get structured study guides.

Related services that your child needs to benefit from or gain access to his or her educational program are then listed in the IEP. These include transportation accommodations (including wheelchair access) and aids and services (such as physical or occupational therapy) that enable your child to participate to the fullest extent possible in the general education curriculum. The law requires that the projected date, the anticipated frequency, and the location and duration of these services and modifications be included in the IEP.

Federal law requires that all students participate in statewide and districtwide assessments of their progress, with modifications and accommodations as appropriate. If the IEP team determines that your child's performance cannot be accurately assessed using general education tests, even with modification, the IEP must include a statement of why the assessment is not appropriate and alternative assessments must be made available. This requirement ensures that your child is progressing toward his or her goals.

Once your child's educational level is determined and the goals, objectives, and needed services are identified, he or she will be assigned to a specific class. The goal is for the IEP team to place your child in a general education classroom in the local public school with supplemental aids and supports. If this is deemed not possible, the team must consider alternative placements or intervention programs but must choose the least restrictive of these options. In accordance with federal and state regulations, each state's Department of Education ranks placement options from least to most restrictive.

The final section of the IEP contains the projected starting dates and duration for services and programs. Your child's programs may last as long as but not more than 12 months. This final IEP section also includes how the school will report your child's progress toward annual goals and how frequently these reports will occur. These reports must be made at least as frequently as are traditional report cards. Finally, the IEP lists the criteria that will determine when your child no longer needs special education services.

After the meeting, the educational staff will take all of the information and plans and generate a written copy of the formal IEP. They then send the program to you with a copy of the procedural safeguards notice explaining all of your rights. Also included is a notice of recommended assignment which asks you to approve or disapprove of the proposed educational program and placement.

The IEP process has a number of important events. Your signature on your child's initial IEP is required before services can begin. But with later IEPs, if you do not return the notice of recommended assignment within 10 days, it is considered approved. Therefore, you should carefully review each IEP when you receive it. If you have minor concerns, you should first call the school and explain your concerns. Sometimes information is misunderstood or conveyed in an unclear way and can be easily corrected. If you have major disagreements, however, you should express your disapproval of the notice in writing. As outlined in the procedural safeguards notice, if there is disagreement about the IEP, a meeting called a *prehearing conference* will be held. If a resolution is not reached, an impartial hearing officer will preside over a due process hearing, a formal proceeding used to resolve differences. The parents and the school typically are supported by attorneys at the hearing. Each side presents evidence, and witnesses provide testimony. The hearing officer renders a written decision that can be appealed. Each state maintains a system of protection and advocacy services at low or no cost to parents. Information about local agencies is included in the procedural safeguards notice. Contacting one of these agencies may help you better understand your rights and the available resources.

PROGRAMS FOR PRESCHOOLERS

Children with disabilities from age 3 to kindergarten age attend preschool programs. Regarding the range of services provided, these programs are much like the programs offered for infants and toddlers (see Chapter 6) but are typically administered by the local public school as opposed to a private agency. Preschool-age children go through the same process for identification, evaluation, and IEP development as school-age children. Preschoolers typically attend programs more often and for longer times during the week than do infants and toddlers. These programs are often part of a neighborhood preschool or child care center or take place in a special classroom in a community center. What is considered the least restrictive environment for a preschooler is different from what is considered the least restrictive environment for a school-age child. For example, a program that works on developmental skills such as language, self-care skills, or fine motor skills may be provided in the home, which may be the least restrictive program for a young child.

SCHOOL ENVIRONMENTS FOR SPECIAL EDUCATION

With the focus on including all children in the general curriculum, there is an emphasis on making accommodations for the student requiring special education services within the general education environment. Even if this is not initially possible and your child enters a self-contained special education class, you should not view this as a decision forever set in stone. This environment is provided only when placement in a general education classroom with adaptations, accommodations, and supports cannot meet your child's learning needs. Even then, the school should look for ways to include your child as much as possible with classmates in general education. The goal of providing needed services in the least restrictive environment is the reason that the IEP is developed for only 1 year of educational programming at a time and the reason that psychoeducational reevaluation must occur at least every 3 years.

In deciding your child's educational placement, you will run into the terms *mainstreaming, integration,* and *inclusion*. In *mainstreaming,* a child with a disability participates in the general curriculum. There may be some modifications in the presentation of the material and/or the form or amount of work the child is required to do, but generally he or she is expected to master the same content as the other students in the class. *Integration* is a term that is used to reflect the student's presence and active participation in the general education classroom primarily for social rather than for academic activities. *Inclusion,* however, means that the student participates in the general education classroom but has different academic goals and receives supports to ensure that he or she achieves these learning outcomes. When thinking about involving your child in a general education classroom, it is important that you have a clear understanding of the learning expectations. More and more students with severe disabilities are being placed in general education classrooms for most of the day. Provided that the necessary supports for learning are available, a child can achieve his or her learning objectives, as well as benefit from the social environment of the classroom.

A related issue concerns who is doing the teaching. Special education teachers have different training from general educators, particularly at the secondary school level, in which instruction is subject specific. As a result, you should not expect that if your child is placed in a general education environment, the teacher will have the same knowledge in modifying curriculum and understanding and planning for your child's needs as would a special education teacher. One way to effectively include a special education student in a general class environment is to develop a collaborative teaching arrangement between a special educator and a general educator. The focus on where your child receives instruction is not nearly as important as ensuring that the program itself meets the learning objectives.

Historically, many children with special needs were placed according to their "label." There has been a dramatic shift, however, and schools are becoming far more flexible and creative in how they provide services and supports. This change has allowed children with disabilities greater participation with typical peers in many different learning environments. In evaluating whether programs can best meet your child's needs, you can look for some of these innovative practices:

- *Collaboration and teamwork among staff who work with your child:* The greatest learning occurs when everyone is working toward the same goals.

- *Integrated instruction:* Many children with special needs require the support of many therapies to achieve their goals. Yet, pulling students out of the classroom to address skills in isolation does not keep your child in the functional environment where he or she needs to practice the skills.

- *Positive reinforcement practices:* When addressing behavioral issues, positive reinforcement practices rather than punishment should be used (see Chapter 11).

- *Multiple methods of presenting materials:* In response to different learning styles, teachers and assistants should be comfortable with presenting materials in different ways, such as on the blackboard, in small groups, and with manipulatives or visual aids.

- *Coordination of strategies throughout your child's day:* Your child will benefit most when his or her teachers and therapists communicate regularly regarding strategies so that these can be applied consistently.

- *Opportunities for practice in functional environments:* Many programs include instruction in daily living skills and self-care skills as they naturally occur, such as practicing putting on a coat prior to going home.

- *A focus on transition to adult life:* Even when your child is very young, it is important that the teachers, assistants, and therapists working with him or her maintain a focus on your child's goal of achieving the maximum possible level of independence.

- *Environments that incorporate fun into the learning:* Look for programs that approach learning as fun by including songs, games, and other activities.

- *Ongoing, open communication between the school and your family:* Due to the nature and complexity of services required by many children with disabilities, far more communication is needed. The responsibility for keeping communication lines open, honest, and professional lies with both your family and the school, but you'll know a school is good at keeping in contact with you if your child's teacher often sends home notes about classroom activities, if school staff genuinely listen when you voice your concerns (even if they disagree with you), and if the people who work with your child ask for and welcome your input.

SUMMARY

The educational process, with its myriad of supports, services, and program options, offers both challenges and opportunities. IDEA mandates that your child receive a free and appropriate education in the least restrictive environment. This educational program may start as early as infancy (see Chapter 6) and continues until graduation from high school or until age 21. Decisions on school placement and curriculum should involve collaboration between you and the school, and monitoring of progress should also be a joint effort. This process is formalized in the annual IEP that outlines the special education services to be provided to your child, their frequency, and their location. Increasingly, the chosen educational option is inclusion within the general education class with supports provided to enable your child to learn. The ultimate goal is for your child to reach his or her academic potential and to learn social skills that will prepare him or her for independence and success as an adult.

Some Questions Answered

How do I get involved with my child's school?

Most schools have active special education parent groups as well as parent–teacher organizations. Your participation and support in both of these provide opportunities and benefits that far surpass those gained from merely attending your child's meetings. You can also volunteer to assist in your child's classroom, and you can take advantage of every opportunity to visit the school depending on your own schedule.

I took my child for a private evaluation. Is the school required to follow all of the recommendations made in the evaluation?

You have the right to have an independent evaluation for your child. The school system will pay for this evaluation if there has been prior approval.

Once this has been obtained, you should make the results available to the school as soon as possible, particularly if the team members are in the process of developing an IEP. The school is required to review these reports or any other input you provide in making a final decision about your child's educational plan. The school is not required, however, to fulfill all of the recommendations as long as they have given them consideration. If you disagree with the IEP, you can request a prehearing conference or go directly to a due process hearing.

My child has severe disabilities, and I just do not see how the statewide test of proficiency will benefit him or how he will be able to take it. What can I do?

You have the right to state at the IEP meeting that you do not want your child to participate in the statewide testing. This will be noted on the IEP. You have the right to deny permission for any evaluation being proposed for your child. You should, however, consider this decision carefully because the test may identify areas of concern that can be treated effectively. Also, starting July 1, 2000, states are charged with developing and conducting an alternative assessment for students who cannot take the statewide test of proficiency even with accommodations. This alternative assessment may provide a better measure for a child with a severe disability.

I really would like to have a copy of all of the evaluations and reports about my child so that I can share them with my child's private therapists. How do I get them?

You have the right to receive copies of all of your child's educational records. You can call the school district headquarters, and they will send you a form to identify which records you want and to whom you want them released. The individual therapists at your child's school cannot release the records directly to you, and your request must be in writing.

I attended my child's IEP meeting, and I agree with the program designed for my child. I just don't like the school that they want to put her in. What do I do?

When you sign your child's IEP, you are approving both the program and the placement. The term *placement* does not refer to a particular school building but rather to the type of classroom environment. School districts are limited at times by the numbers of students, building space, location, and environmental constraints (such as lack of elevators in some buildings). All of these factors affect where a particular class will be located. If you have concerns about the particular school, you need to bring these up at the IEP meeting so that you and the other team members can discuss them, make accommodations, or consider even alternative placements—but the IEP team is not required to make an alternative placement.

I have such a hard time finding baby sitters who really understand my child and know how to care for him. Would it be appropriate to ask his teacher or paraeducator to babysit?

Finding baby sitters who are knowledgeable about the needs of children with special needs is very difficult. Often there are teachers, therapists, paraeducators, and others in the school environment who are willing to babysit. You don't, however, want to put them in the embarrassing position of saying "no," so it might be more appropriate to ask the teacher and the paraeducator if they know people who babysit children with special needs than to ask them directly. In addition, many special education parent groups have resource lists of baby sitters and respite care providers who work well with children with special needs.

13

Identifying Legal
Rights and Benefits

D. Michael Malone

Parenting is a journey filled with many joys and challenges. Although your child's welfare is ultimately your responsibility as a parent, several federal programs are designed to help you support your child's needs. This chapter describes these programs and how your child and family may benefit from them. It discusses several programs that guarantee your child's rights. It also advises about advocating for your child's legal rights and benefits and about estate planning. Finally, the chapter identifies resources that you can draw on to help you become an informed advocate for your child.

Jonathan

Jonathan was born prematurely and had many medical complications before his discharge from the hospital at 2 months of age. His teenage mother, Tina, was not employed and did not have medical insurance to cover Jonathan. With the help of the hospital staff, she applied for Supplemental Security Income (SSI), which also provided Medicaid health insurance. Jonathan was diagnosed with cerebral palsy at 6 months of age. Through the Child Find program in her community, Tina was able to enroll him in an early intervention program in which a physical therapist and early childhood educator visited Jonathan at home weekly. Jonathan continued to require special education programs and to need special equipment when he entered elementary school. Tina used the SSI funding to help purchase a van with a wheelchair lift and to construct a ramp and widen doorways in her house. As school progressed, Tina was generally satisfied with her son's individualized education program (IEP), but sometimes she felt that not all of Jonathan's needs were being adequately addressed. She learned to advocate on his behalf and on one occasion requested a hearing and brought legal representation to obtain services she felt necessary. During Jonathan's early school years Tina went to college and eventually became a realtor. Although her income improved significantly, she was able to maintain Jonathan's Medicaid coverage through a waiver based on his disability rather than her income. When she changed jobs for a better position, Jonathan was covered by a COBRA policy until the new health policy became active. Tina set up a will that both provided financially for Jonathan and identified his grandparents as guardians in the event of Tina's death. Now Jonathan is 14, and although he has significant physical disabilities, he also has many cognitive strengths. He is being evaluated for vocational rehabilitation services to plan for accommodations and training to help him successfully enter the workforce after he finishes his education. Although Tina needed help at first, over time she has become expert in navigating the system to identify Jonathan's rights and benefits and has felt empowered by the experience.

SUPPORTS PROVIDED BY FEDERAL PROGRAMS

The challenges faced by Jonathan and his family are not unique. As a parent of a child with a developmental disability, you are faced with understanding the resultant problems and determining what services and supports your child and family may need. You are also learning about and negotiating with community agencies and programs that may not automatically address your child's needs. This section provides an overview of specific federal programs that offer support to children with disabilities and their families, focusing on the rights and benefits that your child and family are entitled to under each program.

Rehabilitation Act and Amendments

The Rehabilitation Act was designed as a civil rights law to protect people with disabilities from discrimination in areas such as employment, architectural accessibility, and transportation. The law states that its purpose is to "empower individuals with disabilities to maximize employment, economic self-sufficiency, independence, and inclusion and integration into society." Section 504 of the Rehabilitation Act was implemented to protect children with disabilities from discrimination in school programs receiving federal financial assistance. Disability is defined in Section 504 as a physical or mental impairment that substantially limits one or more major life activities. Physical and mental impairments include speech, hearing, visual, and orthopedic impairments, cerebral palsy, epilepsy, muscular dystrophy, mental retardation, emotional illness, specific learning disabilities (including perceptual impairments), brain injury, dyslexia, minimal brain dysfunction (now known as attention-deficit/hyperactivity disorder), and the communication disorder developmental aphasia. Major life activities include self-care, seeing, hearing, speaking, breathing, learning, walking, and performing manual tasks.

Section 504 mandates that your child be provided a free and appropriate public education (FAPE) in the most natural environment possible, such as a general education classroom rather than a resource room. The law also requires your child's school to develop an educational plan that will meet his or her needs. Schools may use the IEP required by the Individuals with Disabilities Education Act (IDEA; discussed later) to meet this requirement (see also Chapter 12). A Section 504 plan, however, is less complex than an IEP, so if your child is eligible for Section 504 but not IDEA, the school may develop and implement the simpler Section 504 plan.

Developmental Disabilities Assistance and Bill of Rights Act and Amendments

The Developmental Disabilities Assistance and Bill of Rights Act (DD Act) was designed to promote the independence, productivity, and inclusion of people with disabilities into all facets of community life. This act (amended in 1999) supports state developmental disabilities councils (DD councils), state protection and advocacy systems (P&As), and university affiliated programs (UAPs) for people with developmental disabilities. The goals of the DD councils are to promote systemwide change to enhance individual capability and advocacy activities and to produce a responsive, family-centered, coordinated, comprehensive system of services and supports for individuals with disabilities and their families. P&As exist to protect the legal and human rights of individuals with disabilities and their families. UAPs are designed to provide interdisciplinary training to students, to conduct community service activities, and to disseminate information and research findings about developmental disabilities. Finally, the DD Act provided the first entirely functional definition of developmental disabilities, removing the need for a person to receive a specific diagnostic label in order to be eligible for services. Each of these programs can serve as a resource to you for information, guidance in networking, and assistance in advocating for your child.

Americans with Disabilities Act

The Americans with Disabilities Act (ADA) is a civil rights law designed to protect people with disabilities from discrimination in employment, public services and accommodations, public transportation, and telecommunications. The ADA was designed to complement the Rehabilitation Act by using the same terms and definitions. The ADA extends the protection of people with disabilities to all public services, programs, and activities (that is, government programs, private businesses, and nonprofit organizations that are open to the public) regardless of whether these services, programs, or activities receive federal financial assistance. Although the ADA does not specifically address the issue of FAPE, Title II of the act states that "no qualified individual with a disability shall . . . be excluded from participation in or be denied the benefits of the services, programs, or activities of a public entity, or be subjected to discrimination by any public entity." This protection applies to students in child care and in private schools that are not administered by religious organizations or entities. Unfortunately, the ADA does not provide for funding of the mandates, procedural safeguards, evaluation or placement procedures, or due-process procedures specifically related to your child's educational rights. The ADA, however, specifies administrative requirements, complaint procedures, and consequences for noncompliance related to services and employment, and it specifies provision of reasonable accommodations for eligible students across educational activities and environments. The determination of reasonable accommodations is specific both to your child and to the program in question. The main test for determining the best accommodation for your child is effectiveness. In particular, the accommodation should provide your child the same *opportunities* as those of children without disabilities in similar situations. The accommodation, however, does not have to ensure your child equal results or benefits. Finally, a program does not need to provide accommodations that represent undue hardship (significant difficulty or expense) or that would fundamentally change the nature of the program. You should consult with a qualified attorney if you have questions about accommodations that are (or are not) planned for your child.

Education for All Handicapped Children Act and Individuals with Disabilities Education Act Amendments

The Education for All Handicapped Children Act, later renamed and reauthorized as the Individuals with Disabilities Education Act (IDEA) Amendments, is the most comprehensive law that supports your child's developmental and educational experiences. IDEA focuses on children and young adults from birth to 21 years of age who experience physical or mental conditions that result in developmental delays in cognitive, physical, communicative, social or emotional, or adaptive development. For children 3–21 years of age, disabilities are specifically defined as mental retardation, hearing, visual, or speech impairment, deafness, blindness, emotional disturbance, orthopedic impairment, autism, traumatic brain injury, other health impairments, specific learning disabilities, deafblindness, or multiple disabilities. Other conditions can be included if they are likely to result in the need for special education or related services and if they fall within one of the categories just named.

IDEA requires that your child receive a free and appropriate public education that includes special education and, if needed, related services (psychological services, speech-language, physical, and occupational therapy, diagnostic medical services, school health services, therapeutic recreation, counseling, social work services, transportation, and parent counseling and training). IDEA provides your child with the right to team-based determination of eligibility and services and the development and use of an individualized family service plan (IFSP) for children younger than 3 years or an IEP for children older than 3 years. Your child has the right to be educated in the least restrictive environment (LRE; see Chapter 12). Your child's school should approach your child's education with the assumption that he or she will be enrolled in the general education classroom with peers who do not have disabilities. Other program options (such as a resource room, a separate class, or a separate school) should only be considered when it is determined that your child's educational needs cannot be met in the general education classroom. Depending on your child's age, the individualized program should also include specific supports for the transition from infant-toddler programs to preschool, from preschool to kindergarten, from middle school to high school, and from high school to postschool opportunities. Finally, IDEA guarantees that you and your child are entitled to written notification regarding identification, evaluation, and placement actions, team and multisource evaluations, periodic review, the right to participate in IFSP and IEP meetings, and the right to impartial hearings if you disagree with the identification, evaluation, or placement of your child.

Supplemental Security Income

The SSI program for children with disabilities can provide your child and family with financial support if you can demonstrate that 1) your child meets the standard of disability and 2) your family meets the established income and asset requirements specified by the Social Security Administration. It is important to understand that the SSI program described here and the Social Security Disability Insurance program are different programs. To meet the SSI standard of disability, your child must have a "medically determinable physical or mental impairment which results in marked and severe functional limitations, and which can be expected to result in death or which has lasted or can be expected to last for a continuous period of not less than 12 months." This standard is supplemented by both a listing of more than 100 disabilities (such as blindness, deafness, cerebral palsy, and mental retardation) and a description of functioning in broad developmental areas. These areas include cognition, communication, motor, social and personal growth, concentration, persistence, pace, and responsivity. Evidence that supports your child's "marked and severe functional limitations" includes medical and school records describing your child's functional abilities. Features that can be considered in determining your child's eligibility include effects of medication, living conditions/environment, need for assistive devices, and school functioning. Information about your child's disability can be obtained from medical personnel, teachers, counselors, therapists, social workers, and others who provide services. Although no specific condition is excluded, keep in mind that your child's eligibility is based on documentation that he or she is experiencing severe functional limitations.

In addition to meeting a disability standard, you must also demonstrate that your family meets an income/asset standard. Several factors are considered in determining income/asset eligibility, including your actual income, the number of dependents in your household, and the total value of certain items that you own (limits of $2,000 for a single person and $3,000 for a couple). If you and your child meet both the disability and income/asset standards, your child may be eligible for as much as $512 per month (as established by the Social Security Administration for the year 2000). This figure varies depending on individual family circumstances. Some states supplement the SSI benefits. All families receiving SSI benefits are required to establish a dedicated bank account into which the Social Security Administration can directly deposit SSI benefits. You can use SSI benefits in a variety of ways to support your child including education, job-related training, personal needs assistance, specialized equipment, housing modifications, medical treatment, and therapy or rehabilitation.

All children who are determined to be eligible for SSI must undergo a periodic continued disability review (CDR), or redetermination, to make sure that they continue to meet SSI eligibility standards. If your child was considered eligible due to prematurity, he or she must undergo a CDR by 1 year of age. If your child's eligibility was determined for a reason other than low birth weight, he or she will undergo a CDR every 3 years until he or she is 18 years of age. When your child turns 18 years of age, your son or daughter's eligibility will be considered in relation to adult standards, which place an emphasis on an individual's ability to work. While your child is receiving SSI, you must provide evidence of his or her limitations and interventions that are being conducted to address those limitations.

Finally, your child's SSI eligibility may automatically qualify your child for Medicaid benefits. Depending upon your specific circumstances, your child may or may not continue to qualify for Medicaid benefits if he or she loses SSI benefits. It is important that you contact your local Social Security Administration office to determine the state regulations related to SSI and Medicaid eligibility.

Medicaid

The Medicaid program is a needs-based program that provides children with special health care needs access to important health services. Families whose income places them at or below 133% of the poverty threshold and whose children meet the disability guidelines established for SSI just discussed qualify for Medicaid benefits. For example, a single-parent household including two children younger than 18 years of age could qualify for Medicaid if the family income is at or below about $17,850. A two-parent household including two children younger than 18 years of age could qualify for Medicaid if the family income is at or below about $22,470. This example is an approximation, and actual eligibility may vary. Some states have raised the standard to as high as 185%, 250%, 300%, or even 400% of the federal poverty level. In most states, your child automatically qualifies for Medicaid if you can establish SSI eligibility.

If you qualify for Medicaid benefits, you can take advantage of the program's early and periodic screening, diagnostic, and treatment (EPSDT) services. This group of services is designed to make sure that all children who are eligible for Medicaid receive necessary health care. EPSDT services include developmental screening services (such as a developmental history, physical and mental assessment, immunizations, laboratory tests, and health education), diagnostic services (such as dental, hearing, and vision services), assistive technology (such as hearing aids, eyeglasses, or communication devices), assistance with transportation and scheduling of appointments, and preventive and corrective treatment (including optional services such as service coordination to help protect your rights, ensure procedural safeguards, and enable access to services authorized in your state; speech, occupational, and physical therapy; rehabilitative services; and private duty nursing). Your child can receive EPSDT services from physicians, nurses, pediatricians, or other qualified health care providers who are certified by your state's Medicaid program. State Medicaid agencies coordinate their efforts to identify and enroll all eligible children with a variety of other social service agencies.

Finally, there are several "safety nets" in the Medicaid program to protect families who are not able to provide necessary health care because of the child's health condition or because of the family's financial status. First, Medicaid waivers have been developed by states to allow families to provide and/or have access to home and community-based care that would not be covered under private insurance. In a waiver program, the state uses both federal and state money to pay for health care for people with health conditions specified in the waiver program. Waiver programs are often more flexible than the federal Medicaid program and may be different from state to state. Before the development of Medicaid waivers, the only option for some parents in gaining access to Medicaid was to have their children institutionalized in approved residential care facilities (such as nursing homes). A waiver program can allow for less costly home and community care. Eligibility for a Medicaid waiver is based only on your child's developmental disability, not your income or assets. The health care coverage provided by these waivers is especially critical if your private insurance does not cover your child's health care needs or if you have exceeded the limits of your private insurance. Second, the program has a presumptive eligibility option through which approved health care providers are allowed to provide temporary Medicaid enrollment for children who appear to be eligible based on age and family income. Third, the Medicaid program now includes a 12-month continuous eligibility option. Should your child's Medicaid eligibility end for any reason, your state can continue your child's coverage for as long as 12 months after the unfavorable determination. Last, the State Children's Health Insurance Program (CHIP) was created to provide health care coverage for families whose incomes are too high to allow them to qualify for Medicaid but are too low to allow adequate coverage through private insurance. Contact your local Medicaid program representative to determine your options related to eligibility and benefits.

Consolidated Omnibus Budget Reconciliation Act

The Consolidated Omnibus Budget Reconciliation Act (COBRA) was written to provide health care support to your child and family in the event that you or your spouse experience a change in employment status that would otherwise result in a loss of group health insurance coverage provided by an employer. The provisions protect only certain employees on the basis of their length of service, the size of the company, and the type of health insurance that the company provides. COBRA defines a number of circumstances as qualifying events that might normally result in a loss of health care benefits for the covered employee, including a shift from full-time to part-time employment, voluntary or involuntary termination of employment, becoming eligible for Medicare, legal separation or divorce, death of the covered employee, and loss of the "dependent child" status as defined in the plan. In such circumstances, you are to be granted a 60-day period during which you can choose to pay for continued coverage under the employer's group health plan. In short, the law is intended to provide your family with a "safety net." Although you can only purchase continued health care benefits for as long as 36 months (depending on the circumstance), the amount that you will pay for premiums during this time is typically less than the cost of purchasing private health care insurance. The continued health care coverage should be identical to what was available prior to the change in employment status. Your employer is obligated to notify you of the COBRA provisions both at the time of your initial employment and at the time of your change in status.

ADVOCATING FOR YOUR
CHILD'S LEGAL RIGHTS AND BENEFITS

The federal programs described so far are designed to ensure that your child's rights are protected and that education, health care benefits, and financial support are provided. In spite of the intent of and protection offered by these federal programs, you may find yourself at odds with your local, state, or federal service system at some point. Conflict between parents and professionals can sometimes be a result of intentional efforts to ignore federal requirements. More typically, however, conflicts are a result of honest mistakes, a lack of sensitivity to or understanding of needs, a lack of knowledge about federal requirements, different interpretations of federal requirements, or differences in opinion regarding options and strategies for meeting your child's needs. All of these situations can be addressed through open communication, the sharing of information, and a willingness to learn about and explore options.

There are several things to consider when advocating for your child. First, you are the expert on your child. Does this mean that you have the technical knowledge that a professional might have? Not necessarily. But you do have the best knowledge about who your child is (his or her interests, abilities, potential, and needs). As the expert, you not only have information that will help the professionals provide the most appropriate supports for your child, but you also have the greatest motivation to see that your child's needs are met. Use that knowledge and motivation to your advantage.

Second, learn about your child's disability and about the services that are available to you and your child. This will not only make you an informed advocate but will also put you in a position in which you do not have to take on faith the information provided by professionals. You will find that you will better understand different perspectives and the full range of options available to you and your child.

Third, foster a positive partnership with professionals through open and honest communication. You can learn about the supports that are available to your child and family, and professionals will learn about your child's needs. As a team, you and the professionals can identify ways to support your child's needs and protect your child's rights. Communication helps you to learn, to share, and to clear up misunderstandings.

Fourth, you should learn to network with other parents and professionals who are experienced and knowledgeable. Seek information that might be useful to you, and don't be afraid to ask a lot of questions. Establish informal relationships for the purpose of gathering information and formal relationships so that you have someone to help you advocate for your child. Choose as an advocate a person with whom you feel comfortable and who has relevant knowledge, resources, and contacts in the community. Finally, discuss the expectations, roles, and responsibilities early in the relationship, and document all in-person, telephone, and written communications. It is also always a good idea to ask for written confirmation from the person with whom you have spoken. Documentation is especially important when decisions are being made because it helps you and the many people with whom you are likely to interact to "stay on the same page" and avoid misunderstandings. Create a file for documentation and keep that file organized in chronological order, up-to-date, and in a handy location.

When Rights and Needs Are Not Being Met

There will be times when you act in good faith, demonstrate patience and proactive communication skills, and provide necessary documentation and still find that your child's rights and needs are not being met. The challenges that you are facing may be directly related to the personal views and actions of the professional with whom you are working (such as lack of knowledge, different interpretation of the situation or program policy, or conflicting personal values and beliefs). The challenges, however, also may be a direct result of program policies or procedures. The person with whom you are working may agree with you but may feel bound by how he or she interprets the program rules and regulations. When you find that you cannot make progress in getting your child's needs met through meetings and discussions with agency personnel, you should first seek informal mediation and voluntary compliance. Solicit the advice and/or assistance of a formal advocate, someone who understands the specific challenges with which you are faced. The guidelines provided by parents who were interviewed (discussed previously) should help you with this process. You should make sure that all people with an interest in or an obligation to your child (the stakeholders) are present during mediation. If informal mediation does not work, you will need to file a formal complaint following the grievance procedures of the program/business with which you are interacting. During a formal complaint procedure, the services of a qualified and impartial mediator should be secured. During this type of hearing, you have the right to have legal counsel present. If mediation is not successful, you can file a formal complaint with the federal agency responsible for administrative oversight of the rights being violated (such as the U.S. Department of Justice for civil rights discrimination, the U.S. Department of Education for IDEA violations, the Social Security Administration for SSI violations, and the Health Care Financing Administration for Medicaid violations). You can also file a civil action lawsuit, which may be necessary if you believe that your child's rights are being violated and that you have exhausted all other options. You should contact state and local consumer organizations (P&As, parent training and information centers, legal aid groups, and the bar association) for direction or advice. You can talk with an attorney whom you know personally and ask for a reference. Make sure that the attorney that you secure to represent your case is knowledgeable about disability law. Finally, choose an attorney who you believe you can trust.

ESTATE PLANNING

Parents often don't give careful consideration to planning for the future when they are investing so much of their energy in making sure that their child's immediate needs are met. Regardless of your financial status, planning your estate is critical for ensuring that your child's needs continue to be met after you are gone. There are a number of issues that you must consider as you plan your estate, including establishing a will. This document outlines your wishes related to your estate, including guardianship, gifts/inheritance, and beneficiaries. The issue of guardianship is critical for all minor children and children over the age of 18 who are not considered fully competent to care for themselves. As a parent, you are your child's natural guardian, the person responsible for your child's care and welfare. In the event of your death, someone else must be appointed guardian of your child. Appointed guardians are often family members or friends whom you can trust to act in your child's best interests. There are three basic types of guardians. A guardian of the person would be authorized to provide consent for your child's activities of daily living. A guardian of the estate would have authority over your child's finances and property. A general guardian would have authority over both personal activities and finances/property. If you fail to appoint a guardian, the state can appoint someone as your child's guardian. Although the decision should be made with the best interests of your child in mind, the state-appointed guardian may not be a choice that you would otherwise approve of. Finally, guardianship for individuals over the age of 18 may be complete or limited in scope depending on the individual's level of competence. In the case of limited guardianship, the courts can decide the scope of the guardian's authority.

After you have written your will, you can modify it as needed to address changes in your financial circumstances and your child's medical and financial needs. When developing your plan, be sure to do the following:

- Design the plan to meet your specific circumstances and the specific needs of your child. Your estate plan should be unique, based on the nature and severity of your child's disability. For example, the type and scope of guardianship will be a function of your child's needs and competence.

- Evaluate your child's current and projected circumstances and need for benefits related to health, productivity/earning potential, and independence.

- Consider your child's current government benefits (such as SSI and Medicaid) *and* your child's potential for needing such benefits in the future. Consider how the plan that you develop may have an impact on your child's eligibility for government benefits. For instance, giving your child a gift of more than $2,000 can make your child ineligible for SSI and Medicaid benefits. Not only could your child lose the cash and medical benefits available through these programs, but he or she could also lose benefits related to supported employment and vocational rehabilitation services, group housing, job coaches, personal attendant care, and transportation assistance.

- Consider developing a special needs trust. A special needs trust is put in the name of a trustee whom you identify and who agrees to manage your child's resources. Because the trust is not in your child's name, he or she can remain eligible for government benefits. Thus, the trust can provide for your child's basic needs without jeopardizing government benefits.

- Write a letter of intent to be included with your will. This document should provide a rich description of your child's history, his or her current status, your personal insights, and your hopes for his or her future. The letter can include the contributions of all relevant stakeholders, including your child, and should be modified as needed. Although it is not a legal document, the letter of intent can provide court personnel and others with guidance in understanding your child and your wishes.

Finally, seek the advice and guidance of a qualified attorney or certified estate planner who is knowledgeable about estate planning and government programs and can provide your child with necessary supports. Your local protection and advocacy office, The Arc (formerly the Association for Retarded Citizens), and the local bar association can help you find a qualified professional.

SUMMARY

A number of federal programs have been developed in an effort to reduce the challenges that your child and family may experience. This chapter has provided an overview of some of these programs and how your child can benefit from them as well as some suggestions for advocating for your child's legal rights and benefits. Finally, it is important that you draw up a will so that your child's needs can continue to be met even after you are no longer able to do so.

Some Questions Answered

How do I find out what my child's rights are under the law?

In most cases, the program or agency with which you are working will provide you with information about your child's rights and benefits. Becoming an informed consumer, however, is always a good idea. Ask questions, do your own research, and talk with other parents. The technological revolution has made information available to you that would have been relatively inaccessible 5–10 years ago. If you are not comfortable with computers, find a friend who is and "surf the net"!

Can I expect everyone to interpret laws in the same way?

People and programs differ regarding values, attitudes, education, understanding, and interpretation of legislation. Your child's and family's experiences will vary depending on the people with whom you interact. Although federal programs are intended to be implemented consistently, the reality is that they are not, and some of this is a reflection of the personnel who are responsible for implementation. As noted previously, there are many reasons for different interpretations. A person might agree with you on one level but may feel bound by program policies or regulations.

What do I do if my child's rights are being violated?

You should first assume that an honest mistake has been made. Seek to clarify the situation. Make sure that you have been included in the process and that your voice is being heard. If you cannot get resolution on your own or with the help of an advocate, you may need to seek formal mediation or, if all else fails, resolution through legal channels.

How do I find an advocate for my child?

Talk with other parents you know, especially those who have preceded you and your child in the system. Talk with professionals you trust and with whom you are comfortable. If necessary, contact local disability-related agencies or your local protection and advocacy office for advice.

I live a pretty modest lifestyle—do I really need an estate plan?

All families, regardless of financial circumstances, should take the time to develop an estate plan. Parents can leave their child with a developmental disability vulnerable if no plan has been developed. The time and stress related to developing a plan are worth the peace of mind and security that it will bring in the long run.

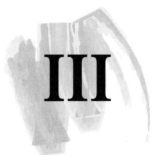

III

Developmental Disabilities

14

Mental Retardation

Mark L. Batshaw

Approximately 1.5 million people in the United States receive services for mental retardation. Most children with mental retardation follow the step-by-step pattern of development described in Chapter 4, gaining skills in a similar sequence but generally progressing more slowly than typical children. How rapidly your child progresses and what level of independence he or she will eventually reach depends on a combination of intellectual gifts, daily living skills, and family supports. This chapter focuses on helping you to understand what the term *mental retardation* means to your child, what testing you can expect for him or her, and what treatment approaches are likely to be useful.

Linda, Sandy, and Billy

Linda was a full-term baby, but during her mother's labor, Linda's heart rate dropped from the usual 160 beats per minute to 40 beats per minute because of a premature abruption (detachment) of the placenta from the uterine wall. The doctors, noting fetal distress, performed an emergency C-section. At birth, Linda did not breathe on her own and required artificial ventilation. Within 2 hours she started to have seizures, which were treated with antiepileptic medication. During her hospitalization, Linda did not suck well, and her cry was weak and high pitched. At 3 weeks of age, she was able to go home but was very irritable, frequently crying for no apparent reason and arching her back. Linda's parents were concerned because she showed little interest in her surroundings.

The pediatrician closely monitored Linda's developmental milestones. At 6 months of age she did not roll over or hold her head up, and she lacked the motor control necessary to keep her hands open. She didn't follow objects with her eyes, although she was able to fix her gaze on her mother's face. She did not smile or make "cooing" noises. In sum, her skills at 6 months were less than those of a typical 2-month-old baby.

The pediatrician told Linda's parents that her development was likely to continue to be delayed but that it was too early to estimate the extent of how much support she would need. Linda was enrolled in an early intervention program; a special education teacher and physical therapist started coming into the home each week to provide therapy. Linda made slow but real progress, and at 2 years of age most of her skills were around a 6-month level. She was able to roll over, sit with support, grasp objects, and transfer them from one hand to the other. She laughed and smiled at her image in the mirror, and her parents were excited that she had begun to babble. At 3 years of age Linda entered a preschool program for children with disabilities. She was diagnosed as having severe mental retardation.

Sandy was the fourth child born to Susan, age 39, and George, age 41. For religious reasons Susan and George chose not to pursue prenatal diagnosis even though doctors often advise pregnant women of Susan's age to have prenatal testing. At the time of birth the doctors told Susan and George that Sandy had the appearance of a child with Down syndrome, a diagnosis that was confirmed when chromosome studies revealed the presence of an extra #21 chromosome (see Chapter 15). Sandy's parents were very upset, but because they had received a diagnosis, they were able to read about Down syndrome and learn what they could do to promote Sandy's development. They also contacted other families that had children with Down syndrome and joined the National Down Syndrome Society. They were also helped by their strong faith and by the support they received from their extended family and their church.

Sandy was a happy baby who fed well, but her development proceeded slowly. She sat at 12 months, walked at 20 months, rode a tricycle at 5 years, and rode a bicycle at 10 years. Sandy's language development was delayed, but she babbled at 12 months, was able to say two or three specific words at 28 months, and began to speak in short sentences when she was 6 years old. Sandy has been in an inclusive classroom in the public school system since that time and enjoys school. Sandy has moderate mental retardation.

Fran had a normal delivery, and her son Billy was a healthy baby. His development seemed typical during the first few years, although in retrospect his parents thought he reached milestones somewhat later than his two older brothers. At age 5, Billy entered kindergarten, but his teacher noticed that he had not gained certain skills that other children in his class had gained, such as knowing colors and the alphabet and printing his name. At his teacher's suggestion, Billy's parents had him evaluated by a developmental pediatrician and a clinical psychologist, and he was diagnosed with mild mental retardation. Billy is doing well in an inclusive education program and is learning many skills that can help him become self-sufficient as he grows older.

WHAT DOES THE TERM *MENTAL RETARDATION* MEAN?

The definition of mental retardation has three parts as described in Table 14.1. First, the diagnosis of mental retardation has traditionally relied on a measure of intelligence called the *intelligence quotient,* or the *IQ score.* People with mental retardation have IQ scores that are significantly below the average of 100, but a certain IQ score alone does not define mental retardation. The second part of the definition of mental retardation is that the IQ score must be accompanied by an impairment in a person's ability to adapt and interact with the environment. Finally, the diagnosis of mental retardation is only given to individuals who have developmental delays that exist prior to age 18. This third part of the definition implies that the damage occurred before birth or during childhood while the brain was still rapidly growing. Table 14.1 also shows the definitions of mental retardation (mental retardation requiring intermittent to pervasive support) that the American Association on Mental Retardation favors because the terms stress how a person can function adaptively with various degrees of support.

The degree of supports that a child with mental retardation requires usually determines how early a diagnosis can be made: The greater the need, the earlier the diagnosis. In addition, the diagnosis becomes clearer once the child has been evaluated for several years and if the child's parents, teachers, and doctors can see a constant rate of development. Having a diagnosis such as Down syndrome for your child permits a more informed discussion of treatment and outcomes based on a group of children with the same disorder.

ASSOCIATED DISABILITIES

Although mental retardation may exist as a sole disability, it may also be associated with other impairments that limit a person's abilities. Associated disabilities, including seizure disorders, cerebral palsy, speech and hearing problems, and visual impairments, are most likely to occur in children who have severe mental retardation (requiring extensive supports). Thus, your child should be tested for these other disabilities so that, if needed, appropriate treatment can be provided.

EARLY CLUES TO MENTAL RETARDATION

Mental retardation may be diagnosed as early as infancy or as late as school age. Sometimes a baby's appearance leads to an early diagnosis, such as with children born with very small heads (microcephaly), those who have physical characteristics typical of a genetic syndrome such as Down syndrome, or those who have physical differences suggestive of other genetic syndromes.

In addition to physical appearance, other, less obvious traits may alert a pediatrician to check for developmental delay, such as when a baby is very irritable and inconsolable or when a baby is "too good," lying without com-

Table 14.1.   Diagnostic criteria for mental retardation

- Significantly subaverage intellectual functioning: an IQ score of approximately 70 or below on an individually administered IQ test (for infants, a clinical judgment of significantly subaverage intellectual functioning)

- Concurrent deficits or impairments in present adaptive functioning (i.e., the person's effectiveness in meeting the standards expected for his or her age by his or her cultural group) in at least two of the following areas: communication, self-care, home living, social/interpersonal skills, use of community resources, self-direction, functional academic skills, work, leisure, health, and safety

- Onset before 18 years of age

. . . .

Degree of severity reflecting level of intellectual impairment:

Mild mental retardation (requiring intermittent support)	IQ level 50–55 to approximately 70
Moderate mental retardation (requiring limited support)	IQ level 35–40 to 50–55
Severe mental retardation (requiring extensive support)	IQ level 20–25 to 35–40
Profound mental retardation (requiring pervasive support)	IQ level below 20–25

plaint for hours. Difficulty feeding may indicate that the baby does not suck and swallow well, another possible indication of developmental delay. A high-pitched or strident cry, little recognition of parents by 3–4 months of age, lack of reaction to sound, and an inability to follow objects visually are other markers for developmental delay. There may also be abnormalities in muscle tone, with either too much or too little tightness in the muscles. As described earlier, a significant delay in reaching certain developmental milestones may also alert you or your child's pediatrician to a problem. These milestones include smiling at 2 months, babbling at 6 months, sitting at 7 months, saying single words at 12 months, and walking by 15 months. Often it is the combination of a number of these findings rather than an isolated problem that raises concerns for families and health professionals.

IQ TESTING

There are many tests available that yield IQ scores. Some of these are questionnaire-type tests administered in combination with achievement tests by the teacher to all children in the class at the same time as a way of screening for learning differences. These tests, however, give only an approximation of your child's abilities and are not performed by a psychologist. Language skills and other cognitive abilities are not tested, resulting in an IQ score that may differ significantly from a score obtained using individual IQ tests. Therefore, a child who may have a significant developmental lag should be given an individual IQ test.

There are different psychological tests designed for children of different ages. The three most commonly used individual tests are the Bayley Scales of Infant Development, the Stanford-Binet Intelligence Scale, and the Wechsler intelligence scales. The Bayley takes about 1 hour whereas the others take 2–3 hours to complete, during which time a clinical psychologist will evaluate a number of aspects of your child's intellectual abilities.

The Bayley Scales

The Bayley Scales are generally used for infants and toddlers younger than 2 years of age. You will probably stay in the room with your child during the test, and your child will be expected to play with various objects or perform certain tasks. For example, a 6-month-old ought to be able to reach for two blocks, transfer them from hand to hand, and bang them together. At 12 months a child should be able to place a round peg in a pegboard. Tasks for an 18-month-old include imitating a crayon stroke and pointing to body parts on a doll. At 2 years the child is asked to put together three-piece puzzles, and at 2½ years the child is asked to follow prepositional commands such as "Put the doll *under* the chair."

Language skills are the single best predictor of intelligence. Because language does not emerge as a major skill until about 18 months of age, the Bayley Scales are primarily based on the observation of visual-motor skills and therefore have limited predictive value. Any testing performed with a child younger than 2 years of age is not as accurate as are tests given later in childhood, when the child has a greater repertoire of behaviors that can be sampled. More than half of infants tested before 2 years of age will have Bayley Scales scores that differ by more than 10 points from their adult IQ scores. Despite these limitations, the Bayley Scales are a good predictor of intelligence for infants whose performance differs significantly from average. These children will show a significant delay not just in one area of intelligence but in most or all areas.

Stanford–Binet Intelligence Scale

Beginning at around 2 years of age, the Stanford-Binet Intelligence Scale is often used. It comprises 15 subtests that assess four areas: verbal abilities, abstract/visual thinking, quantitative reasoning, and short-term memory. In this and other psychological tests given to older children, your child is examined while you are not in the room, as you may be a distraction or may unintentionally "help" your child answer the questions. You may be able to watch the testing through a one-way mirror without being observed by your child.

In contrast to the Bayley Scales, the Stanford-Binet Intelligence Scale relies heavily on verbal responses to questions. For example, a 2½-year-old is presented with a group of pictures and is asked to name them. The quality and quantity of words your child puts together into phrases give the examiner an assessment of spontaneous language skills. At 3½ years of age, your child is asked, "Tell about the pictures," and is also asked questions that require more complex reasoning, such as discriminating *similar* versus *different* objects. At 4 years of age, your child is asked relational questions such as "If brother is a boy, sister is a _____ ." At 5 years, your child is given incomplete drawings and is asked to describe what is missing. The expectation is that expressive language and receptive language (your child's understanding of what is said) will increase in complexity as your child grows. Nonlanguage reasoning skills (spatial ability and so forth) are also measured using puzzles and crayons.

Wechsler Scales

Although the Stanford-Binet test can be used throughout childhood, the most commonly used tests after 3 years of age are the Wechsler series of intelligence scales. The WPPSI–R (Wechsler Preschool and Primary Scale of Intelligence–Revised) can be used until your child is 6 years of age. The WISC–III (Wechsler Intelligence Scale for Children–Third Edition) is used for children ages 6–16 years. The WAIS–R (Wechsler Adult Intelligence Scale–Revised) is given to adolescents and adults.

Similar to the Stanford-Binet, the Wechsler scales test both language abilities and visual-perceptual (eye–hand or performance) skills. The tests are divided into six verbal and six performance subtests, none of which requires reading or spelling. The verbal subtests include information, comprehension, arithmetic, similarities, vocabulary, and digit span (memory of a number sequence). The performance subtests include picture completion, picture arrangement, block design, object assembly, coding, and mazes. The overall scores on verbal and performance subscales tend to be within a few points of each other in children who have mental retardation. This, however, is not always the case; two children with the same IQ score may have very different profiles of subscale strengths and weaknesses. When planning your child's educational program, it is important to know his or her unique combination of strengths and weaknesses.

Other Intelligence Tests

Although the Bayley Scales, the Stanford-Binet Intelligence Scales, and the Wechsler are the most commonly used psychological tests, many other tests are also available. Some are particularly useful in testing children with hearing or visual impairments. For example, the Leiter Scale is used with deaf children or those with a significant communication disorder. The Leiter Scale does not depend on language but rather relies on nonverbal reasoning abilities. With blind children, only the verbal portion of the Wechsler test is used.

Because mental retardation involves a deficit in adaptive (self-care) as well as cognitive skills, it is common to test these abilities as well. A common interview, called the Vineland Adaptive Behavior Scales, may be given to you to assess your child's social and self-care skills. The interview measures your child's communication skills, daily living skills, socialization, and motor skills. Although it is common for similar scores to be obtained on IQ and social-adaptive scales, some children will do better on one or the other. Knowing this is important in planning your child's educational, recreational, and social programs.

MEDICAL TESTS

There is not a standard procedure for medical testing of all children with mental retardation. The specific tests given really depend on the likely cause and the degree of the impairment. Less than one quarter of children with mild mental retardation have an identifiable biological cause of the disability, whereas more than two thirds of children with mental retardation requiring extensive supports have a specific cause of the disability (see Table 14.2). Thus, doctors are more likely to recommend tests for your child if he or she has a more significant delay because a cause is more likely to be found. This investigation is particularly important as many of the causes are genetic and a diagnosis may permit prenatal diagnosis in future pregnancies (see Chapter 26). In these instances, one or more of the following tests may be performed: a chromosome study, a DNA test for fragile X syndrome, metabolic studies of blood and urine samples, a brain wave test (EEG, or electroencephalogram), and a brain imaging study (MRI, or magnetic resonance imaging, scan). The specific tests performed will depend on the possible diagnoses your child's physician is considering. In addition to these medical tests, your child should receive a hearing and vision screening to confirm that a sensory impairment is not causing or contributing to the disability.

TREATMENT APPROACHES

Although mental retardation has no cure, many things can be done to help your child reach his or her potential. Multidisciplinary therapy, in which several different specialists work together with you and your child for a prolonged period of time, has proved particularly effective. This therapy often is directed at a number of aspects of your child's life: education, social and recreational activities, behavior and emotional issues, and associated disabilities. Each of these aspects of care is discussed in detail in the sections that follow.

Education

Education is the single most important discipline involved in the treatment of children with mental retardation (see Chapter 12). Many children with disabilities are placed in inclusive programs in neighborhood schools. In choosing a school program, your major concern should be that your child be in a class that he or she enjoys and that helps effective learning to occur. The program should be relevant to your child's needs and address his or her individual strengths and difficulties. Children who are placed in classes in which the level is too high often feel continually frustrated, whereas those placed in programs that are not stimulating enough may be bored. In either case, the child will not learn effectively and may develop behavior problems. The ideal program should stretch your child's abilities while enabling him or her to achieve as much as possible.

Leisure and Recreation

Besides education, you should consider the social and recreational needs of your child. He or she needs friends and the opportunity to play with other children outside of school, just as much as any other child. Encourage friendships with typically developing neighbors and schoolmates who have a similar disability. There may also be programs at local parks and recreation areas that can give your child a chance to learn a sport, develop a skill, burn off some energy, meet other children with similar interests, or simply have fun and relax. For the older child, social activities are very important and may include dances, trips, dating, and recreational events.

Encourage your child's participation in sports as it offers many benefits, including weight management, development of physical coordination, maintenance of cardiovascular fitness, developing social supports, and improvement of self-image. Inclusive sports programs work well for many children, and participation in the Special Olympics could also be considered.

Behavior Problems

Whereas behavior problems are learned, emotional disorders (discussed more in the next section) tend to be part of a child's biological makeup. Behavior problems include temper tantrums, self-stimulatory behavior (such as rocking or twirling), restricted food preferences, and refusal to go to bed (see Chapter 11). They may represent attempts by your child to gain attention or avoid frustration. The behavior therapist and educator can work with your child and can help you identify ways to deal with difficult behaviors.

In contrast, depression is an example of an emotional/psychiatric disorder. Emotional disorders are generally treated by a psychiatrist, a clinical psychologist, or a social worker. Children with emotional disorders may also have behavior problems. For example, a child with depression may show his

Table 14.2.   Identifiable causes of severe mental
retardation (by percentage)

Chromosomal	35
Multiple congenital anomalies	16
Early pregnancy problems	11
Perinatal insults	10
Single-gene defect	10
Postnatal brain damage	5
Other	13

or her unhappiness by having temper tantrums or by not eating. Therefore, it is important to determine whether your child has a behavior problem, an emotional disorder, both, or neither.

Behavior problems can be especially hard to sort out in children with mental retardation. You must keep your child's developmental age in mind when assessing the appropriateness of behavior. For example, an average 4-year-old who gets into everything may be considered hyperactive, but for a 4-year-old with moderate mental retardation, exploratory behavior may not be unusual.

Some medical issues can adversely affect your child's behavior, and addressing them will probably improve matters. The identification and correction of a hearing or vision problem may decrease frustration arising from the sensory impairment (see Chapters 20 and 21). Treatment of previously undetected seizures (see Chapter 18) or treatment of esophageal ulceration due to gastroesophageal reflux (see Chapter 7) will provide relief and decrease irritability. Sometimes the short-term use of medication to treat a sleep disturbance or constipation can help irritability.

Behavior problems can also result from the frustration or boredom caused by an inappropriate educational program, so this program should be evaluated and changed if necessary. Changing the school environment, however, is often not the whole answer; behavior management techniques or medications are frequently needed. Behavior management involves encouraging appropriate behavior and discouraging inappropriate behavior. This therapy is especially useful for children who are noncompliant, aggressive, or show self-stimulatory/self-injurious behavior. Although behavior therapy is often used to address problem behaviors, these same methods can be used to stimulate the development of daily living skills (see Chapter 7).

Although behavior management techniques are often effective, medication is sometimes needed to help manage behavior problems. Stimulant medications such as Ritalin (methylphenidate), Dexedrine (dextroamphetamine), and Adderall (dextroamphetamine and levo-amphetamine), which are beneficial in controlling hyperactive and inattentive behaviors in children with typical IQ scores, are often effective in treating children with mental retardation who also have attention-deficit/hyperactivity disorder (ADHD). The antihypertensive drugs (used to treat high blood pressure) Catapres (clonidine) and Tenex (guanfacine) may also be helpful in decreasing hyperactivity, although they have little effect on attention problems. For aggression and self-injurious behavior, psychiatric drugs such as Haldol (haloperidol) and Risperdal (risperidone) may be useful. They are discussed further in Chapter 10. These drugs should be used cautiously, starting with a trial period, during which time you and your child's teachers keep a record of attention, behavior, and activity levels. A doctor should monitor closely how your child responds to the medication, and the medication should be continued only if it is shown to be effective and has few side effects. Reassessments, at least yearly, should occur to determine if the medication needs to be continued.

Emotional/Psychiatric Disorders

Individuals with mental retardation are at an increased risk for psychiatric disorders, especially if there is a family predisposition. Individuals with both mental retardation and a psychiatric disorder are said to have a *dual diagnosis*. As emotional/psychiatric disorders can affect so many aspects of life, it is imperative that the disorder be diagnosed rapidly and that treatment be multidisciplinary. Guidance can be offered by social workers, psychologists, psychiatrists, and service coordinators (case managers) as well as by other professionals. Distinguishing typical from atypical emotional responses, however, is equally important. It is not atypical to have occasional outbursts in response to certain situations.

Confusion also results from situational anxiety that is very common and may be misinterpreted as a significant emotional problem. Going to the doctor may be stressful for your child, especially if he or she has had previous bad experiences or is fearful of what may happen there. This can be avoided by explaining to your child in advance what will occur and how it will affect the normal routine. It is helpful to expose your child to many different experiences while providing the support needed to develop his or her coping mechanisms.

There are many individuals who are competent to diagnose and treat psychiatric problems in individuals with developmental disabilities such as mental retardation. Counseling may take the form of teaching you parenting skills and helping you understand the underlying emotional problem. Concrete and simple supportive therapy, nonverbal methods such as play therapy, and group therapy involving the child with or without the family have all proved helpful. Psychotherapy (talk therapy) is often effective for individuals with good communication skills but is less so for individuals who have difficulty expressing themselves verbally. Music and dance/movement therapy have recently been suggested to be effective in treating some emotional problems but have not undergone scientific scrutiny. Relaxation and biofeedback techniques have also proved helpful for some people. If depression is a concern, drugs such as the selective serotonin reuptake inhibitors Prozac (fluoxetine), Paxil (paroxetine), or Zoloft (sertraline) and the tricyclic antidepressants Norpramin (desipramine) and Elavil (amytriptiline) can be helpful (see Chapter 10).

Evaluating and Treating Associated Impairments

The final aspect of treatment involves determining whether your child has other, undetected impairments, such as hearing loss, visual impairment, or seizure activity. Because these associated disabilities can affect school performance, early identification and treatment is essential. Yearly vision and hearing testing may be appropriate, and an EEG should be performed if you or the doctor suspects that your child has had seizures. In addition, general yearly reassessments ensure that your child has a correct school placement and that he or she has no new medical problems.

Treating the Rest of Your Family

Although we have focused on your child, treatment must also take into account the rest of your family. How are you doing? Do you have enough time for yourself and your other children? What are your feelings about your child with disabilities? How are your other children faring? The answers to some of these questions may be distressing and may indicate the need for professional counseling for members of your family from a psychologist, a psychiatrist, or a social worker. This could take the form of family counseling or individual psychotherapy, depending on the problem and the coping strategies of your family. Take care of yourself by using summer camps, respite care, and baby sitters so that you will not feel overwhelmed by your child's care needs. There are also family support networks such as the National Parent-to-Parent Support and Information System (see the Suggested Readings and Resources for Chapter 1 at the end of this book).

SUMMARY

A person with mental retardation has impairments in intellectual and adaptive skills and requires some level of supports, varying from intermittent to pervasive. A person with mental retardation may live independently or may require supports throughout his or her life. Early diagnosis is important, no matter what your child's abilities may be, so that interventions can give your child the best possible start in education and provide your family with the knowledge and supports needed to help your child reach his or her full potential.

It is difficult to predict your child's potential when he or she is very young or is being evaluated for the first time. Prediction becomes more accurate over time and following reevaluations. For example, if a physician has followed your child for 2–3 years and each year your child gains 6 months of new skills instead of 12 months, the physician can predict your child's abilities with some confidence.

As a general indicator of your child's eventual mental age, assume that intellectual growth is complete by about 16 years of age, and then multiply your child's current IQ score as a percentage of the average score (100) times 16 years. Thus, a child with an IQ of 60 might be expected to have the intellectual abilities of a 10-year-old (approximately 60% of 16) as an adult. In this case, you could expect your child to attain the abilities to do functional reading and arithmetic and to live independently. Keep in mind, however, that your child's future is not solely a function of intellectual gifts and adaptive abilities. It is significantly influenced by the home and school environment and by your child's and your own motivation and efforts. It is true that historically the employment of people with mental retardation has been limited, but there are now many supported employment programs and on-the-job supports leading more individuals with mental retardation to find and keep jobs (see Chapter 28).

Some Questions Answered

Will my son catch up to other children his age?

The gap between your child's skills and those of typical children of the same age is likely to widen rather than narrow as your child grows older. Consider two 4-year-old children, one with an IQ score of 100 and the other with an IQ score of 50. Each year, the child with an IQ score of 50 will gain only half of the skills and abilities mastered by the typically developing child. By 14 years of age, the child with an IQ score of 100 will have a mental age of 14 years, whereas the child with mental retardation will have a mental age of about 7 years. As noted previously, however, IQ score is not the whole story. A child's abilities can also be influenced positively by good adaptive (self-care) skills, strong motivation, effective teaching, and a supportive family.

Are errors likely to be made in IQ testing?

Serious errors are uncommon but possible. They are most likely to occur when testing an infant who may be ill or a child who has an unrecognized hearing or visual impairment. Children with hearing or visual impairment may score much lower than their abilities would allow unless they are given special IQ tests that take into account their sensory impairment. A severe motor impairment such as cerebral palsy or muscular dystrophy may also interfere with a child's finishing within the time limits on standard IQ batteries.

If your child is simply tired or unhappy, however, his or her IQ score should not be significantly affected. Psychologists know how to get the best performance from your child. If there are concerns about the accuracy of the tests, the psychologist may request that you return for a second visit so the results can be checked. If your child is found to have a significant developmental delay, the psychologist will probably suggest a retest in a year or two. If the second test shows a similar delay, the diagnosis is likely to be correct.

My child had a mental retardation screening test during the newborn period, and it was normal! How can she have mental retardation?

Newborn screening is performed for a number of rare inborn errors of metabolism that can cause mental retardation. The specific diseases tested for in the United States vary from state to state but generally include phenylketonuria (PKU), hypothyroidism (a congenital deficiency of thyroid hormone), galactosemia (an inborn error of sugar metabolism), and maple syrup urine disease (an inborn error of protein metabolism). These genetic disorders have an incidence of between 1 in 6,000 and 1 in 300,000 births. Thus, they account for very few of the total number of children with mental retardation. The importance of this test is that it can identify certain diseases that, if left untreated, lead to mental retardation. Early treatment of these diseases can often prevent the occurrence of mental retardation. A normal result on this screening test only means, however, that your newborn did not have one of these illnesses; it does not ensure that your child has typical intelligence.

If my child has mental retardation, why was his brain wave test normal?

An EEG measures brain wave patterns; it is used to evaluate the possibility of a seizure disorder. Many children with typical intelligence have abnormal EEG patterns, and many children who have mental retardation have typical EEG readings. An EEG is not a test for mental retardation.

His brain imaging scan was also normal. What does that mean?

CT (computed tomography) and, more commonly, MRI (magnetic resonance imaging) are brain imaging techniques that look for major structural brain abnormalities. Most causes of mental retardation, however, involve microscopic or biochemical changes in the brain and cannot be seen on these scans. Thus, the scan may be normal or show only mild abnormalities even in the presence of severe mental retardation.

Will my child's physical growth be normal?

People with mild retardation generally reach the genetic growth potential of their parents. Certain genetic forms of mental retardation, such as Down syndrome, however, are associated with short stature. Children with severe mental retardation (requiring extensive supports) also tend to be short. In addition, these children may mature physically later, their secondary (permanent) teeth tend to come in later, and their growth spurt begins later. The beginning of menstruation may be delayed in girls.

What will my daughter's life span be?

The vast majority of individuals with mental retardation have typical life expectancy. Only those people with the most complex or severe disabilities (such as Down syndrome or profound mental retardation) have a shortened life span, and even they now usually live into adulthood.

Are medications helpful in treating mental retardation?

No drug has been found to improve intellectual functioning in individuals with mental retardation. As mentioned before, medication may be helpful, however, in treating associated behavior and psychiatric problems or seizure disorders. The improvement in these associated problems may improve cognitive functioning as well. Medication may also help your child focus on other matters, such as working on self-care and community living skills. Your child's environment, supports, and motivation will also influence his or her life outcomes.

What are the chances of our having a second child with mental retardation?

Generally the chance of having a second child with mental retardation is less than 10%. For certain genetic causes of mental retardation, however, the recurrence risk is higher. When you are considering having other children, you may find it helpful to visit a genetic counselor who can go over with you information relevant to your situation (see Chapter 26).

15

Down Syndrome

Nancy J. Roizen

Down syndrome is the most common genetic cause of mental retardation and occurs in about 1 in 800–1,000 births. The syndrome is named for Dr. John Langdon Down, who in 1866 published the first complete physical description of Down syndrome, including facial features (see Figure 15.1), and noted the resemblance among individuals with the syndrome. In 1959, researchers discovered a chromosomal abnormality, an additional #21 chromosome, among individuals with Down syndrome (see Chapter 26 for more information on chromosomes). Since the late 1970s, more and more individuals with Down syndrome have become active in their communities, and communities have welcomed their inclusion. This chapter describes the developmental, physical, and medical characteristics of children with Down syndrome and offers guidance on how you can optimize your child's experience and potential.

Mick

Laurie and George have two young daughters. When Laurie was 28 years old, she enjoyed an easy third pregnancy. Labor began 2 days after the expected date, delivery was uncomplicated, and Laurie and George's son Mick was born.

The doctors noticed that Mick looked different from other newborns. His head was small and flattened at the back. Mick's eyes were slanted upward, and there was a fold of skin over the inner corners. Their doctors told Laurie and George that this combination of physical traits suggested that Mick had Down syndrome. Later the doctors confirmed the diagnosis by performing a chromosomal analysis and finding an extra chromosome #21 in Mick's white blood cells. Laurie and George didn't understand. They were young, there had been no sign of trouble during pregnancy, and they had no family his-

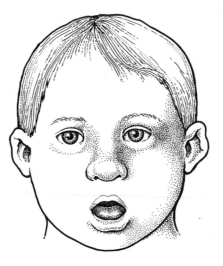

Figure 15.1.   The physical features of a child with Down syndrome include a small head with flattening of the back of head and face. The nose is recessed, and there is an upward slant to the eyes with folds at the inner corners. The ears and mouth are small, as are the hands and feet. The fingers are short and stubby, with incurving of the pinky. There is often a crease extending all the way across the palm. The neck is short and broad, and the skin may appear mottled.

tory of Down syndrome. They wondered what had happened and what the future held for Mick and their family.

CAUSES OF DOWN SYNDROME

It is still unclear how the extra chromosome actually causes the characteristics of Down syndrome, but this is likely to become clearer because the gene contents of chromosome #21 were identified in 2000. It is suspected, however, that the additional information contained in the third #21 chromosome alters the normal genetic blueprint. This extra chromosome results from a phenomenon called *nondisjunction,* in which the chromosomes do not separate as expected during cell division and two copies of chromosome #21 are passed on to a daughter cell (see Figure 15.2). This abnormality can occur during the maturation of either the egg or the sperm. As discussed in Chapter 26, when a developing sperm or egg cell divides, each of the resulting cells should have one copy of each of the 23 chromosomes. But in nondisjunction, one cell gets two copies of one chromosome, whereas the other cell gets none. The cell that lacks a chromosome usually dies, but the cell with an extra copy can become fertilized. As a result, the fertilized egg has three copies of one chromosome rather than the usual two. This condition is called *trisomy.* The most likely chromosome to have an extra copy is #21 (see Figure 15.3), which is the reason that Down syndrome is sometimes called *trisomy 21.*

OTHER CAUSES OF DOWN SYNDROME

Although 95% of all children with Down syndrome have trisomy 21, there are other causes of Down syndrome. *Mosaicism* and *translocation* are responsible for the remaining 5% of children with Down syndrome.

In mosaicism, the abnormal cell division occurs during the development of the embryo. As a result, only some of the embryo's cells are affected. The child has a "mosaic" of normal and abnormal cells, with as many as 75%–80% of the cells being unaffected. Children with mosaic Down syndrome may have fewer of the facial characteristics and medical problems than do children either with trisomy 21 or with translocation and developmentally may be more advanced. The characteristics of children with mosaic Down syndrome, however, may vary widely, and these children may be indistinguishable clinically from children with trisomy 21.

In translocation, one of the parents is usually a carrier of an unusual chromosomal rearrangement. Although the parent appears unaffected, he or she has only 45 chromosomes because part of the missing #21 chromosome is

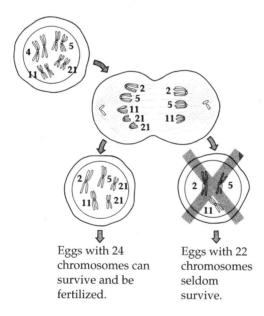

Eggs with 24 chromosomes can survive and be fertilized.

Eggs with 22 chromosomes seldom survive.

Figure 15.2.   Nondisjunction. During division of the sperm or egg, a mistake can occur in which there is unequal division. One of the new cells ends up having an extra chromosome, and the other cell has one chromosome less than usual. In this figure, the process is simplified and shows only four pairs of chromosomes. As a result of nondisjunction, one daughter cell has five chromosomes and the other has three. The cell with one less chromosome does not survive. The egg or the sperm with the extra chromosome, however, can survive and be fertilized, leading to the birth of a child with 47 rather than 46 chromosomes. The most common chromosome affected by nondisjunction is the 21st, leading to Down syndrome.

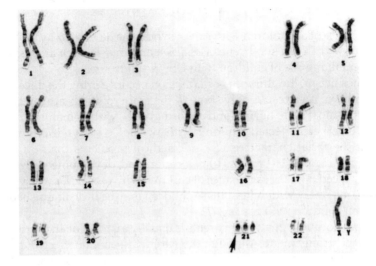

Figure 15.3. Karyotype, or chromosomal pattern, of a male child with Down syndrome. There are 47 rather than 46 chromosomes, with three copies of #21. There is also one X and one Y chromosome, indicating that this child is a boy.

attached to the arm of another chromosome, usually the #13. In effect, this person has the information of all 46 chromosomes carried on only 45 chromosomes. When this parent passes on a sperm or an egg containing the translocated #13/21 chromosome as well as the normal #21, the resulting embryo will have 46 chromosomes but three copies of #21: a copy from each parent and a third copy attached to the #13 chromosome. The infant will have Down syndrome.

It is important to know whether your child's Down syndrome is caused by a trisomy, mosaicism, or translocation because the risk of recurrence in future children differs, depending on the nature of the genetic anomaly. For a young couple with a child with trisomy 21 Down syndrome, the recurrence risk for trisomy 21 or mosaicism is about 1 in 100, as compared with about 1 in 2,000 for other young couples. When translocation is the cause, however, the risk is about 1 in 50 for male carriers and 1 in 10 for female carriers. Therefore, all children with Down syndrome should have a chromosomal analysis (blood test) to identify which abnormality has caused the disorder. If your child has a translocation, both parents' chromosomes should also be studied to determine who is the translocation carrier. You may then wish to seek genetic counseling for planning future pregnancies. In addition, other family members who may be at risk for carrying a translocation can be notified.

THE EFFECT OF PARENTAL AGE

Both the mother's and father's age affect the likelihood of their having a child with Down syndrome because the cells of older people are more likely to divide unequally. At birth a woman's ovaries contain all of the eggs that she will ever have. During childhood, the eggs are immature and have 46 chromosomes, but between adolescence and middle age about 500 of these eggs will ripen sequentially and be released at monthly intervals. During this ripening process, the cell splits to become a mature egg with 23 chromosomes. In older women, the egg cells have been present for a prolonged period of time and are more likely to divide incorrectly. Nondisjunction is also more likely to occur in the sperm of older men. In men, however, new sperm cells are produced constantly and are therefore less likely to undergo nondisjunction than are eggs of women the same age. Overall, 95% of all trisomy 21 occurs as a result of nondisjunction in women.

PRENATAL SCREENING AND DIAGNOSIS OF DOWN SYNDROME

The goal in screening for Down syndrome is to identify a small group of pregnant women who are at enough of a risk of carrying a fetus with the syndrome that they should be offered prenatal diagnostic testing. The first screening item is age; prenatal diagnostic testing is offered to pregnant woman 35 years of age or older. Although only 5%–8% of pregnant women in the United States are 35 years of age or older, 20% of children with Down syndrome are born to women in this age group. Amniocentesis or chorionic villus sampling (CVS) (see Chapter 26) is offered to all of these women as well as to women who have already had a child with Down syndrome.

If a pregnant woman is younger than 35 years of age, her blood will be tested to determine whether prenatal diagnostic testing is recommended. The blood screening involves measuring three chemical markers and is performed in the second trimester of pregnancy. A formula is then used to calculate the woman's risk. If a pregnant woman is found to be at high risk of carrying a fetus with Down syndrome, she is offered amniocentesis or CVS.

PHYSICAL FEATURES OF CHILDREN WITH DOWN SYNDROME

A syndrome is defined by a set of physical characteristics that occur together. In Down syndrome, the pattern is so well known that your doctor may share suspicions about the diagnosis with you at birth. Distinctive facial features, a single crease near the top of the palm, and a large space between the big and first toe all are clues that may lead the pediatrician or the obstetrician to recommend a chromosomal analysis for your child. The facial features include flattening of the face and back of the head, eyes that slant upward, a fold of skin at the inside corner of the eye, known as an *epicanthal fold*, flattening of the bridge of the nose, a small nose, and a short, broad neck with extra tissue at the nape (see Figure 15.1). It is important to note that children with Down syndrome may have only a few of these features.

GROWTH OF CHILDREN WITH DOWN SYNDROME

Newborns with Down syndrome are slightly smaller in height, weight, and head circumference than are typical newborns and are somewhat more likely to be premature. Following birth, the growth patterns of most children with Down syndrome do not follow the typical curve. This makes it important for the pediatrician to plot your child's growth on charts specific for children with Down syndrome (see http://www.brookespublishing.com/gcharts). In the first 2–3 years of life, children with Down syndrome may be slim or light for their height. Your child's doctor may recommend increasing caloric intake for your child. Yet, this advice must be balanced with the consideration that there is a high incidence of obesity in children with Down syndrome beginning as early as 3 years of age. This is related to the fact that children with Down syndrome need fewer calories than other children do to maintain their body weight. Prevention of obesity after 2 years of age requires a lifestyle for your child that includes daily exercise, good eating habits, and a reduced fat and calorie diet.

INTELLECTUAL ABILITIES

There is a great diversity in the behavior, cognitive abilities, medical problems, and physical development of children with Down syndrome. As with their peers, for children with Down syndrome, the rate of gaining intellectual skills depends on many factors, including educational opportunities, environment, genetic background, health, and personal traits. For example, although almost all children with Down syndrome have some degree of mental retardation, the mental retardation may range from mild to severe. There is an apparent slowing in development over time. At 6 months of age, children with Down syndrome have fairly typical development. By 4 years of age, however, their average IQ score is around 45, and by 11 years their average IQ score is about 37. Between 11 and 21 years, there is no further change in IQ score. It is not clear what causes this pattern. Many individuals appear to function at a higher level in daily situations than would be expected based on test scores. Perhaps testing does not adequately capture the potential of children with Down syndrome. Or, perhaps a neurological process interferes with development, or maybe medical problems such as hearing or vision impairments bring about this effect. Right now no one knows. Language and gross motor skills, however, are the slowest to develop in children with Down syndrome, whereas self-help and hand–eye coordination skills show the fastest progress.

Individuals with Down syndrome older than 35 years of age may have a gradual loss of memory and cognitive abilities. If this occurs, the first possible causes to think about are treatable conditions such as hypothyroidism (a disorder involving the underproduction of thyroid hormone, which regulates the body's metabolism) and depression; however, occasionally the memory loss may be due to Alzheimer's disease. Whenever an adult or a child with Down syndrome has a loss of memory or cognitive abilities, he or she should go to the doctor for a complete medical evaluation because effective treatment may be available.

PERSONALITY CHARACTERISTICS AND BEHAVIOR

Although children with Down syndrome have a reputation for being happy and lovable, they are certainly just as capable as typically developing children of having difficult temperaments. It is important that you establish clear boundaries for your child and are consistent in using them. For ideas on coping with difficult behavior, you may want to consult your child's pediatrician (see also Chapter 11). In terms of psychiatric disorders, autism (see Chapter 23) is found somewhat more frequently in children with Down syndrome than in typical children, but mania, eating disorders, and schizophrenia occur less frequently. If your child has behavior or mental health issues, he or she should be evaluated and treated by a specialist (psychiatrist or psychologist).

IDENTIFYING YOUR CHILD'S HEALTH CARE TEAM

Because your child with Down syndrome is likely to have some health problems that are specific to children with Down syndrome and others that are common to all children, he or she will probably need both a general pediatrician and pediatric specialists. Your child's general pediatrician should be comfortable in caring for a child with special health and developmental needs and be willing to seek consultation with and follow-up monitoring by specialists. Developmental pediatricians who specialize in managing the interdisciplinary care of children with disabilities or who direct specialized Down syndrome clinics may also be an option. In addition, your child may be referred to specialists dealing with cardiac, hearing, and vision problems. Ideally, evaluations should be performed by pediatric specialists who are accustomed to caring for children with special needs. Following each evaluation you have the right to request copies of all health reports so that you can keep a complete file for your child. Also, make sure that you understand the recommendations and plans for follow-up care. In addition, your child's pediatrician can refer you to the local parent support group, where parents of older children with Down syndrome can tell you about services and help you with advocacy issues.

MEDICAL PROBLEMS IN
CHILDREN WITH DOWN SYNDROME

Children with Down syndrome are more likely to have certain medical problems than typically developing children are, and you may find the list of possible problems to be overwhelming and anxiety provoking. The problems are usually manageable and fall into three groups. The first group includes heart, hearing, vision, and thyroid problems. These occur so often that all children with Down syndrome need monitoring, evaluation, and/or treatment for them. The second group encompasses medical problems that occur somewhat more commonly in children with Down syndrome than in the general population and require a watchful eye. This group includes leukemia, malformations of the bowel, neck subluxation (partial dislocation), and seizures. The third group involves medical problems, such as gum disease and obesity, that require preventive care.

Medical Problems that Always Require Evaluation

Because about half of all children with Down syndrome have congenital heart disease that places them at risk for developing damaging increased blood pressure in the lungs, all children with Down syndrome should have an echocardiogram (an ultrasound test examining the structure of the heart) performed soon after birth. The three most common defects involve an opening between all four chambers of the heart (endocardial cushion defect), an opening between the two lower chambers (ventricular septal defect), and an opening between the two upper chambers (atrial septal defect). If your child needs corrective surgery, it may be reassuring to you to know that the outcome is usually good.

Approximately two thirds of all children with Down syndrome develop hearing loss or impairment in childhood. This may result from fluid in the middle ear from an infection or from a structural abnormality, from dysfunction of the auditory nerve, which conveys sound to the brain, or a combination of these two factors (see Chapter 20). The goal of medical care and monitoring is for the child to retain optimal hearing through early diagnosis and treatment. At birth or within the first few weeks of life, your child should have a hearing test so that any permanent and significant hearing loss can be corrected if possible using a hearing aid. Even if the newborn hearing test is normal, your child's pediatrician should watch for middle-ear fluid and hearing loss, which are commonly associated with middle-ear infections. This should be checked for at least every 6 months for the first 3 years of life and annually thereafter. Your child's physician should aggressively treat middle-ear fluid buildup medically or surgically to prevent permanent hearing loss. Surgical treatment involves the placement of small tubes that allow the fluid to drain from the middle ear to the outer ear.

About 60% of children with Down syndrome have vision problems that need to be monitored or treated. Of children who have a normal examination by the general pediatrician, 35% will still be found to have an eye problem by an ophthalmologist. The incidence of eye conditions in children with Down syndrome increases with age throughout childhood. Therefore, your infant with Down syndrome should be evaluated by a pediatric ophthalmologist within the first few weeks of life, with follow-up evaluation occurring every 1–2 years (see Chapter 22).

Many of the signs of hypothyroidism, such as slow growth and development, floppiness (loose muscle tone), and dry skin, are frequently found in children with Down syndrome. Approximately 4% of children with Down syndrome are born with hypothyroidism or develop the condition because of thyroiditis (inflammation of the thyroid gland) during early childhood. Beginning in the preteen years, the incidence gradually increases until 10%–20% of adults with Down syndrome have hypothyroidism. Hypothyroidism can jeopardize a child's short- and long-term growth and development and can cause other health problems. All children are screened at birth for thyroid problems, but children with Down syndrome also need a thyroid blood test annually throughout life to determine whether they need thyroid supplements.

Medical Problems that Require Vigilance

Children with Down syndrome have a somewhat greater risk for several medical problems that warrant vigilance, even though some of these problems, such as leukemia and diabetes, are rare. These problems also include bowel obstruction, infections, seizures, sleep apnea, and subluxation of the neck and other bone and muscle problems.

About 4% of all children with Down syndrome are born with an obstruction of their bowel. The blockage must be corrected with surgery to permit the normal passage of food and solid waste. In addition, despite diet changes and medication, some children have constipation that is caused by Hirschsprung disease (enlarged colon); this condition requires surgery to remove the enlarged section of the bowel.

About 1 in 250 children with Down syndrome develops diabetes, about seven times the rate in typical children. If your child begins showing symptoms suggestive of diabetes—increased fluid/food consumption, frequent urination, and tiredness—a doctor needs to check for the disorder.

Approximately 1 in 150 children with Down syndrome develops leukemia, representing a risk 10 or 15 times greater than that of the general population. The beginning of leukemia may be marked by easy and excessive bruising, paleness, fatigue, fever, and multiple infections. Early identification and treatment can be effective.

Between 6% and 13% of children with Down syndrome develop seizures, at least 10 times the usual occurrence risk. Seizures may appear as convulsions with shaking and tensing of the body or less frequently as a lack of progress in gaining developmental skills or as the loss of skills. A rare type of seizure called *infantile spasms* is a particular concern (see Chapter 18). Seizures are generally responsive to antiepileptic medication.

Because of a combination of certain facial structures, smaller diameter of airway passages, and decreased muscle tone in the mouth cavity, children with Down syndrome have a greater chance of developing obstructive sleep apnea (brief stoppages of breathing during sleep) that can decrease oxygen flow to the brain and other organs and can stress the heart. If your child snores or appears to stop breathing while sleeping (making long pauses between snores), your child's physician should make further evaluations. Treatment many involve removing the tonsils and adenoids or providing oxygen while sleeping.

Because children with Down syndrome have loose ligaments (tissue that connects bones to bones), they are prone to dislocating or subluxing (partially dislocating) multiple joints including the hips, knees, and shoulders. Of most concern, however, is the possible subluxation of your child's neck, with slippage of the first vertebra into the second (atlantoaxial subluxation). This can injure the spinal nerves and result in neurological impairments. When your child is about 3 years of age, an X ray should be done to determine the alignment of his or her neck vertebrae. About 15% of individuals with Down syndrome have X ray results that indicate a possibly unstable neck, but only 1% of children develop neurological symptoms. The most frequent symptom of subluxation is a decrease in motor skills and weakness. Less frequently, there is neck pain, stiff neck, or loss of bowel and bladder control. The identification of subluxation or the presence of symptoms requires immediate evaluation. Treatment may involve surgery to realign the vertebrae.

Medical Problems that Require Preventive Care

Obesity and dental problems are common in children with Down syndrome and are best treated by prevention. Obesity is discussed in the section on growth. Regarding dental care, many children with Down syndrome don't get their first tooth until after their first birthday (a first tooth at 1½ years is typical). Your child's teeth should be cleaned twice per day because children with Down syndrome are prone to very early gum (periodontal) disease. Advanced gum disease may require dental surgery and can mean that your child will lose permanent teeth. Preventive dental care is effective and requires brushing twice daily and professional cleaning by a dentist at least every 6 months (see Chapter 8). Typically, children with Down syndrome have malocclusion (misalignment of teeth) that requires orthodontic treatment.

ALTERNATIVE MEDICAL THERAPIES

As noted previously, standard medical treatment for children with Down syndrome includes surgical correction of cardiac and gastrointestinal malformations, monitoring and treatment of hypothyroidism, and management of vision, hearing, and other problems. Because of the absence of a medical "cure" for Down syndrome, however, many alternative therapies have been proposed. These have included mixtures of vitamins, minerals, and hormones, cell therapy (injections of cells from the brains of lamb fetuses), and most recently, Piracetam, a stimulant available in Europe. Scientific studies of vitamin, mineral, and cell therapies for children with Down syndrome have not shown improvement in appearance, developmental functioning, growth, or health. Piracetam has been associated with improved writing in children with dyslexia, but a controlled study of children with Down syndrome indicated no improvement in intellectual development. None of the alternative therapies has proved effective in scientific studies. You need to carefully examine information on alternative therapies, discuss the therapies with your child's physician, and balance the possible costs and benefits to your child and family.

ENHANCING YOUR CHILD'S DEVELOPMENT AND EDUCATION

Because Down syndrome is likely to be identified before or just after your child is born, he or she has the chance to receive early intervention services (see Chapter 6) starting in the first few months of life. Early intervention programs are designed for children younger than 3 years of age and focus on improving your child's rate of early development. Most early intervention therapists have worked with many children who have Down syndrome and are aware of their usual therapy needs. In general, the development of children with Down syndrome is similar to that of typical children but occurs more slowly. In addition to focusing on your child's development, early intervention services can provide emotional support and link you to a parent group.

For more on general education issues, you may want to read Chapter 12. Feeding and speech, however, are two issues that affect school experiences for children with Down syndrome. Your child may have difficulty feeding because of low muscle tone or may have difficulty making the change from baby food to solids. A feeding specialist can be helpful with these issues (see Chapter 7). Speech-language therapy is especially important for many children with Down syndrome, whose development of expressive language (speech and writing) lags behind their other skills. In elementary school, middle school, and high school, your child may continue to need speech-language therapy to focus on the clarity of his or her speech.

Kenny

Kenny is a 21-year-old who, among other accomplishments, has spoken to many first-year medical students about his life. This is an excerpt from one of his talks:

"But, in most ways, I am like you. I have fun going out with my friends. I like to eat out, and I have a girlfriend named Linda. I want to work as a teacher's aide with special children. I am training to do this. Now I'm happy person, but I had a pretty hard time when I was a kid. Children can be sort of mean, and I looked and acted different. Other kids made fun of me and some-times hit me. No one ever chose me to play games. Sometimes they just treated me like I wasn't there. My brother helped sometimes, but then they would start calling him names, too.

"My parents are great. They tell me I'm a good kid, and they love me. They spend lots of time with me and are my friends. I like being with regular people, but I am really happy with other kids like me. In school I had most of my classes with my friends, but I had gym and art with the other kids. I was in a Cub Scout troop and the Special Olympics—I won a lot of medals! Now I'm older, and I understand people more. I live with four kids in a group home. We have a counselor who helps us cook, takes care of our money, and breaks up fights. I finish school this year and then start working full time. I feel good about myself now."

Kenny's experiences reflect his strengths and those of his family. Some children with Down syndrome will not attain Kenny's level of sophistication and understanding. He is high functioning with only mild mental retarda-tion, but, equally important, his family gave him their love, acceptance, guid-ance, and independence. Kenny's perception of himself as a good and useful member of society is within the reach of many children with Down syn-drome.

LONG-TERM PROGNOSIS FOR
CHILDREN WITH DOWN SYNDROME

Life expectancy and quality of life for people with Down syndrome continue to improve. Because of improved health care, at 30 years of age, 79% of indi-viduals with Down syndrome who do not have congenital heart disease are surviving and 50% with heart defects are living. In the past, most adults with Down syndrome were placed in institutions. Today, most adults with Down syndrome live with their parents or semi-independently in supported living environments. They participate in volunteer work, are employed in sup-ported work environments, and enjoy social and recreational activities. Sup-ported employment opportunities often offer a living wage and benefits such as dental, disability, and health insurance (see Chapter 28). Your child can work on self-care skills, relationships, responsibility, and social skills in reli-gious organizations, scouting, and Special Olympics. Sports offer opportuni-ties for fitness, physical development, and socialization and a chance to be a fan. Group sports such as T-ball and soccer are especially good while your son or daughter is young, and individual sports such as biking, skiing, swim-ming, and tennis provide lifetime recreation and socializing experiences. Early planning and development of skills needed for independent living will help your child to succeed. You can support your child in learning important communication, decision-making, and self-care skills and can work with pro-fessionals to prepare your child for a life in the community.

Some Questions Answered

What can I do to improve my child's language development?

There is wide variation, but a child with Down syndrome generally says his or her first word at around 1½ years of age and uses two-word phrases a year later. Communication is the main purpose of language, so focus on communicating with your child as you interact. Because your young child will spend much time with you, you have many chances to do this during everyday activities such as dressing, preparing meals, or going to the park. Take advantage of these times to speak to your child constantly about what you are doing together and especially about what catches his or her interest at the moment. You need to give the message that speech and language are a good way for your child to get attention. You can do this by responding to vocalizations with attention and a verbal response. Daily "reading" from a picture book, even for only 5 minutes, gives the powerful message that reading and books are part of each day and are fun. As your child approaches 2 years of age, if he or she has not as yet developed the language skills to communicate basic needs and wants, use of sign language in conjunction with speech is recommended. These methods will help your child to communicate while he or she learns verbal communication skills. Also, try to keep distracting background noise in your home down by turning off the television and radio when no one is using them.

How can I facilitate my child's friendships?

As with any child, your child with Down syndrome will have friends who come and go. The efforts that you put into developing your child's communication and social skills will help your child to make and keep friends. In addition, provide opportunities for your child to interact with many children, including relatives, neighborhood children, and classmates, and to participate in community activities such as sports and religious classes. You can help your child learn the first step in approaching other people by suggesting things to do and say. Short play dates that include only one other child can be good experiences and give you and your child a chance to talk about the activity later. You should include as possible friends both children with and without special needs.

16

Genetic Syndromes

Gretchen A. Meyer

Ricardo and Maria were thrilled at the birth of their only daughter, Isabel. But though Isabel looked healthy, her facial features were unlike those of her brothers and were somewhat unusual. Her ears were small and low set on her head, her eyes slanted downward, and her fingers were short, with the pinkies curved inward. At Isabel's 2-month well-baby checkup, Ricardo and Maria were told that their daughter had a heart murmur. They began to wonder if any of these unusual things were connected. At 12 months of age, Isabel was not yet sitting on her own and made few recognizable sounds. Her limbs were "floppy" due to low muscle tone. She was diagnosed with developmental delay. Because of the combination of unusual features, heart murmur, and developmental delay, Isabel's physician suggested that Ricardo and Maria take their daughter to a genetic specialist, who told them Isabel might have a genetic syndrome. They were worried and anxious. The word *syndrome* was frightening. What would this mean for Isabel?

WHAT ARE GENETIC SYNDROMES?

Children with developmental disabilities occasionally have physical features that are unusual. Their appearance may differ noticeably from that of other family members. For example, they may have differences in the shape or position of the ears, eyes, roof of the mouth, fingers, toes, or even genitalia. Groups of children often share common physical features that experts recognize as a pattern. When a pattern of traits has a single cause, the condition is known as a *syndrome*. Down syndrome is the best known example of a genetic syndrome (see Chapter 15).

Syndromes are often named after the physician or scientist who first described them. Occasionally they are named for the type of physical abnormality or the location of the chromosomal defect. You can find catalogs and reference books in libraries that describe a large number of the identified syndromes. Some syndromes are caused by the presence of an additional chromosome (such as Down syndrome), others are caused by losses of a small part of a chromosome (such as deletion #22q11.2 syndrome), and still others involve a specific mutation or error in one of the hundreds of genes that are contained in a chromosome (such as Williams syndrome). The underlying causes of some syndromes are yet to be discovered. In most instances, a mutation occurs *sporadically*, meaning neither parent chromosome carries a similar error. When a chromosomal abnormality or a single-gene mutation does exist on a parent chromosome, however, there is an increased risk that future children will inherit the genetic error. This is one way in which certain syndromes can run in families (see Chapter 26). It should be noted that genetic errors generally occur randomly and that there is little that anyone can do to make them more or less likely to occur. Thus, you should not be concerned that you have done something to "cause" your child's genetic disorder.

Advances in medical science have helped researchers and doctors identify and describe an increased number of syndromes. Although there are many (albeit rare) genetic syndromes, this chapter highlights several genetic syndromes because they are common or they explain certain genetic principles. It should be emphasized that not all individuals with a specific syndrome are alike; all of the descriptions in this chapter are generalizations, and each has exceptions.

DISORDERS OF CHROMOSOME NUMBER

As noted in Chapter 26, some infants are born with an extra copy of one of the 22 pairs of nonsex chromosomes. The most common example is Down syndrome, in which there are three copies of chromosome #21 instead of two. The two other common trisomic syndromes are trisomy 13 and 18, involving an extra #13 or #18 chromosome, respectively. In each of these cases, there are 47 chromosomes in each cell rather than the typical 46. The presence of the extra chromosome, containing hundreds of extra genes, alters the typical development of the fetus by mechanisms we do not yet understand.

Trisomy 13

Trisomy 13 is a genetic syndrome that occurs when three copies of chromosome #13 are present within an individual's cells. It is found in approximately 1 in 8,000 newborns. Children with trisomy 13 have severe mental retardation, cerebral palsy, and severe congenital abnormalities. At birth, they are often small in length and weight and their heads are disproportionately small and/or misshapen. The ears are set low, and the mouth is small. They often have cleft lip and palate and various types of heart defects. These infants have difficulties with feeding and breathing and may have seizures. Many children with trisomy 13 do not survive infancy, and those who do survive have significant disabilities and require extensive support. Parents are encouraged to seek support in helping to deal with these most difficult issues.

Trisomy 18

Trisomy 18 is similar to trisomy 13 in severity and occurs in 1 in 6,600 newborns. As with children who have trisomy 13, children with trisomy 18 are very small at birth, have low-set ears, and most often have life-threatening heart defects. Their hands are clenched, and the index and middle fingers usually overlap, giving a crossed appearance. The outcome is similar to that of children with trisomy 13.

Sex Chromosome Disorders

Other examples of abnormalities in the overall number of chromosomes include errors in the number of sex (X and Y) chromosomes. Typically, a male has one X and one Y chromosome, whereas a female has two X chromosomes. The most common female sex chromosome abnormality is Turner syndrome. In this syndrome, the female has only one X chromosome, that is, a total of 45 instead of 46 chromosomes in each of her cells, resulting in an XO pattern of sex chromosomes. This occurs when a sperm or egg with only 22 chromosomes instead of the typical 23 joins with a normal sperm or egg with 23 chromosomes. This is the only case in which a cell with too few chromosomes can develop into an embryo that can survive to birth.

In Klinefelter syndrome, the most common male sex chromosomal abnormality, the opposite situation occurs. In this syndrome, the male has an extra X chromosome resulting from an egg or sperm containing 24 chromosomes joining with a normal cell with 23 chromosomes. The result would be a fetus with 47 total chromosomes and a sex chromosome pattern of XXY. Because this individual has a Y chromosome, he will be a male. Other sex chromosome abnormalities do exist but are extremely rare.

Leslie

Leslie had always been shorter than her two sisters had been when they were her age. She experienced learning difficulties in school, although with special assistance she never failed a grade. As a toddler she had repeated ear infections necessitating the placement of ear tubes to drain fluid from the infection on two occasions. By the age of 14, Leslie had not begun to mature sexually. On the basis of her physical appearance, lack of sexual development, and short stature, a diagnosis of Turner syndrome was suspected. Chromosomal analysis confirmed that she was missing one X chromosome.

The outcome for Leslie and others like her is quite positive. She was given hormones to stimulate both growth and sexual development and grew to be 5 feet tall. After high school graduation Leslie married and took a position in sales. She and her husband have adopted two children and are enjoying a life filled with family, friends, and interesting careers.

Turner Syndrome   Turner syndrome is found in about 1 in 5,000 female births. Girls with the syndrome are very short, reaching an adult height of less than 5 feet. Research indicates, however, that long-term treatment with growth hormone may increase final height by as much as 3 inches. Characteristic physical features of girls with Turner syndrome include a lowered hairline, a broad chest with widely spaced nipples, and a short neck with extra skin at the nape (giving a webbed appearance). Twenty percent of the girls diagnosed with Turner syndrome have a narrowing of the blood vessel leaving the heart (coarctation of the aorta) that may require surgical correction. The ovaries of girls with Turner syndrome do not function normally, resulting in sexual immaturity and sterility. Treatment with estrogen replacement, beginning in adolescence, brings about the appearance of sexual maturation, although most individuals with Turner syndrome remain infertile. These girls usually have IQ scores in the typical range; however, they tend to have learning disabilities, particularly in visual-perceptual skills and mathematics.

Klinefelter Syndrome   Occurring in approximately 1 in every 500 live male births, Klinefelter syndrome is the most common disorder arising from an error in the sex chromosomes. Boys with Klinefelter syndrome tend to be taller and thinner than their peers and have some underdeveloped secondary sexual characteristics (such as a lack of facial hair and a voice that does not deepen after adolescence). In many cases, the diagnosis is made only when puberty does not begin around the expected age. The presence of an additional X chromosome decreases male sex hormone production, but treatment with testosterone beginning in adolescence is helpful. Older boys and adults may have enlarged breasts (gynecomastia), small penises, and small testicles. Body hair may be sparse. Most men with Klinefelter syndrome are sterile because their sperm do not develop normally. Intellectual ability ranges from typical to mild mental retardation. Language development may be particularly delayed, and behavior problems are not uncommon. Boys with Klinefelter syndrome generally grow up to lead lives indistinguishable from their peers.

DISORDERS OF CHROMOSOME STRUCTURE

The genetic syndromes discussed previously are caused by too few or too many chromosomes in a child's cells. An error in the number of chromosomes, however, is only one type of defect in the genetic blueprint. Even when the chromosomes are present in the correct number, rearrangements may alter the structure of the genetic material inside. This may happen spontaneously, or the tendency to have rearrangement may be inherited. The rearrangement causes a scrambling or loss of the gene's message. Small pieces may break off the ends of two different chromosomes and exchange positions. This type of abnormality is called a *translocation*. A breakage resulting in a missing piece of a chromosome or missing genes is known as a *deletion*.

When a chromosomal error is present, it is noted in the following way: First, the number of the chromosome involved is listed followed by a *p* or *q*, indicating whether the mutation is located on the short (p) or the long (q) arm of the chromosome. Then, the site on the chromosome of the mutation is indicated. Banding sites (which look like stripes) appear when the chromosomes are stained and viewed with a microscope. Thus, deletion #22q11.2 indicates that a deletion error exists at numeric banding site 11 on the long arm of chromosome #22. Some of these deletions are large enough to be seen with a microscope; others (called *microdeletions*) are very small and can be identified only by special staining techniques, the most common of which has the whimsical acronym FISH (fluorescent *in situ* hybridization). Whereas the loss of a chromosome involves approximately 1,000 genes, a deletion may affect 100, and a microdeletion less than 10 genes. There is not always a direct relationship between the number of genes lost (or gained) and the severity of the syndrome. Certain genes are so important that a defect in even one can lead to severe problems.

Nancy

Nancy was born with a cleft palate and a serious heart defect that required surgery when she was 2 days old. She did not have unusual facial features and, in fact, looked like her two older sisters did at birth. Because of the presence of the cleft palate and the heart defect, however, Nancy's physicians performed a FISH study and found a small deletion on her #22 chromosome. Careful review of the medical history of immediate family members revealed that Nancy's mother, Alice, had a nasal speech quality, a mild heart murmur, and had experienced learning difficulties in mathematics as a child. Alice, too, was tested and found to have the same deletion as was seen in her daughter. Doctors told Alice that the disorder was inherited as a dominant trait (inherited by the child when at least one parent has the trait) and that the risk of recurrence in each subsequent pregnancy would be 50% (see Chapter 26).

Deletion #22q11.2 Syndrome

Deletion #22q11.2 syndrome results when a small piece of the long arm of the #22 chromosome has been altered or deleted. During the 1990s, the variety of clinical abnormalities that can occur as a result of this deletion were delineated. Syndromes previously known as *DiGeorge syndrome* and *velocardiofacial syndrome* have now been linked to a deletion at this site. It is believed this deletion may be present in 1 out of 5,000 live births and, after Down syndrome, may be the single most common cause of genetic heart malformation.

Children with deletion #22q11.2 syndrome may have certain facial features including a small, open mouth, small, narrow-set eyes, a flat bridge of the nose, and, occasionally, a bulbous tip of the nose. A child with the syndrome may also have long, slender fingers. Abnormalities of the palate range from none to a completely cleft palate. Often, the palate has no apparent cleft but does not rise and fall typically, resulting in a nasal speech quality. Shortly after birth, there may be evidence of a mild immune deficiency because of the underdevelopment of the thymus (an organ that produces antibodies for fighting infection). More than 80% of children with deletion #22q11.2 syndrome have congenital heart problems. Although the overall cognitive abilities of children with the syndrome generally fall in the typical range, these children almost universally have learning disabilities. In fact, a particularly distinct pattern of nonverbal learning disability, including difficulty in mathematics, has been noted in these children.

Kevin

Kevin smiled and laughed often and had a winning, lively personality. He was a small boy with an unusual appearance; he had a small, upturned nose, full lips, a small chin, and puffiness around his eyes. He talked a great deal, and his language was more eloquent than his age might suggest and had an animated quality. His understanding of language, however, was below age level. Furthermore, although he could launch into a detailed discourse on a subject that interested him, he was quite slow to learn how to hold a pencil, recognize shapes, or perform simple arithmetic. Since birth, he had a unique type of heart defect known as *supravalvular aortic stenosis*. It caused a heart murmur, and he was examined regularly by a cardiologist. Over time, Kevin's difficulty with learning in nonlanguage areas became more noticeable. Kevin's worried parents had him tested by a clinical psychologist who told them that Kevin's cognitive abilities fell into the range of moderate mental retardation. In addition, the psychologist recognized Kevin's facial features and personality to be suggestive of Williams syndrome. Laboratory analysis confirmed the psychologist's suspicion.

Kevin required special education throughout his school years. Although he now requires a moderate amount of assistance with his finances and job skills, he lives with a group of young adults with similar disabilities. He enjoys reading, sings in a performing chorus, is an accomplished pianist, and has countless friends who appreciate his lively conversation and good humor.

Williams Syndrome

Williams syndrome is caused by a deletion in the long arm of chromosome #7. It occurs in 1 in 10,000 live births and is seen equally in males and females. In most cases, the mutation occurs sporadically. Children with Williams syndrome tend to look so much like one another that they appear to be siblings. They are generally short, with characteristic facial features that include the small, upturned nose, full lips and cheeks, and fullness around the eyes as described in Kevin's story. In the newborn period, babies with the syndrome may have a heart murmur and a problem with the metabolism of calcium. Many children with Williams syndrome have a particular talent in musical endeavors and may have perfect pitch. Their hearing is often exceptionally sensitive. As toddlers, however, children with Williams syndrome often experience sleep and behavior disturbances.

Fragile X Syndrome

Fragile X syndrome is the most common inherited cause of mental retardation in boys, with an occurrence of approximately 1 in 1,000 children. It is an X-linked disorder in which most boys with the syndrome have a characteristic pattern of physical, cognitive, and behavior impairments; a fraction of girls who are carriers show less severe symptoms. Boys with fragile X syndrome may have a typical physical appearance with a long face, large ears, double-jointedness, and (after puberty) large testes. They may have mental retardation, communication disorders, and attention-deficit/hyperactivity disorder (ADHD); girls have borderline typical intelligence, learning disabilities, and a high risk of psychiatric disorders (such as depression and anxiety disorder) and disorders on the autism spectrum. Fragile X syndrome is caused by an expansion of a triplet base pair repeat (see Chapter 26) that creates a fragility of the X chromosome and inactivates a gene known as *FMR1*. This gene is normally responsible for the production of FMRP, a protein important in early brain development. Although there is currently no specific treatment for this disorder, special education, behavior management techniques, social skills training, and behavior control medications can improve the outcome of children with fragile X syndrome. Life span is typical, and prognosis is most related to the degree of mental retardation, associated behavioral/psychiatric problems, and the effectiveness of the child and his or her family in coping with this disorder.

SINGLE-GENE DEFECTS

A single-gene defect is usually a metabolic disorder, such as Tay-Sachs disease, in which a mutation or error in a single gene leads to the absence of an enzyme or the production of a defective enzyme that is needed for normal body metabolism. This results in the buildup of a toxin and brain damage. Children with single-gene defects usually look typical, and their biological problem is chemical rather than an abnormality of physical structure. It was formerly thought that single-gene defects did not produce syndromes. Researchers are now learning, however, that single-gene defects can in fact produce complex genetic syndromes that have structural abnormalities and are inherited as recessive or dominant traits (see Chapter 26). One syndrome caused by a single-gene defect is holoprosencephaly.

Holoprosencephaly

During early development of the embryo, the brain must undergo a complex series of foldings and division. An error in this procedure means that a child is born with a brain that is not divided into two hemispheres; this syndrome is called *holoprosencephaly.* The syndrome occurs in 6–12 per 1,000 newborns. There are a range of abnormalities in this disorder, but most children with the syndrome have an unusual facial appearance, narrow-set eyes, and mental retardation. It turns out that the underlying defect is a mutation in a gene with the eccentric name *sonic hedgehog.* This gene directs a phase of brain development, and in its absence the brain's hemispheres do not divide.

NONTRADITIONAL INHERITANCE: IMPRINTING

As noted in Chapter 26, a phenomenon known as *imprinting* can result in different genetic syndromes depending on whether or not the defect is in the chromosome inherited from the mother or the one from the father. Classic examples of this phenomenon involve Prader-Willi syndrome and Angelman syndrome.

Joey

After Joey was born, he had extreme difficulty with feeding by mouth and required tube feeding for several months. He was "floppy" because of low muscle tone, and he began crawling and walking later than his parents had expected. Joey had unusual facial features, including almond-shaped eyes, and he had small hands and feet relative to his body size and height. His genitals were somewhat underdeveloped.

When Joey was 3 years old, he began to overeat and gained weight excessively. His parents had difficulty controlling his voracious appetite as he foraged for food. By the time Joey was in elementary school, he was markedly obese. In addition, he had difficulty with learning and had unpredictable, noncompliant behavior. Joey was seen by a genetic specialist who diagnosed him as having Prader-Willi syndrome. Testing showed a characteristic deletion on the long arm of the paternally derived chromosome #15.

Joey and his parents have been working closely with his physician, therapists, and a dietary specialist for several years. Through a program of regular exercise and healthy eating, he has kept his weight in reasonable control. He attends his local high school where he receives special education services. He will soon begin working with a job coach to investigate his options for future employment.

Prader-Willi Syndrome

Prader-Willi syndrome was first described in 1956 but has only recently been linked to a deletion on the paternal chromosome #15 (#15q11-13). Newborns with the syndrome are floppy because of low muscle tone, particularly in the neck and trunk. In nearly all cases the child has difficulty with nipple feeding to the point that he or she needs to be tube fed. Generally, the need for tube feeding gradually abates and muscle tone improves. There may be mild underdevelopment of the genitalia. Characteristic facial features include almond-shaped eyes, a narrow forehead, and a narrow nose. Often, children with this syndrome have fair hair and blue eyes.

After the second or third year of life, children with Prader-Willi develop a severe overeating problem. They gain excessive weight and often become obese. Many times their desire for food is so intense that they steal or hoard food. A behavioral nutritional program is essential during this stage. The exact reason for the overeating is not well defined but is thought to be related to underactivity of the *hypothalamus*, a brain region that helps control appetite.

In addition to overeating and obesity, children with Prader-Willi syndrome have varying degrees of cognitive impairment and behavior disturbance. Mental retardation can vary from mild to moderate, and the minority of children with typical intelligence almost always have learning disabilities. During adolescence, delays in the start of puberty and in the appearance of secondary sexual characteristics may require treatment with hormones.

Emma

Emma, like Joey, showed evidence of developmental delay during the first months of life. Although she did not have trouble with feeding, she did have some delays in learning to crawl and walk. She eventually learned to walk at the age of 5, although her gait was jerky and unbalanced. In fact, her movements were described as "puppet-like." What particularly troubled Emma's parents was that, even after the age of 3 years, Emma was not developing any functional use of language. Her facial features included a large mouth with prominent chin. Emma was diagnosed with seizures at the age of 2 and was treated with antiepileptic medications. Laboratory analysis confirmed a deletion on the #15 chromosome, and a diagnosis of Angelman syndrome was established. Although distraught over the severity of their child's disability, Emma's parents were relieved to learn that there was an explanation and that her disorder had a name.

Angelman Syndrome

Like Prader-Willi syndrome, Angelman syndrome is caused by a small deletion on the #15 chromosome. In Angelman syndrome, however, the child is missing a piece of the chromosome #15 that came from the mother. Children with Angelman syndrome have only subtle differences in appearance compared with typical children, at least in the first year or two of life. Although children with the syndrome are later noted to have light skin and hair coloring, this is not generally noted at birth. Children with Angelman syndrome tend to have a large mouth with a protruding tongue and a large, prominent jaw. Their teeth may be widely spaced, and their heads are long. The diagnosis of Angelman syndrome is often suspected in the presence of a severe delay in language, coupled with one or two of the physical features just mentioned.

Children with Angelman syndrome characteristically have a happy demeanor with frequent outbursts of laughter. They are overexcitable and extremely active, and they often have sleep problems. Seizures occur in more than 90% of children with the syndrome and generally begin between 1 and 3 years of age. Although the seizures may be initially quite severe and difficult to control, they usually become milder and easier to manage later in childhood (see Chapter 18).

DISORDERS INFLUENCED BY GENETIC AND ENVIRONMENTAL FACTORS

In some syndromes, a group of malformations appear together (for example, a cleft lip, palate, and misshapen ears) but the cause is felt to be *multifactorial* (caused by an unknown combination of genetic and environmental factors). Examples of multifactorial associations include the CHARGE association and the VATER association.

CHARGE Association

The spectrum of malformations that are seen in the CHARGE association vary widely. However, the acronym CHARGE arose because most individuals with the association have three or more of the following features: an abnormal cleft, or coloboma, in the iris or retina of the eye, a heart defect, blockage of the nasal passages (choanal atresia), growth retardation and delayed cognitive development, genital abnormalities, and ear malformations. Surgery is generally required in the first few days of life to correct the structural defects of the baby's heart and nasal passages. In rare instances, the severity of the malformations causes death in the newborn period. In most cases, a child with CHARGE association who survives the newborn period requires extensive medical and educational support throughout childhood. The exact cause of this syndrome is unknown but is thought to be multifactorial. There have been reports of CHARGE association recurring within a family, which suggests a genetic component. Surgical treatments for many of the malformations are available and quite successful.

VATER Association

Another group of malformations that tends to occur together make up what is known as the VATER association. This group of malformations includes vertebral (spinal) abnormalities, a heart defect (often a *v*entricular septal defect, or a hole between the two lower chambers of the heart), blockage of the anus (*a*nal atresia), abnormal connection between the *t*rachea (windpipe) and *e*sophagus (swallowing tube) called a tracheoesophageal fistula, abnormalities of the forearm bone (*r*adial defects), and kidney malformations (*r*enal abnormalities). The VATER association occurs sporadically. Chromosomes are usually normal, and no specific genetic error has been identified. Though most children with VATER association will have some difficulty feeding and gaining weight in infancy, their growth is ultimately normal. Similarly, although developmental delay is common in the first few years of life, cognitive abilities of children with the association are usually within the typical range when measured during later childhood.

DISORDERS OF UNKNOWN INHERITANCE

Although many new disorders are being identified each year, more than 750 syndromes have not yet been linked to a specific genetic error. In many syndromes, a genetic defect is strongly suspected, but the precise abnormality has not yet been found in the laboratory. One example is Noonan syndrome.

Noonan Syndrome

Noonan syndrome is a relatively common multiple malformation syndrome. It is thought to occur in 1 in 1,000–2,500 live births. Children with Noonan syndrome have distinct facial features consisting of widely spaced eyes, drooping eyelids, and low-set ears. Their foreheads are often sloping, and their ears may be thick and angled toward the back of the head. Newborns with Noonan syndrome often have excess skin at the nape of the neck, as is seen frequently in Turner syndrome. Children with Noonan syndrome are usually short in stature and have broad chests. Approximately 50% have a cardiac defect noted shortly after birth, usually a narrowing of the valve leading from the heart to the lungs (pulmonary stenosis). Occasionally, there is underdevelopment of the genitalia.

Approximately one third of infants with Noonan syndrome have feeding difficulties and, as a result, will have poor weight gain. Later, low muscle tone may lead to a mild delay in motor skills; a child with Noonan syndrome typically walks alone at the age of 21 months. Although cognitive skills may be typical in some instances, at least one third of children with Noonan syndrome have some degree of learning disability or mental retardation. Hearing loss is frequent, and hearing testing should be a routine part of the evaluation of a child thought to have Noonan syndrome.

Early researchers noted a similarity in appearance between children with Noonan syndrome and girls with Turner syndrome. Children with Noonan syndrome, however, do not have the chromosomal abnormality characteristic of Turner syndrome. The underlying cause or genetic defect is still unknown, although most experts agree that a genetic abnormality is likely. Although Noonan syndrome occurs sporadically most of the time, there have been some instances in which the syndrome occurred twice or more in one family, further supporting the theory that a genetic defect is involved. The variability of this syndrome is so wide that mild versions frequently go unrecognized.

Isabel

Ricardo and Maria did take Isabel to see a genetic specialist. After a full evaluation, including chromosomal analysis, no specific syndrome could be identified. This is not uncommon. Often a genetic specialist will conclude that a child has "a pattern of malformations that is not recognized." Though genetic research is expanding knowledge regarding syndromes rapidly, much remains to be learned. Ricardo and Maria have been advised to have Isabel reevaluated yearly. It remains possible that over time, more clinical or scientific evidence will become available, making a definitive diagnosis possible. Regular medical checkups as well as teamwork among parents, physicians, and therapists will be important in helping Isabel reach her full potential.

SUMMARY

This chapter has discussed a few of the more common genetic syndromes that are recognized in children. A combination of unusual physical features in a child can often be attributed to a single cause, which may include an error in the child's genetic blueprint. When a genetic syndrome is suspected, a genetic consultation should be arranged. A proper diagnosis helps the family as well as the child fully understand the condition and often permits the family to find out the recurrence risk (see Chapter 26). A diagnosis also may guide a parent in a search for appropriate treatment and for other families who have children with the same disorder.

Some Questions Answered

How can I tell whether my child's disability is genetically inherited?

If your child has a developmental disability, certain situations make it either more or less likely that the disorder has a genetic basis. For example, meningitis can cause brain damage in an infant, yet this is an infectious rather than genetic cause of disability, and the risk of recurrence in future children is no greater than in the general population. Similarly, if your child's disability was caused by brain injury, there is no reason to suspect a genetic cause.

If a close member of your family has had a similar disorder, however, it is much more likely that the disorder had a genetic basis. (Close family members are mother, father, brothers, sisters, aunts, uncles, and first cousins.) A disability in more distant relatives is usually not an indication of an inherited disorder. The risk of certain genetic diseases is higher if you and your spouse were related prior to marriage, such as first or second cousins. Often, however, the child in question is the only member of the family with the genetic disorder.

Certain signs and symptoms in a child may also suggest a genetic disorder. If your child's appearance is different from that of other family members, and if he or she has unusual physical features or a malformation in a major organ system, your child may have a chromosomal disorder. A progressive worsening of your child's condition, rather than a stable or improving situation, may also indicate an inherited disorder. You should ask your child's doctor about these possibilities and about whether your child should be referred to a genetic specialist for further counseling or tests.

Why do I need to know if a genetic syndrome is the cause of my child's developmental disability?

You may be reluctant to pursue a genetic evaluation and may be fearful of the term *syndrome.* There are some important benefits, however, to identifying a definitive diagnosis. First, you may feel relief after learning, at long last, that there is a name and explanation for the various aspects of your child's disability. It may allow you to move past the search for what is "wrong" and to focus, instead, on a quest for appropriate treatment. Second, some genetic syndromes involve complications that require medical or surgical attention. Third, a proper diagnosis can provide important information to you, your children, and other members of your family regarding prognosis and recurrence risk in future children.

My child has been diagnosed with a genetic syndrome. What treatment is available?

There is currently no "cure" for any of the genetic syndromes. Many treatments, however, are available, and the selection of treatments depends on the features of the particular syndrome. When a genetic syndrome is accompanied by delays in development or learning, therapy and educational programs can be invaluable in helping your child achieve meaningful goals. In addition, hormone treatment is needed for physical health in some genetic syndromes. (If your child requires hormone treatment, you should seek advice from an endocrinologist.) Furthermore, some syndromes caused by a deficiency in the body's metabolism can be treated with dietary restrictions or supplements. Scientific research may yield treatments in the future designed to alter or repair the error in a child's genetic blueprint (see Chapter 26). A specialist in genetic syndromes of children can advise you if any of these treatments become available.

Spina Bifida

Catherine Shaer

Spina bifida, also known as *meningomyelocele*, is a complex birth defect of the spinal cord and brain. Affecting 1 of every 1,000 pregnancies, spina bifida is the second most common birth defect resulting in disabilities. Until the early 1950s, infants with this condition rarely survived for more than a few months or years. Now, because of medical and surgical advances, most children with spina bifida can live long, relatively healthy lives.

Ralph

During the fourth month of pregnancy, Judy's doctor suggested that she have a routine serum alpha-fetoprotein (AFP) test to screen for certain birth defects, especially spina bifida and Down syndrome. The results were back within the week and showed that the level of AFP in Judy's blood was abnormally high, suggestive of spina bifida. Judy's obstetrician explained that although the screen is positive in about 5% of women, only a fraction of these women are actually carrying a child who will be born with spina bifida. The test was repeated, and Judy's AFP level was still elevated, which meant that it was more likely that her baby would have spina bifida. The diagnosis was confirmed by a fetal ultrasound (sonogram) that showed a large opening in the lower portion of her son's spinal column.

After a great deal of thought and family discussion, Judy and her husband Ed planned for delivery and early treatment at a university hospital with experience in caring for infants with spina bifida. The remainder of the pregnancy was uneventful, and at birth Ralph was vigorous and pink. There was, however, a large, bubble-like mass containing the underdeveloped spinal cord in the middle of his back. A pediatric neurosurgeon closed the spinal opening on the second day of Ralph's life and 5 days later surgically implanted a thin tube called a *shunt* to control the buildup of fluid within his brain.

Ralph was able to go home at 2 weeks of age. The plan for follow-up included both visits with his primary care doctor and with the specialists at the multidisciplinary spina bifida program: a team of medical, surgical, and allied health professionals, including physical and occupational therapists, social workers, and nurses. Ralph was also enrolled in an early intervention program through which he received therapy on a regular basis. In addition, his parents worked with him daily to carry out the treatment plan that Ralph's physical therapist and teacher developed with them. Although Ralph's motor skills were delayed, his verbal skills and winning personality charmed fam- ily and friends. Uncharacteristic fussiness alerted his parents to an episode of shunt failure when he was 9 months old. The shunt, which had become blocked, was replaced, and Ralph was home within just a few days.

He did well, stayed healthy and out of the hospital, and began to walk with braces by his second birthday. Although he did not have control of his bowels or bladder, he started on a catheterization program when he was 4 years old and now, at the age of 6, needs minimal assistance with the pro- cedure. He has been working on a bowel control program for several years, and he is making slow but steady progress.

WHAT IS SPINA BIFIDA?

There is a spectrum of abnormalities of the spine and spinal cord that falls under the umbrella term *spina bifida*. This chapter addresses the more serious meningomyelocele form of spina bifida. Meningomyelocele is one of a broader group of conditions called *neural tube defects*, which occur when a portion of the central nervous system (the brain and spinal cord) fails to develop completely in the first month of pregnancy. When the top portion of the tube is incomplete, anencephaly (incomplete development of the brain) occurs. When the abnormality occurs in a portion of the spinal cord, spina bifida results. The vertebrae, which normally surround the spinal cord, are also incompletely formed, and the incompletely developed spinal cord pro- trudes through the opening in these bones. A meningeal sac, made from the tissues, or meninges, that usually envelop all parts of the central nervous sys- tem, often forms on the back and contains the undeveloped portion of the spinal cord and spinal fluid. Spina bifida can occur at any level of the spinal cord (see Figure 17.1) but is most commonly found from T1 to L5.

CAUSES, PREVENTION, AND PRENATAL DIAGNOSIS

Researchers have discovered that women who take the B vitamin called *folic acid* prior to becoming pregnant and during the first trimester have a signifi- cantly reduced risk of having a baby with a neural tube defect. As much as 70% of neural tube defects can be prevented when folic acid is taken as described. How folic acid works to prevent neural tube defects is not well

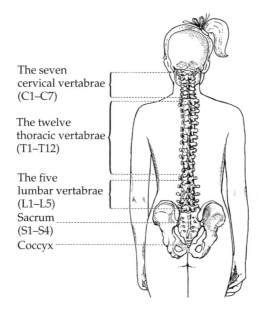

The seven
cervical vertabrae
(C1–C7)

The twelve
thoracic vertabrae
(T1–T12)

The five
lumbar vertabrae
(L1–L5)

Sacrum
(S1–S4)

Coccyx

Figure 17.1. Levels of the spine. This drawing shows the various levels of the spinal column. Spina bifida can occur at any level.

understood. Whether or not fertile women of childbearing age are planning a pregnancy, it is recommended that they take 0.4 mg (400 micrograms) of this vitamin every day because it is difficult to take in this amount even with a balanced diet.

Although the inheritance of spina bifida is not well understood, genes do play a role. A defect in a specific gene has been shown to cause spina bifida in mice. It is unclear whether defects in this gene can also cause spina bifida in humans, but it is known that once a family has had one child with a neural tube defect, their risk of having a second child with this disorder increases as much as fivefold—although the risk of recurrence is still no more than 5%. Others with an increased risk of having children with a neural tube defect include people with relatives who have had a child with this condition, individuals who have spina bifida themselves, people of English or Irish descent, and women taking certain antiepileptic drugs, especially Depakote or Depakene (valproic acid) and Carbatrol or Tegretol (carbamazepine). In these special cases of increased risk, the recommendation is for women planning pregnancies to take a higher daily dose of folic acid. If you are in a high-risk group, consult a genetic counselor to discuss your individual situation and to get specific guidelines on folic acid supplementation (see Chapter 26).

Spina bifida can be diagnosed prenatally in most cases. AFP, a substance found in the blood and spinal fluid of all developing fetuses crosses the placental barrier and makes its way into the mother's bloodstream. A blood test called *maternal serum alpha-fetoprotein* (MSAFP) can be used to measure the level of this protein. When the spinal cord is open, larger amounts of AFP leak from the exposed nervous tissue into the amniotic fluid, and higher levels are found in the blood of women carrying a fetus with spina bifida. Obstetricians use this test to screen for neural tube defects in the 16th–18th week of pregnancy. The test is not specific for spina bifida, however, and if the MSAFP level is high, the test is usually repeated and a diagnostic sonogram is performed to visualize the spine and spinal cord. The sonogram can usually detect an open spinal cord and sac if present. Amniocentesis, a procedure in which amniotic fluid is withdrawn from the womb for study, can also be done to further evaluate the level of AFP and is more accurate than the MSAFP because the levels in amniotic fluid are much higher than in maternal blood.

If the prenatal diagnosis of a neural tube defect has been made, your family is faced with the difficult decision of whether to continue the pregnancy. This is a very complex and personal issue that is influenced by a number of factors, and there is no easy or "right" answer (see Chapter 26). Even if pregnancy termination is not an acceptable option, it is best to diagnose a neural tube defect before the baby is born. Early detection allows your family to begin to learn about this very complex condition and to select and meet with the doctors and other health care professionals who will help care for your baby. Parents also can begin to talk with other families of children with spina bifida.

HOW SPINA BIFIDA AFFECTS THE BODY

Messages pass up and down the spinal cord, carrying information between the brain and all areas of the body. When formation of the spinal cord is incomplete, messages cannot be sent to or received from areas below the spina bifida defect. As a result, several body systems cannot function properly. The main areas affected are the central nervous system (brain and spinal cord), the genitourinary system (kidneys and bladder), and the musculoskeletal system (muscles and bones).

Effects on the Central Nervous System

The most obvious abnormality of the central nervous system is the open, incomplete portion of the spinal cord protruding through the unfused vertebrae. After delivery, it is important that the opening be closed; this is usually done by a pediatric neurosurgeon between 24 and 72 hours after birth. Although the surgery will stabilize the condition of the spinal cord, it will not restore function to damaged or undeveloped nerves, and the child will have some degree of paralysis below the level of the damaged spinal cord.

In addition, virtually all children with this condition have abnormalities in the structure of the back of the brain, which together are called *Arnold Chiari II malformation* (Chiari II). Instead of resting at the bottom of the skull, the base of the brain (brain stem) sits abnormally low and extends into the neck. This downward protrusion acts like a cork sitting in the neck of a bottle and obstructs the natural flow of spinal fluid. Fluid builds up within the ventricles (fluid-filled chambers) of the brain, causing a condition called *hydrocephalus.* Virtually all children with spina bifida have hydrocephalus, and 80%–90% of these children require a shunt to control the condition. This thin silicon tube is implanted in the ventricles and allows the fluid to flow out, usually into the abdominal cavity. When a baby is born with spina bifida and severe hydrocephalus, the back surgery and shunt placement may be done at the same time. More often, however, the shunt is not placed until several days after the back closure. In some infants, significant hydrocephalus develops very slowly, and determining whether a shunt is needed can take months.

Although shunt technology has dramatically improved over the years, there continue to be problems with these devices. Children can outgrow the shunts, or the devices can become clogged at either end, break, or become infected. The signs of shunt failure vary with age and from individual to individual, but the most common ones are listed in Table 17.1. As a parent, you may often be the first to suspect a shunt malfunction and in such cases should contact your neurosurgeon or spina bifida coordinator immediately. Modern diagnostic tests such as ultrasound, CT (computed tomography), or MRI (magnetic resonance imaging) scan can be used to evaluate your child's shunt function. There is no "usual" number of episodes of shunt failure during a lifetime. Some children have more than a dozen replacements in the first few years of life, whereas others never have a problem with the device. If shunt failure occurs, your child's neurosurgeon will determine whether all or part of the malfunctioning shunt needs to be replaced. If a problem with shunt function is detected early, the replacement procedure is usually straightforward, and your child will be back to normal within days. This underscores the importance of being alert for signs of failure such as irritability, persistent vomiting, headache, and lethargy.

A rarer but quite serious complication is an infection of the shunt. Although a shunt infection can sometimes be treated without removal of the device, the more usual course is to remove the shunt, treat your child with intravenous antibiotics, and place a new shunt once the infection has resolved.

It is natural for you to worry about the shunt at first, but with time you will become familiar with your child's temperament and be better able to differentiate between episodes of usual fussiness and a possible shunt malfunction. If there is any question of a shunt failure, you should call your child's pediatrician or neurosurgeon for advice.

In addition to causing the structural problems that lead to hydrocephalus, the Chiari II malformation can cause other complications. The brain stem rests low in the skull in a much smaller and cramped space than it was meant to occupy. As a result, the brain stem becomes distorted and, in some cases, underdeveloped or damaged. Your child may then have one or more of a number of symptoms, including choking or gagging on food or drink,

Table 17.1.   Signs of shunt failure

Age	Signs of shunt failure
Birth to 1 year	Full or bulging fontanel (soft spot)
	Enlarging head size
	Crossed eyes (new or worsening)
	Irritability
	Vomiting
	Increased sleepiness
	Swelling along the shunt tract
	Excessive spitting up (gastroesophageal reflux)
	Noisy breathing (stridor)
2–3 years	Increased head size
	Irritability
	Temperament changes
	Persistent headache
	Vomiting
	Seizures
	Swelling along the shunt tract
	Crossed eyes (new or worsening)
4 years to adult	Personality changes
	Deterioration in school or job performance
	Persistent headache
	Pain at the spina bifida repair site
	Swelling along the shunt tract
	Changes in vision

uncoordinated eye muscle movements, apnea (abnormally long pauses while breathing), paralysis of the vocal cords (leading to a harsh noise with breathing called *stridor*), and weakness in the hands or arms.

In many cases, symptoms caused by the Chiari II clear up over time without any specific treatment. At other times treatment can be simple and straightforward, such as the use of special feeding techniques if your child experiences a lot of gagging and choking. When symptoms are severe, however, your child's pediatric neurosurgeon may recommend a surgical procedure called *posterior fossa decompression*. The operation is designed to relieve pressure on the brain stem by enlarging the space it occupies. This is a complicated operation, the risks can be significant, and, in some cases, your child may still have symptoms even after the brain stem has been well decompressed. Therefore, the decision as to whether your child will undergo posterior fossa decompression should be made only after you have discussed the options with your child's pediatric neurosurgeon and understand the potential risks and benefits.

Later Spinal Cord Complications

Once the opening in your child's back is closed, his or her neurologic functioning usually will not worsen. If your child shows a decrease in strength, a change in sensation, or a deterioration in bowel or bladder function or if he or she develops an unexplained deformity such as a new curvature of the spine, one of several problems of the spinal cord should be suspected. A condition called *tethered cord* can occur at any time during childhood or early adulthood and, if unrecognized, can cause additional damage to your child's spinal cord and nerves. Tethering is caused by crowding of the spinal cord by meningomyelocele tissue that could not be removed at the time of the initial surgery or by scar tissue that forms around the spinal cord in the area of the original surgery. In either situation, the spinal nerves can become stuck and, as your child grows, the spinal cord cannot move and grow as it should. This can result in stretching and thinning of the cord, causing additional damage to the spinal cord and nerves.

In some children with spina bifida, abnormal pockets (syrinxes) of fluid form inside the spinal cord. Syrinxes can collect anywhere along the spinal cord and, similar to a tethered cord, can cause compression with associated nerve damage and deterioration of function. When a tethered cord or a syrinx is suspected, an MRI scan is usually done to allow doctors to view an image of the spinal cord and surrounding structures. If either of these conditions is found, your child's neurosurgeon should be consulted regarding the best course of treatment. Tethered cords can be surgically released, and syrinxes can be treated with small shunt-type devices that drain fluid from the pocket, usually to an area beneath the tissues surrounding the spinal cord.

Effects on the Musculoskeletal System

Because typical nerve development and function do not occur at or below the level of the spinal cord defect, the higher up the neural tube defect, the higher the level of paralysis. Physical examination and diagnostic testing, when needed, can pinpoint your child's level of function.

It is important to know that children with spina bifida who have partial or even complete paralysis of the legs can usually walk with the use of assistive equipment such as braces, canes, crutches, and walkers. Even children with minimal paralysis often are fitted with braces in early childhood to support and protect the developing muscles and joints. Although each child is different, Table 17.2 shows the type of equipment that children with varying levels of spina bifida use to get around.

Many muscles work in pairs to balance joints and keep bones aligned. Children with spina bifida often have one member of a muscle pair working better than the other. This imbalance can lead to a variety of problems including dislocated joints, misshapen bones, and curvature of the spine. Some of these problems are present at birth, whereas others develop over time. Early involvement of an orthopedic surgeon experienced in the care of children with spina bifida is important. This specialist will determine if your child can benefit from exercises, splints, or casts or if corrective surgery is required. Your child may need several orthopedic procedures over a number of years to achieve the best possible body alignment and the highest degree of motor function.

Spinal Curvature and Humps

Abnormal alignment of the backbones or vertebrae presents a special problem. Curvature of the spine (scoliosis) can develop in your child for a variety of reasons. The vertebrae themselves may be deformed, but more commonly a lack of muscular support allows the bones to fall into a C- or S-shaped curve. As mentioned in the section Later Spinal Cord Complications, a tethered cord or a syrinx can also cause scoliosis.

Mild scoliosis usually is treated with a special brace called a *body jacket* that fits around your child's chest and abdomen and supports the spine. If the curve progresses and a tether or a syrinx is not an issue, spinal fusion may be necessary. With spinal fusion, the position of the vertebrae is surgically corrected as much as possible and the bones are then fused together to maintain the correction. When vertebrae are fused, however, they can no longer grow. For that reason, spinal fusion is usually not done until after puberty, when your child will have gained all or most of his or her expected height.

A humpback, also known as a *gibbous* or *kyphotic deformity*, can occur if your child has a mid- to high thoracic level of spina bifida (see Figure 17.1). Muscular support to the spinal column is very weak, and children with this condition usually have it at birth. Management of a gibbous deformity can be difficult because the skin over the hump is very thin and fragile. To allow maximum growth of the spine, surgery is often not done on the hump until the teenage years. Some orthopedic surgeons do advocate early surgery, however, and you can discuss this option with your child's health care team.

Effects on the Genitourinary System

Virtually all babies with spina bifida are born with normal kidneys. Unfortunately, this is not the case for the bladder. The nerves that serve the bladder are located in the lowest region of the spinal cord. Almost all spina bifida occurs above this level, so very few children with spina bifida will have normal bladder function. In all likelihood, your child will not feel a full bladder,

Table 17.2.   Prognosis for walking

Spina bifida level[a]	Equipment usually needed
T12 and above	Brace above waist to walk for short distances
	Walker or crutches
	Wheelchair for most activities, even in childhood
L1	Long leg braces with a band around the waist
	Crutches
	Wheelchair for any distances, walks for exercise only
L2–L3	Long leg braces (up to thigh or waist) with crutches
	In later years, wheelchair for long distances, may walk for exercise only
L4	Usually above- or below-knee braces, possibly also crutches or a cane
	Wheelchair at older ages, usually by adolescence
L5–S1	Short leg braces to help with foot position and to push off
	Possibly crutches or a cane
S2–S4	Frequently walks without aids (braces or crutches)
	Possibly shoe inserts

[a]See Figure 17.1 for a diagram of the levels of the spine.

will not be able to control the flow of urine, and may not be able to empty the bladder completely. In addition, high pressure in the bladder may force urine backward toward the kidneys in a process called *reflux.* These problems can lead to urinary tract infections and, over time, kidney damage. Regular consultation with a pediatric urologist familiar with these issues and evaluation of bladder and kidney function as needed will usually allow these problems to be detected early, preventing significant kidney damage.

Although maintaining well-functioning kidneys is critical, it is socially important for your child to achieve some control over bladder function so that he or she can leave diapers behind. Most children will learn to empty their bladders with a catheter, a flexible straw-like device that is inserted into the bladder to drain urine and is removed when the bladder has been emptied. This procedure, called *clean intermittent catheterization,* or *CIC,* may be started in infancy in children with reflux but is usually begun between 3 and 5 years of age and is done every 2–4 hours during the day. Although most children will need assistance at first, they will be able to catheterize themselves independently by the age of 7 or 8 years. With the aid of catheterization and, in some cases, medication, most children can be socially dry. A number of surgical procedures have been developed to improve continence for those for whom CIC and medication is not adequate. Your child's urologist can advise you as to whether such surgery is right for your child.

Effects on the Bowel

As with the bladder, the bowel receives messages from nerves originating at the bottom of the spinal cord. Therefore, your child will probably not feel the need to have a bowel movement, nor will he or she be able to control the passage of stool.

The normal pattern of digestion starts with food entering the stomach and, after being churned with digestive juices, moving into the small intestine where nutrients and minerals are absorbed into the bloodstream. Stool, which is liquid at this point, then moves into the large intestine where water is reabsorbed and becomes more solid as it moves toward the rectum. In individuals with spina bifida, intestinal muscle contractions are often decreased, causing the liquid stool to move very slowly through the system. Too much water is reabsorbed, resulting in firm, hard stools or constipation that can cause a partial or total blockage of the large intestine. Diarrhea can also occur when liquid stool leaks around the blockage. It is important to keep your child's stools soft beginning at an early age because once a pattern of constipation develops, it can be very difficult to reverse. If severe constipation develops, strong laxatives, enemas, and, occasionally hospitalization for a bowel "clean-out" may be needed. Feeding your child a diet rich in high fiber foods such as grains, fruits, and vegetables will help the stool retain water as it passes through the intestines. A variety of commercial fiber agents such as Per Diem, Kondremul, Metamucil, Citrucel, and Fiber Con can be helpful when used routinely.

A number of programs can help children with spina bifida achieve bowel continence, but none of these will be effective if the stool is hard. One of the most commonly used methods is called *habit training,* in which the goal is for the child to have a stool at the same time each day. Enemas or suppositories are used daily to cause the child to pass stool at the designated time. Eventually, your child should have a bowel movement at the same time each day without the use of these medications. It takes time, patience, and a great deal of dedication to keep up this routine for extended periods of time, but the rewards of a well-functioning bowel program are tremendous for your child and you in terms of both physical and emotional well-being.

OTHER MEDICAL ISSUES

Because spina bifida affects so many body systems, the potential for other medical problems is high. Some individuals will experience few, if any, of these problems; others will experience many of them.

Skin Problems

Spina bifida usually causes loss of sensation below the level of the spinal lesion. There may be partial or complete loss of normal skin sensitivity to pain, touch and temperature in the buttocks, legs, and feet. As a result, your child is at increased risk for injury to the skin from many sources, including extremes of temperature and pressure. Care must be taken to protect your child's skin from frostbite in cold weather, from burns caused by such common sources as hot bath water, radiators, and sun-baked asphalt, and from pressure points where skin contacts braces or a wheelchair for prolonged periods. In addition, rug and floor burns can occur if your child's legs and feet are left uncovered when crawling. Damaged skin must be treated early, or deeper layers of the skin can become involved, possibly causing serious infections of the underlying muscles and bones. Areas lacking good sensation also heal more slowly than areas with full feeling, so persistence and patience are needed when treating a skin breakdown.

To avoid these problems, you should examine all skin daily for signs of irritation and take prompt action to treat any damaged areas. Your child should be encouraged to gradually assume the responsibility for checking the skin so that by adolescence he or she can do this independently. A mirror may be used to view hard-to-see areas such as the bottoms of the feet and the buttocks.

The most important thing you can do once a pressure sore has developed is to remove all sources of pressure and irritation. In addition, there are many products that can accelerate the healing process. Because this is a very specialized area and new products are always being introduced, it is best to consult a physician or a nurse with experience in treating pressure sores.

Fractures

Bones become strong when they are used, but children with spina bifida who get around by using braces, crutches, or wheelchairs do not bear weight fully on their legs. This leads to the development of osteoporosis (thin bones). These weak bones can break with even minor injury. This disorder tends to be more of a problem for children with spina bifida at the high lumbar or thoracic levels (see Figure 17.1). Because of the decreased or absent feeling in the legs, your child may be unaware of an injury. As a result, swelling, deformity, or fever may be the only signs of a broken bone.

Seizures

Seizures (epilepsy) occur in approximately 1% of all children. This figure rises to about 1 in 20 individuals with spina bifida. The risk of developing a seizure disorder is greatest for children who have had central nervous system infections or many episodes of shunt failure. Most seizure disorders are successfully managed with conventional antiepileptic medication (see Chapter 18).

Early (Precocious) Puberty

The age when puberty begins varies from child to child, but it usually starts between 10 and 11 years of age in girls and between 12 and 14 in boys. Puberty can start as early as 7 or 8 years of age, however, in children with abnormalities of the central nervous system, including those with spina bifida and hydrocephalus. The predominant side effect of precocious puberty is short stature. Typically, a major growth spurt occurs during puberty, but when puberty begins early, the total number of growing years is reduced and affected individuals are often shorter than typical. In addition, younger children are often unprepared for the emotional and physical changes that accompany this stage of development. Medications can be used to delay the start of puberty, but a full medical evaluation should be done if the child shows signs of precocious puberty.

Latex Allergy

Children with spina bifida are at high risk for developing an allergy to latex (natural rubber). Symptoms of latex allergy are frequently limited to a runny nose, itchy eyes, and hives, but life-threatening reactions can occur. It is best to minimize your child's exposure to products containing latex from birth, with the hope that by avoiding latex, your child will not develop this allergy. Synthetic, nonlatex, catheters should be used for CIC, and only nonlatex gloves should be used for medical, surgical, and dental procedures. Contact with rubber balloons, balls, and other rubber toys should also be avoided at home, at school, and during any physical or occupational therapy.

Obesity

Many children with spina bifida, especially those who are nonambulatory, become overweight. You may be tempted to overfeed your baby in an attempt to compensate for the challenges and physical hardships he or she faces. Although this is done out of love, excess weight will make it even harder for your child to become active and independent. Your child's pediatrician and medical specialists can answer any questions you may have about your child's diet.

A good diet alone is not enough, however. Recreational activities such as swimming, horseback riding, and wheelchair sports can play an important role in maintaining your child's cardiovascular fitness and an appropriate weight.

Sexual Function

Children with spina bifida will undergo all of the usual physical changes that come with adolescence. Similar to the nerves that control the bladder, however, those responsible for sexual sensation and function come from the lower portion of the spinal cord. So, most individuals with spina bifida will have some degree of sexual dysfunction. Girls with spina bifida most often will not have full sensation in their genitalia. Although their fertility is unaffected, women with high levels of paralysis may have severe curvature of the spine, small abdominal cavities, and other physical problems that make it difficult for them to carry a child for a full 9 months. A gynecologist with experience in high-risk pregnancies should be consulted when decisions about childbearing are made. Every young woman with spina bifida should have a yearly gynecological examination, beginning with puberty.

The situation is a bit different for males with spina bifida. They may have difficulty achieving and maintaining an erection (impotence), and ejaculation may not always occur. As a result, men with spina bifida may have difficulty fathering children. Many new techniques and treatments are available for the treatment of impotence as well as infertility. Programs specializing in the treatment of individuals with paraplegia can be good resources for treating impotence and confirming fertility status of an individual, as well as investigating other options for having children such as in vitro fertilization and adoption.

Although there are special challenges to be addressed, people with spina bifida can have deeply satisfying intimate relationships. It is interesting to note that sensitivity is often dramatically increased above the level of paralysis, resulting in nontraditional erogenous zones. A number of books address the issue of sexuality and can help individuals solve basic problems such as positioning and dealing with incontinence. As with any child, one of your jobs as a parent will be to help your son or daughter recognize and fulfill his or her sexuality.

SOCIAL AND EDUCATIONAL CONCERNS

The medical and surgical issues that have been covered so far in this chapter are, of course, critical to your child's achieving and maintaining a state of good health and maximizing physical function. Of equal importance, however, are the psychological, social, and educational factors that determine how independent a life an individual with this complex condition will be able to achieve.

Social Concerns

Many infants and children with spina bifida have frequent hospitalizations that can interfere with their social development. In addition, it is natural for you to try to shield your child from the pressures, demands, and disappointments of life. Although watching your child struggle with simple tasks such as dressing, picking up dropped objects, or getting in and out of bed can be difficult, it is best to let him or her try and to help only when necessary. Give your child chores that are appropriate for his or her age and abilities. Teach your child that he or she is responsible for the consequences of his or her actions, and give your child opportunities to make choices and decisions, such as what to wear to school or how to spend free time. It is also important to encourage your child's social relationships with children who do or do not have disabilities.

At some point your child will likely express frustration and anger at the disability. In particular, adolescents with spina bifida may have more difficulty in maintaining social relationships than do their peers without physical disabilities, and some degree of depression is not unusual. It may be possible for you to help your child over the rough spots, but professional help should be considered especially if you have concerns about a persistent depression, a change in school performance, or social isolation in your child.

Educational Needs

Although the IQ scores of most children with spina bifida fall within the typical range, the scores cluster at the lower end of the scale. Learning disabilities are common and can be significant. In general, your child's verbal abilities are likely to be significantly better than his or her visual motor abilities. This results in a pattern of poor short-term memory, weak organizational skills, and difficulty with tasks that require eye–hand coordination. Mathematics is often the most challenging subject. Your child's educational needs can be met in a variety of settings (see Chapter 12).

Federal and state laws, including the Americans with Disabilities Act (ADA) of 1990, require that individuals with disabilities be given the opportunity to live, work, and go to school in the least restrictive environment and that reasonable accommodations be made to help these people gain access to and benefit from their educational environments. This means that services such as physical, occupational, and speech-language therapy as well as assistance with self-care needs such as clean intermittent catheterization must be available to your child in the school environment.

The identification of your child's motor, cognitive, and learning problems should not, however, await school entry. It is important that a developmental specialist assess your child's abilities as early as possible, usually in the first 6 months of life. Early intervention services are mandated in all states, and health care professionals or your county's Department of Education or Health Department can provide you with information on getting services for your child (see Chapter 6).

PROSPECTS FOR FUTURE TREATMENT

Over the past few decades, major strides have been made in the treatment of children with spina bifida. Researchers are currently working on a variety of innovative and potentially revolutionary treatments. Studies in animals suggest that closing the spinal defect before birth minimizes damage to the nervous system. The thought is that over time, the amniotic fluid bathing the open spinal cord may have a corrosive effect. In fact, a few neurosurgeons have operated prenatally on spina bifida defects in a very small number of human fetuses, with mixed results. Although motor function seems to have been improved in some children, the miscarriage rate is very high, greater than 50%. Prenatal shunting of hydrocephalus is another procedure that neurosurgeons have been evaluating. Again, although there have been some successes, the procedure is fraught with technical difficulties and, at this time, most experienced neurosurgeons look on it as an experimental procedure. Work is also being done, primarily in animals, on nerve transplantation and regeneration.

SUMMARY

Spina bifida is a complex condition requiring ongoing assessment and management by a variety of medical and surgical specialists in collaboration with allied health professionals including physical and occupational therapists, educational specialists, and social workers. A multidisciplinary team specializing in the care of children with spina bifida is usually the best source of state-of-the-art care.

Some Questions Answered

Spina bifida is such a difficult medical condition that I don't know how to get the medical care my child needs. Where do I begin?

Spina bifida is indeed a complex medical condition and is best managed by a team of specialists. There are dozens of programs around the country, most in children's hospitals and other academic medical centers, that bring together a broad spectrum of health care professionals who work as a team to provide the most up-to-date treatment. Although each team is unique, most have a nurse coordinator, neurosurgeon, orthopedic surgeon, physical therapist, and urologist who can evaluate your child on a regular basis and work together to help your child fulfill his or her potential. The Spina Bifida Association of America in Washington, D.C., posts a listing of these spina bifida programs on its web site (http://www.sbaa.org). In addition, your child should have a primary care physician close to home who can provide routine

Table 17.3.   Tests of various body systems for individuals with spina bifida

Test	Interval	Purpose
Head CT (computed tomography) scan	As newborn, then yearly or as indicated	To assess ventricular size and and shunt function
MRI (magnetic resonance imaging) scan	Occasionally in newborn period or when Arnold Chiari II malformation, syrinx, or tethered cord suspected	To visualize brain and spinal cord most effectively
Renal/bladder sonogram	As newborn, then every 1–2 years	To assess kidney size, evaluate bladder drainage, check bladder size
Voiding cystourethrogram (VCUG)	As newborn, then every 1–2 years	To evaluate bladder size and shape, look for backflow of urine from bladder to kidneys
Renal scan	In first year, then as needed	To view kidney size and function as well as any damage from infection
X rays of the spine, legs, hips, or feet	As newborn, then as needed to assess bone growth and better visualize other bony abnormalities	To detect problems early as a key to early treatment

care such as immunizations and physical examinations as well as be available for acute illnesses.

What should be done to prevent complications of spina bifida?

Although it is not possible to predict every complication in every child, a variety of tests can be done to monitor your child's condition and that may detect changes or problems before damage occurs. Table 17.3 lists tests that are used to assess the function of various body systems. The timetable for performing these tests is intended as a reference only because each child's situation and needs are different.

18

Epilepsy

Steven Weinstein

Tonic-clonic (grand mal) seizures are frightening to watch. Your child's apparent struggle to breathe may make you think your child is swallowing his or her tongue. Blue lips may make you worry that your child is receiving insufficient oxygen and may suffer brain damage. Shaking and lack of muscle control are frightening to watch and may lead you to assume that your child is in pain. Finally, you may interpret sleepiness after the seizure as proof that your child's brain has been harmed.

Actually, all of these observations lead to unfounded fears; typical tonic-clonic seizures do not damage your child's body or brain (unless your child is injured during a fall). What you really see during the seizure are breathing difficulties caused by abnormal muscle control, resulting in the mouth being clenched tight and the chest muscles moving inappropriately. Your child cannot swallow his or her tongue because it is attached to the floor of the mouth. Studies in animals suggest that a seizure must last for more than 30 minutes for any irreversible changes to occur in a developing brain. Furthermore, studies in children suggest that seizures must be even longer before they will harm the brain, and although a seizure seems to last forever, more than 90% of tonic-clonic seizures last less than 5 minutes.

There is a theory that the chemical events leading up to any seizure may cause subtle changes in brain neurochemistry and structure that could increase the likeliness of future seizures. Although this "kindling phenomenon" has been found in animals, it has not been conclusively found in humans. In general, you can think of a seizure as a synchronous electrical discharge in the brain. This may help alleviate some of your fears about what is happening during even the most frightening of events. Similarly, the deep sleep that follows a seizure is only the result of extinguishing the preceding "firestorm" in the brain.

Almost 1 in 10 people will have at least one seizure in their lifetime. Just because your child has a single seizure, however, does not mean he or she will develop epilepsy. Epilepsy affects only 1% of children. It is diagnosed when there have been two or more spontaneous seizures, that is, seizures that are unrelated to fever in a young child, brain injury, drug exposure, or any other immediate cause. Furthermore, the diagnosis of epilepsy does not necessarily imply that your child has cognitive or motor abnormalities. In fact, most children with epilepsy have typical intelligence, and the seizures themselves rarely cause brain damage. Children with other developmental disabilities, however, are at greater risk of developing epilepsy than typically developing children are.

You will, of course, want to know why the seizure happened, and your child's pediatrician or the emergency room physician will perform tests to try to identify a cause. For approximately half of children who have had a seizure, no explanation for the seizure can be found. In fact, an unknown cause should be considered a good sign because identifiable disorders that cause seizures are often more dangerous and less treatable than hidden (idiopathic) causes. When a seizure disorder is diagnosed, your child may be placed on an antiepileptic medication to decrease the risk or intensity of subsequent convulsions. No one can guarantee, however, that the medication will completely control the seizures or be without side effects. Because no one can predict whether your child will outgrow the seizure disorder you will also need to live with a degree of uncertainty.

In an attempt to prevent future seizures, you may be tempted to overprotect your child. Restricting activities and experiences, however, limits your child's social and physical interactions with peers. This may cause your child to be "vulnerable"—making him or her ill-equipped to deal with the disorder and to succeed as an independent adult. We encourage you instead to set aside your fears and challenge your child to reach his or her full potential.

WHAT SEIZURES ARE

Brain cells, or neurons, are like batteries; they generate electricity. The electricity is produced by chemicals inside the neuron and is influenced by neighboring structures. The neurons are linked together into networks that allow electrical charges to build up and discharge to produce an output signal such as a movement or a thought. Take reading this chapter as an example. Your network for vision (in the occipital or back lobe of the brain) combines with your language area (usually the left temporal or middle lobe) and area for motor control of eye movements (frontal lobe) to permit reading. Each network performs distinctly different but simultaneous activities. The interconnections also permit the production of new memories and the drawing-upon of old memories (middle temporal lobe).

A seizure is an electrical event that is not chaotic brain electricity but rather an excessively synchronized discharge of a network in one area or throughout the brain. People who have had seizures report having hallucinations or displaying unusual behaviors at the beginning of a seizure and sometimes notice an "aura" before a seizure. The aura results from the abnormal discharge confined to a small area of the brain. The type of aura is related to the function normally associated with that area of the brain. Examples include visual disturbances from the occipital lobe, twitching from the frontal motor areas, and intense emotions from the middle temporal region.

The abnormal discharge may spread to other areas of the brain and lead to more complex behaviors and, finally, with maximal brain involvement, to a generalized tonic-clonic seizure (previously called a *major motor* or a *grand mal convulsion*). The seizure usually ends spontaneously, presumably because protective influences in the brain not only may extinguish the seizure but also may decrease brain electricity in general. This inhibition of brain activity often leads to incontinence and subsequent sleep during the postictal (postseizure) state. It is during this time that you may think your child is lifeless because he or she may be difficult to arouse and may have shallow breathing. Following the seizure, a strong inhibition of the part of the brain from which the seizure arose may result in momentary blindness or weakness (called *Todd's palsy*). This may make you think your child has had a stroke, but full recovery occurs within hours or, on rare occasions, within days. The point is that seizures look much worse than they are; they are generally not life threatening and almost never cause brain damage. Realistic concerns about seizures include potential injury from falls, social stigma, and possible effects of seizures and/or antiepileptic drugs on learning.

CAUSES OF SEIZURES

Everyone's brain can produce a seizure given the proper stimulus. What distinguishes those individuals who have seizures from those who do not is the nature and location of the brain stimulus as well as a genetic predisposition for having seizures. Together, these factors determine a person's likelihood of having a seizure.

Brain cells include neurons, nerve cells that perform the function we normally think of as brain activity, and the more numerous supportive glial cells. There is a delicate balance between chemicals that are released when neurons "talk" to each other, with the glial cells fine-tuning that "conversation." If there is an imbalance in the amount of chemicals released, a defect in their uptake, or the production of abnormal signals in the "receiving" neurons, there is a greater likelihood for seizures to occur. These chemicals all are under genetic control, and as a result some people are at a greater risk for developing seizures.

Injury to the brain also increases the probability of seizures by disrupting the normal circuitry. For example, a severe lack of oxygen, brain infection such as meningitis or encephalitis, severe head trauma, and brain tumors all are associated with increased risk of seizures. These seizures may occur at the time of injury or may develop later.

Some seizures are clearly provoked and do not count toward the diagnosis of epilepsy. For example, in a child between the ages of 6 months and 5 years, a high fever may produce febrile convulsions. Other causes of isolated seizures include abnormalities in the body's metabolic balance, head trauma such as from falls or from sports injuries, migraine headaches, and toxic substances such as medications or illicit drugs. If such stimuli are avoided, it is unlikely that spontaneous seizures will occur. Everyday events do not usually induce seizure activity. Although sleep deprivation, infections that are not in the brain, and stress are commonly reported as triggers for seizures, they are mostly reported by individuals who are later found to have a seizure disorder.

SEIZURE TYPES

There are a number of seizure types; each has different symptoms and responds to a specific class of antiepileptic medication (see Table 18.1). The first distinction in diagnosing the type of seizure is whether the electrical discharge starts in one area or starts throughout the brain. Seizures starting in one area are called *partial seizures*. If your child's consciousness is impaired during the seizure (that is, if he or she is confused or is unable to understand or has no memory of the event), the seizure is called a *complex partial seizure*. Partial seizures in which consciousness is maintained are called *simple partial seizures* or *auras*. Seizures arising simultaneously throughout the brain are called *primarily generalized seizures,* and consciousness is usually impaired during these. Your child's doctor must distinguish between these seizure types to ensure that the diagnosis is made appropriately and the correct medication is prescribed. Therefore, the appearance of the seizure at its onset is the most important information you can provide to your child's physician.

The most dramatic and frightening type of seizure is the tonic-clonic seizure. During this kind of seizure, your child will typically stiffen, then all of his or her extremities and face will shake. Your child's mouth will be clenched tight, and he or she will appear to be struggling to breathe, often with blue lips. The tonic-clonic seizure usually lasts less than 5 minutes and is followed by a period of deep sleep that may last a few hours. If the seizure does not stop in 15–20 minutes, it is called *status epilepticus.* And if it continues beyond 30–60 minutes without effective treatment, which rarely occurs, there is at least the possibility of damage to brain cells.

Partial seizures can start with a variety of sensations or movements depending on where the seizure focus lies. These auras may include visual, auditory, or smell hallucinations, abnormal sensations in the belly or head, feelings of fear, or twitching movements. Almost any behavior that is not usually present in your child's repertoire may be an aura. If there is a single

Table 18.1. Types and characteristics of seizures

Type of seizure	Characteristics
Partial	
Simple partial seizure (formerly called a *focal motor* or *focal sensory seizure*)	Stereotyped sudden sensation or movement—the same sudden sensation or movement during every seizure (such as sudden feeling of pain, perception of a foul odor, or feeling of nausea); does not affect consciousness
Complex partial seizure (formerly called a *psychomotor seizure* or *temporal lobe epilepsy*)	Unusual stereotyped behaviors, such as staring, fumbling with clothes, lip smacking, and automatic hand movements, accompanied by a change in or loss of consciousness
Partial with secondary generalization	May begin as a partial seizure and progress to include a generalized response
Generalized	
Atonic (formerly called *drop attacks*)	A sudden loss of muscle tone, usually resulting in a fall and in most cases also including a loss of consciousness
Myoclonic	Generalized jerking of extremities, lasting less than 5 seconds, usually with a brief period of unconsciousness that can go unnoticed; may occur in clusters
Absence (formerly called *petit mal*)	Loss of consciousness, usually lasting less than 15 seconds, with no other visible change; may involve blinking or lip smacking
Generalized tonic-clonic (formerly called *grand mal*)	Tonic phase involves generalized stiffening of muscles usually lasting less than 1 minute, followed by a clonic phase of rapid jerking. The individual is unconscious during both phases and will not remember the seizure afterward.

From Kuntz, K.R. (1996). Seizures. In L.A. Kurtz, P.W. Dowrick, S.E. Levy, & M.L. Batshaw (Eds.), *Handbook of developmental disabilities: Resources for interdisciplinary care* (p. 398). Gaithersburg, MD: Aspen Publishers, Inc.; ©1996; adapted by permission.

focus, the seizure aura should seem almost identical every time. Many children with partial seizures, however, do not have an aura or are unable to connect its occurrence to the onset of a seizure. If the seizure spreads and becomes complex, your child may stare, make fumbling motions with his or her hands, wander aimlessly, and be less responsive to the environment. Partial seizures occur far less frequently (usually less than once per day) than do absence seizures, last longer (30 seconds to 5 minutes), and often bring on a postictal state of drowsiness. Typical startle responses, temper tantrums, anxiety attacks, and tics (involuntary jerky movements) can be confused with partial seizures.

Perhaps the least dramatic seizure is the absence, or petit mal, type. This is an event that usually lasts less than 10 seconds, during which time your child has an altered state of awareness. Your child may show a number of behaviors, including staring into space, abnormal eye movements and eyelid fluttering, and changes in posture. Your child is unaware of surroundings during the seizure and cannot remember what happened in those few seconds. There is no postictal state, so your child will immediately resume the interrupted behavior. This could place your child at risk for injury, for example, if he or she is crossing the street or swimming. Your child cannot begin new tasks, answer questions verbally, or process information during the seizure. If untreated, these seizures typically range from 10 to 100 or more per day, often occurring during difficult tasks or drowsiness. Some individuals with absence seizures describe their life as being like a movie with critical scenes cut out. Absence seizures must be distinguished from drowsiness, daydreaming, being engrossed in an activity (such as watching television or playing on the computer), and attention-deficit/hyperactivity disorder.

Myoclonic seizures are uncommon and appear as sudden jerks, usually involving the upper body and head and infrequently involving the extremities. Myoclonic seizures often occur with other types of seizures and are a sign of significant abnormalities of brain function; unlike other seizure types, mental retardation is common in people with myoclonic seizures. When these seizures occur in clusters in young infants and in the presence of a particular brain electrical pattern called *hypsarrthymia,* they are called *infantile spasms.* If myoclonic seizures occur in isolation and without background abnormalities shown on an EEG (electroencephalogram), then the disorder may not require therapy. Usual infant behavior such as jerks while falling asleep, sudden movements during sleep, and startle reflexes, none of which are linked to EEG abnormalities, can seem to resemble myoclonic seizures.

Other seizure types exist but are sufficiently rare that they are beyond the scope of this chapter. Your child, however, could have more than one seizure type. This is important to note because treatment for one type of seizure does not protect against all types. Also, a mixed seizure pattern suggests a more severe brain abnormality and a poorer prognosis both for treatment and cognitive outcome.

DIAGNOSIS

The diagnosis of a specific seizure type depends on an accurate description of the behavior during an episode. Seizures have a sudden beginning, followed by the development of specific signs and symptoms during the event, and an abrupt ending. These signs reflect changes in brain electricity. They start with an excessively synchronous discharge in one area, spread to other brain regions, and then turn off.

Although it is difficult to be an objective observer of a seizure when your child appears to be in acute danger, attention to details is important. You should note whether your child is awake or asleep at the onset of the event. Was there a provoking event (such as watching cartoons or prolonged physical exercise), or did you notice "automatic" behaviors (such as repetitive buttoning or eyelid fluttering) and changes in consciousness (no response to being called by name, being pinched, or being shaken) when the seizure began?

An assessment of brain electricity can be made with an EEG. This test can identify the presence of a population of neurons that are generating abnormal electricity. The belief is that these neurons are capable of producing seizure activity under the right conditions. The EEG is performed by pasting electrodes (electronic contacts) to the scalp, amplifying brain-generated electrical signals, and recording these onto paper, a computer disk, or a videocassette. The recording provides a sampling of electricity over multiple areas of the brain during both wakefulness and sleep. The EEG allows for an assessment of overall brain wave activities, as well as the detection of abnormal signals (shown by spikes and sharp waves) associated with seizures. Because seizures are most likely to occur between sleep and waking, you may be asked to keep your child awake most of the preceding night and/or to allow him or her to be given a sedative such as chloral hydrate to ensure a sleep period during the testing. It is standard practice to flash a bright light and to have your child breathe rapidly to bring out other electrical abnormalities linked with specific seizure types.

The EEG is an imperfect tool for identifying whether a "spell" is a seizure. For the test to be most useful, the abnormal electrical signals must match the behavior that the doctor is concerned about. Furthermore, a normal EEG does not necessarily rule out a seizure disorder, and an abnormal EEG may not mean epilepsy. For example, complex partial seizures frequently have their focus deep within the brain, so the EEG may be normal because of the long distance the abnormal electrical signal must travel to reach the surface of the skull, where it can be detected. Frequently occurring spells can be clarified by capturing the event during prolonged (overnight or 24-hour) EEG recordings with or without simultaneous videotaping. In circumstances in which the exact localization of the seizure focus must be identified, such as during evaluation for possible surgery, a video EEG is mandatory.

Although the EEG is useful in defining the nature of a seizure, it does not always explain why the seizure occurred at a particular moment or whether it indicates an underlying brain disorder. When your child has a first seizure or if your child with epilepsy has an increasing number of seizures or a change in the nature of seizures, your child's physician may recommend obtaining a brain imaging test such as a CT (computed tomography) or MRI (magnetic resonance imaging) scan to detect an underlying anatomic abnormality. In the presence of fever or under other special circumstances, a lumbar puncture (spinal tap) may be done to rule out an infection of the brain. Not every child with a first seizure needs all of these tests, but occasionally an extensive evaluation is required.

WHEN A SEIZURE OCCURS

There are actually only a few things you need to do and certain things you should not do when your child has a seizure. If your child is falling to the floor, try to break the fall and turn your child on his or her side so that if there is vomiting, he or she will not inhale it into the lungs, which could cause pneumonia. The seizure will almost always stop within a few minutes; however, if it lasts more than 10 minutes, you should call 911 so that your child can receive oxygen and be taken to an emergency room to receive intravenous medications to stop the seizure. Please do not attempt to restrain a limb from jerking, pry open and place anything in your child's mouth, or perform mouth-to-mouth resuscitation, as these efforts may lead to bitten fingers, loose teeth, and the most concerning complications, vomiting and aspiration of the stomach contents into the lungs.

If your child has a seizure disorder associated with frequent or prolonged convulsions that is difficult to control, you may be taught to give a rectal dose of Valium (diazepam) to stop the cluster or long seizures at home. Other Valium-like drugs can be placed under the tongue or given by injection. By administering these drugs, you may not need to take your child to the emergency room. You should, however, notify your child's doctor if you need to use this emergency medication because a change in the long-term medical solution may be needed.

If your child is at risk for seizures, certain preventive measures can be taken. One is controlling fevers that can stimulate seizure activity. Although Advil (ibuprofen) and Tylenol (acetaminophen) do not treat an underlying infection or seizure disorder, they will suppress the fever and its tendency to induce seizures. Another example is to help your child avoid excessive fatigue or emotional distress if these tend to increase the occurrence of seizures in your child.

USE OF ANTIEPILEPTIC MEDICATION

The standard treatment of epilepsy includes daily medication. It should be emphasized, however, that antiepileptic drugs do not cure seizure disorders, they only suppress seizure activity. The drugs may be so effective that seizures seem to all but disappear. In the past, doctors felt that once a person started taking seizure medication, he or she needed to continue taking it for life. Now, it is known that many individuals can discontinue medication following a period of stability. As your child matures, changes in gene expression result in the turning on or off of specific chemicals in the brain. This may explain why seizures first appear at one age and may disappear later in life. This concept of a dynamic brain makes sense given that we acknowledge that infants are different from toddlers (and that everyone acts differently from teenagers).

The goal of any therapeutic intervention is to use the best medication in the smallest dose possible so as to control seizures and minimize side effects. There are now many choices of medication, each with potential benefits and side effects. In deciding which medication your child will try, his or her doctor will consider the type of seizure, the age of your child, and the risks and benefits of specific medications. In considering side effects, it is helpful to remember that medications inhibit seizure activity by entering the brain to alter chemistry. These changes may affect other activities as well, producing sedation or hyperactivity, improved or worsened behavior, and so forth. Often these effects are dose related. Your child, however, may not need to live with side effects that extend beyond the first few days of starting a drug or following dosing increases because alternative therapies exist. Chapter 10 discusses various antiepileptic drugs that have been found to be useful in treating different seizure types, and these are listed in Table 10.8.

Recommended blood levels are available for many of the antiepileptic drugs to help your child avoid adverse effects. It is often difficult to predict, especially in children, the relationship between the dose swallowed and the amount of medication that actually reaches your child's bloodstream and ultimately the brain and other body organs. Ranges have been established regarding the amounts that are generally safe and effective for the various antiepileptic drugs. The doctor will usually want to check drug levels in your child's blood a few times a year or more frequently when the dosage is first started or changed. Some drugs can cause abnormalities in the function of certain other body organs, most commonly the bone marrow and liver. Therefore, a complete blood count (CBC) and liver function tests may be obtained together with the drug level to ensure that these organs are functioning properly.

For many years, few new antiepileptic drugs were developed, and there were few surprises regarding side effects because the drugs had been used by many patients for prolonged periods of time. These drugs included Dilantin (phenytoin) and Luminal (phenobarbital). They were not completely effective, especially against complex seizure disorders, and often had unpleasant side effects. They were supplemented by Carbatrol or Tegretol (carbamazepine), Depakene or Depakote (valproate), Zarontin (ethosuximide), and Klonopin (clonazepam), but many children had incomplete seizure control or experienced side effects. Since the mid-1990s, however, there has been an explosion of new drugs. The driving forces for the development of these novel drugs have been advances in our knowledge of brain chemistry and the ability of scientists to synthesize drugs that mimic these brain substances. These new medications include Lamictal (lamotrigine), Neurontin (gabapentin), Felbatol (felbamate), Topamax (topiramate), Gabatril (tiagabine), Trileptal (oxcarbazepine), and Keppra (levetiracetam). They are often very effective and appear to have fewer side effects. Because they have not been used for an extended period of time, however, their long-term impact and full range of side effects remain to be defined. In deciding whether to try one of these newer drugs, you, your child, and your child's doctor should keep in mind that newer does not necessarily mean better. The choice of which drug your child should receive will depend on the age of your child, the kind of seizure, and which side effects you and your child are willing to accept.

ALTERNATIVE THERAPIES

Alternative antiepileptic therapies are also available. Although they may sound "natural," they must also manipulate the chemistry of the brain to be effective in controlling your child's seizures. As a result, so-called natural substances are not always safer or more effective than manmade chemicals. The ketogenic diet that involves an intake of nutrients that reverses the normal ratio of fat to carbohydrate and protein is one example of a natural therapy that may be helpful in treating certain seizures. The diet appears to be beneficial not because of the large amount of fat but rather because of the severe restriction of carbohydrates and protein. The brain is forced to switch from one form of metabolism to another. Like antiepileptic drugs, the ketogenic diet does not cure epilepsy and requires that your child be seizure-free for a period of time before he or she can stop the diet. In terms of herbal and vitamin therapy, unless there is an underlying rare inborn error of metabolism that is responsive to vitamin supplementation, the therapies are unlikely to be effective in reducing the seizures.

SURGICAL TREATMENT OF SEIZURES

Surgical therapy is available for the most serious seizures. Surgery can be effective because of removal of the area where the seizures are starting, or it may alter the nature of the seizures so that they are less disruptive to your child and family. In the past, surgery has been the last resort because of the risks involved, because it is irreversible, and because it is hoped that the child with the most serious seizures might outgrow epilepsy. However, when the medications do not work, when there are too many side effects, or when your child's quality of life is unacceptable, surgery should be considered.

Surgical treatment for certain partial forms of epilepsy are often safe and curative if the specific region of the brain causing the seizures does not perform vital functions. This is most commonly done in cases of treatment-resistant temporal lobe epilepsy, with cure rates as high as 85%. A team consisting of a neurologist, neuropsychologist, psychiatrist, nurse, social worker, and neurosurgeon will typically review all that is known about your child and his or her seizure history. They will decide whether there are sufficient reasons to do the surgery and will assess the risks of any procedure. Parents and children must participate in the decision to go ahead with epilepsy surgery. The greatest concerns during the operation include rare bleeding and the need for transfusion, stroke from a damaged blood vessel, infection, and the possibility of the removal of the part of the brain necessary for sight and memory. If there are no problems during the procedure, however, your child might be able to go home in a matter of days to recuperate during the next month.

A new surgical procedure in which no tissue is removed is the insertion of a *vagal nerve stimulator*. An electrical probe is surgically placed in the neck directly upon the vagus nerve, which runs from the brain to the organs in the chest and belly. A battery is implanted under the skin, and electrical stimulation is provided to the nerve from time to time. How this procedure works and for which seizures it works best is still under investigation. About 30%–40% of individuals who undergo this procedure have at least a 50% reduction in their seizures, but a total elimination of seizures is rare. Periodic hoarseness, swallowing difficulties, and discomfort are common but usually tolerable consequences of the stimulator.

SAFETY ISSUES

Regardless of the interventions used to control the seizures, the goal is for your child to lead as typical a life as possible. Some activities, however, should be done in moderation. For example, college students who experience seizures should avoid "all-nighters" because sleep deprivation and the resulting daytime drowsiness may bring on seizures. Physical exhaustion may also precipitate a seizure. Certain activities are fine in certain instances and not in others. Diving is fine as long as your child's seizures are under control. Swimming is fine if supervised; play at heights, such as on a jungle gym, is probably not a good idea. Operating automobiles is legally permitted if seizures are under good control.

Check with your pharmacist for any interactions between other drugs and the antiepileptic medications prescribed for your child. All drugs affecting function of the central nervous system, such as antihistamines, should be used with caution, illicit drugs should never be used, and alcohol should be avoided. Generally, no particular dietary restrictions or nutritional supplements are required. In general, you can depend on your own common sense as to what activities should be restricted, but try to limit as little as possible.

CO-EXISTING DEVELOPMENTAL DISABILITIES

Because seizures are a sign of brain dysfunction, it is not surprising that epilepsy frequently occurs along with other disorders of brain cell function. In general, the greater the brain abnormality, the higher the risk for developing seizures. Mental retardation and cerebral palsy are both associated with seizures, and the risk is particularly high in children who have both of these developmental disabilities. In terms of acute medical conditions, if your child has a minor head trauma (as in a fall) the risk of developing a seizure disorder is low, even if a seizure follows the injury. If there has been a severe brain injury, however, such as in a car accident, your child's risk of developing a seizure disorder and having other developmental disabilities is higher.

Children with newly diagnosed epilepsy frequently may show subtle signs of school underachievement, learning difficulties, and behavior disturbances. These reflect preexisting brain dysfunction and are most evident when seizures are under poor control or when side effects of medication are present. Once the seizures are under control and the medication is adjusted properly, these symptoms often improve. Your child however, may have significant and persistent social and emotional problems relating to the embarrassment and isolation that seizures may cause.

Sheila and Simon

Sheila has simple febrile seizures. These are frequently genetic in origin and do not require extensive medical evaluation. The treatment usually involves aggressive management of the fever, but antiepileptic medications are rarely required. Studies have shown that children with this kind of seizure usually develop typically in elementary school regardless of the number of febrile seizures they experience during early childhood.

As part of the evaluation for his seizures, Simon had an EEG and MRI scan. The EEG showed a spike-and-wave pattern originating in the temporal lobe, and the MRI scan showed evidence of scarring of the temporal lobe, which often can be related to prior seizures. Simon's cognitive and behavior problems cannot be attributed simply to the epilepsy because they were present before the seizures recurred. Simon's seizures have been difficult to control medically, but he recently had surgery to remove the scarred region, which has resulted in marked improvement of his seizures. He now takes a single antiepileptic drug. His parents are more confident about his leaving the relative safety of the home with his seizures under good control, and Simon also seems to be gaining more confidence.

SUMMARY

Seizures are commonplace in children. When unprovoked and recurrent, they constitute epilepsy. Although frightening, they are rarely dangerous, but they may call attention to other cognitive and behavioral problems that the child is experiencing. Medications are available but should be used only when the risks of the seizures outweigh the side effects of the therapy. Treatable triggers should also be sought and addressed. A significant number of children will outgrow their epilepsy, especially if they have no other disabilities.

Some Questions Answered

If my child has had febrile seizures, does she have epilepsy?

Febrile seizures occur frequently in children younger than 5 years of age. They appear to happen when the fever rapidly peaks. The seizure is usually tonic-clonic and lasts less than 5 minutes. Although your child may have multiple provoked episodes, these do not qualify as epilepsy and she will probably outgrow the seizures before school entry. There is little reason to treat febrile convulsions with antiepileptic drugs unless they are very frequent.

Do seizures cause brain damage?

Assuming a seizure has not lasted for hours and that adequate care has been provided in the emergency room for a prolonged seizure, brain damage is unlikely to occur. If there are cognitive or behavior problems, it is more likely that an underlying brain disorder is the cause rather than the result of both the seizures and the associated disabilities. Another possibility is that side effects of the antiepileptic medications may be contributing to these problems.

How will my child's doctor choose an antiepileptic drug?

The drug is primarily chosen on the basis of the seizure type. Not all antiepileptic drugs work well with all seizure types. There are usually a number of drugs, however, to choose from that work equally well for a seizure type. The choice is based, then, on the doctor's previous experience with the drug, the cost of the drug, and the possible side effects.

When can my child stop taking seizure medication?

Whether and how long it will take for your child to "outgrow" a seizure disorder is unknown. But there is consensus that at least 2 years of no seizures is sufficient time to attempt weaning antiepileptic medications for most children. There is a greater risk of recurrence if the medication is stopped sooner. Yet, there seems to be little advantage in waiting longer than 2 years, as the outcome for remaining seizure free does not change that much after 2 years of no seizures.

Will I have to compromise between seizure control and side effects of medication for my child?

Hopefully your child will not have to continue taking seizure medication that produces severe side effects, but when the seizures are resistant to treatment, high doses or multiple medications may be needed. Both of these approaches increase the frequency of side effects that may interfere with your child's learning and behavior. Therefore, you may have to choose between complete control of seizures with side effects or partial control with fewer side effects. This choice is necessary with less than one quarter of children with seizure disorders.

Is everything that looks like a seizure really a seizure?

Actually there are a number of conditions that mimic seizures. Breathholding is the most common example in infants. When angry, frustrated, or in pain, a young child may cry and then hold his or her breath for up to a minute. There may be associated blueness of the lips, back arching, and loss of consciousness. The EEG, however, is normal, and a child grows out of this behavior by preschool age. Certain sleep disorders, such as night terrors, can also resemble a seizure. The child with this disorder awakens 1–3 hours after falling asleep, cries out, and appears disoriented. This episode only lasts a few minutes and ends with the child's returning to sleep. Again, the EEG is normal. Motor tics, which involve brief repetitive movements, can also mimic seizure activity. Your child may have facial twitching, head shaking, blinking, or shoulder shrugging, all of which resemble myoclonic seizures but, unlike seizures, are not associated with altered consciousness and can be voluntarily suppressed for a period of time. Finally, certain behavior disturbances can look like seizures. Uncontrolled rage and self-stimulatory or self-injurious behaviors can appear as complex partial seizures, but again there are no EEG abnormalities.

Cerebral Palsy

Louis Pellegrino

The brain goes through its most dramatic growth and development before birth and during early childhood; damage to the brain during these periods can cause a disorder called *cerebral palsy*. Cerebral palsy is formally defined as a nonprogressive motor impairment syndrome caused by a problem in the developing brain. If your child has cerebral palsy, his or her brain has difficulty controlling muscles and directing movement. Some disorders such as muscular dystrophy are caused by abnormalities of the muscles themselves, and some conditions such as polio are caused by disorders among the nerves running from the spinal cord to the muscles. Other conditions in which abnormalities of the spinal cord itself, such as spina bifida, cause dysfunction of muscles (see Chapter 17). In cerebral palsy, however, the brain itself rather than the muscle or spinal cord is the source of the motor dysfunction.

HOW COMMON IS CEREBRAL PALSY?

Cerebral palsy occurs in about 2 in 1,000 children. It is less common than attention-deficit/hyperactivity disorder, or ADHD (which occurs in 2–9 in 100 people), but much more common than many relatively rare but frequently discussed genetic, metabolic, and neurologic conditions. (For example, phenylketonuria, or PKU, a metabolic condition that is tested for in most state newborn screening programs, occurs in about 1 in 14,000 births). About half of children now diagnosed with cerebral palsy were born prematurely. The greater the prematurity, the greater the risk for developing cerebral palsy.

Etta

Etta, now 2 years old, was born prematurely. Her parents, concerned that she was not yet walking, took her to her pediatrician for an evaluation. In other areas, her development seemed to be on target. She began using single words at 12 months and now says about 100 words. She is starting to put words together into short phrases. She points to all of her body parts when asked and enjoys having tea parties with her dolls and stuffed animals. She uses a spoon and fork to feed herself and is showing some interest in toilet training.

Etta began crawling at 8 months but did not sit independently until 10 months. Her parents remember that it was hard for her to sit because her legs seemed "stiff" (increased muscle tone), and she couldn't seem to get them to stay under her in the sitting position. When she started to pull to stand at 15 months, her parents noticed that her legs always seemed to be extended and crossed or scissored and that she stayed up on her toes. She is now cruising but still has trouble bending at the knees and still toe walks.

Her pediatrician noticed these same characteristics and could not flex Etta's feet back past the flat position. Etta's knee-jerk reflex (a deep-tendon reflex, tested by tapping on a muscle tendon with a rubber hammer) was exaggerated, and her legs began to tremble (called *clonus*). The doctor also noticed that her right eye had a tendency to turn inward, giving her a crossed-eye appearance (called *strabismus*).

Etta's cognitive and social development seems to be appropriate for her age and does not point to a larger pattern of developmental delays (known as *global developmental delay*) associated with mental retardation. Her pediatrician confirmed her parents' impression that Etta's legs are very stiff (or *hypertonic*). In addition, the increased deep-tendon reflexes and clonus suggests that Etta has a specific kind of hypertonia known as *spasticity*. Sometimes, most of the muscles are involved, but often only some of the muscles (in Etta's case, the muscles of the legs) are affected. Etta's parents also report that their daughter can use a spoon and fork with some difficulty but prefers to finger-feed. She also dislikes playing with crayons and puzzles because of difficulties with fine motor coordination. The pediatrician reexamined Etta's arms and found that although her muscle tone was normal, the deep-tendon reflexes in her arms were a bit brisk. This suggests that Etta has motor control problems in the arms that are similar to but much less severe than those in the legs. This would be unusual for most spinal cord problems, which tend to involve the lower parts of the spine and do not usually affect arm function. Etta's pediatrician feels comfortable that she meets most of the criteria for cerebral palsy.

CAUSES OF CEREBRAL PALSY

Cerebral palsy, like other developmental disabilities, has more than one cause. It is convenient to classify some of these causes based on whether the onset was before birth (prenatal), around the time of birth (perinatal), or during the early years after birth (postnatal). It is particularly important to note that birth injury is thought to be the cause of cerebral palsy in only about 10% of individuals. Most of the time, prenatal factors are the cause of cerebral palsy.

TYPES OF CEREBRAL PALSY

Over the years, doctors have developed a number of different classification systems to help define the subtypes of cerebral palsy (see Figure 19.1). Although all people with cerebral palsy have a primary problem with control of motor function, different brain regions may be involved, producing different patterns of motor impairment. For the purposes of this chapter, three primary types of cerebral palsy are defined: spastic, dyskinetic, and ataxic.

Spastic Cerebral Palsy

Spastic cerebral palsy is the most common subtype, representing 70%–80% of all occurrences of cerebral palsy. It is also the subtype most often associated with prematurity. One of the most characteristic features of spastic cerebral palsy is that it often affects one region of the body more than another. If your child has *spastic diplegia,* the legs are mainly involved. If *spastic hemiplegia* is diagnosed, only one side of your child's body is involved. If *spastic quadriplegia* is diagnosed, the entire body (including all four limbs) is affected. Spastic cerebral palsy is also characterized by tightness of affected muscle groups (*hypertonicity*) that is usually associated with briskly increased *deep tendon reflexes* (such as the well-known knee-jerk response). Because specific muscle groups tend to remain consistently tight in an individual over time, accumulated stresses across specific joints tend to be more problematic for a person with spastic cerebral palsy than a person with another subtype. As a result, if

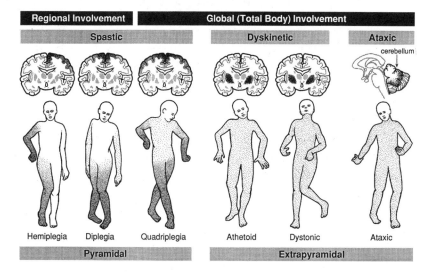

Figure 19.1.   How types of cerebral palsy are classified. Overlaps in terminology used are shown. For spastic subtypes, signals from the *cortex* of the brain are disrupted. For dyskinetic subtypes, deep brain structures called the *basal ganglia* are involved. For ataxic cerebral palsy, the *cerebellum* is involved.

your child has spastic cerebral palsy, he or she is more likely to have dislocations and contractures requiring orthopedic intervention such as surgery (discussed later in this chapter).

Dyskinetic Cerebral Palsy

Although spastic cerebral palsy can sometimes involve the entire body, dyskinetic cerebral palsy always does. *Dyskinetic cerebral palsy* represents about 15%–20% of all occurrences of cerebral palsy. If your child has this form of cerebral palsy, on different days or even at different times of the day, his or her muscles will alternate between feeling loose (hypotonic) and rigid (hypertonic). In some cases, this form of cerebral palsy is associated with involuntary or dyskinetic movements. When a person has rapid, jerky movements or slow, writhing movements (together known as *choreoathetosis*), then he or she has *athetoid cerebral palsy*. When a person has unusual posturing of the head, trunk and limbs, then he or she has *dystonic cerebral palsy*. The various forms of dyskinetic cerebral palsy have been especially associated with hypoxia during birth (lack of oxygen) and more recently with certain birth defects (inborn errors of metabolism).

Ataxic Cerebral Palsy

Ataxic cerebral palsy affects only about 5% of all individuals with cerebral palsy and is characterized by problems with voluntary movement. If your child has this diagnosis, he or she may experience problems with balance, the timing of movements, and tremor of the limbs (especially the hands) during voluntary movements. Ataxic cerebral palsy is thought to be linked with problems with the part of the motor control system that is centered in the cerebellum (see Figure 19.1) and has also been associated with a number of genetic syndromes.

Mixed Cerebral Palsy

Children who have severe brain injury, such as from head trauma or an anoxic (lack of oxygen) episode may have signs both of spastic and dyskinetic cerebral palsy; the type of cerebral palsy they have is called *mixed cerebral palsy*. This form of the disorder usually has the least favorable prognosis in terms of the development of functional motor skills such as sitting independently, crawling, walking, or reaching.

IMPAIRMENTS AND MEDICAL
PROBLEMS ASSOCIATED WITH CEREBRAL PALSY

Although cerebral palsy is defined strictly in terms of motor impairments and functional mobility, it is frequently associated with other developmental and medical problems. More than half of children with cerebral palsy also have associated impairments that can limit potential if unrecognized or untreated. These concerns range from cognitive and sensory impairments to seizures and nutritional issues.

Cognitive Impairments

About half of children with cerebral palsy also have mental retardation. Those who do not have mental retardation may have milder cognitive impairments, including learning disabilities.

Vision and Hearing Impairments

If your child has cerebral palsy, he or she may experience some associated visual problems. Etta's pediatrician had noted that one of her eyes turned in. This is called *esotropia*. When an eye turns out, the condition is called *exotropia* (see Chapter 22). *Strabismus* is the general term used to describe these imbalances of the muscles controlling eye movements. When one eye has difficulty focusing, the other eye tends to become dominant, as the brain gradually loses the ability to interpret information from the affected eye. Permanent vision loss can result from this imbalance, in a condition known as *amblyopia*. Amblyopia can be prevented, either by the use of a patch to wear over the unaffected eye (to force the "weak" eye to focus) or by surgery to correct the strabismus.

Children with cerebral palsy have an increased incidence of nearsightedness (*myopia*), problems with the retina resulting from retinopathy of prematurity (an eye condition often found in premature babies) and leading to visual impairments or blindness (see Chapter 5), and visual field defects (loss of vision in segments of the visual field). Given the many visual problems associated with cerebral palsy, it is important that your child have an ophthalmologic evaluation. After this initial evaluation, even if no problems are found, it is recommended that testing be done at frequent intervals.

Children with cerebral palsy are also at increased risk for hearing loss. Even severe hearing loss may not be recognized until 2–3 years of age because of the focus on the motor impairment. Your child should have a formal audiological assessment in infancy, with regular retesting after that. Various hearing tests are available, so it is possible to test hearing in all children regardless of age or developmental status (see Chapter 20). Even modest sensory impairment can significantly influence your child's ability to communicate or walk, adding to the problems of the cerebral palsy itself.

Seizure Disorders

Many children with cerebral palsy, especially those with more severe forms, are prone to the development of a seizure disorder (epilepsy; see Chapter 18), so you should watch for seizures. If you suspect that your child has had a seizure, a pediatric neurologist should examine your child. Seizures are usually treatable with antiepileptic drugs, but a brain wave test (EEG, or electroencephalogram) will be performed to diagnose the condition, and then treatment decisions can be made.

Gastrointestinal and Nutritional Problems

Many children with cerebral palsy don't grow as much as other children. The most common reason for poor growth is inadequate nutrition. Your child with cerebral palsy may not get enough to eat for several reasons. He or she may have trouble controlling the muscles involved with chewing and swallowing (see Chapter 7). Feeding is thus a slow, labored, inefficient process, so it is difficult to ensure that your child has taken in adequate calories. Children with cerebral palsy also have difficulty with the transport of food from the esophagus, to the stomach, to the intestines. A particular issue is the backing up of stomach contents into the esophagus, known as *gastroesophageal reflux (GER)*. Chronic regurgitation of acidic stomach contents into the esophagus leads to irritation, inflammation, and eventual scarring of the lining of the esophagus. Eating food tends to aggravate these symptoms, so children with GER often eat less.

Another gastrointestinal problem your child may experience is constipation. In addition to toileting and hygiene difficulties caused by constipation, the condition frequently reduces your child's appetite, further aggravating nutritional difficulties. Varied approaches to constipation and other nutritional problems, such as medications, dietary changes, and behavior management techniques, are discussed in Chapter 7.

Respiratory Problems

Your child may be prone to respiratory problems related to control of the upper airway. The *upper airway* includes the nasal passage, the mouth, the back of the throat (*pharynx*), the voice box (*larynx*), and the windpipe (*trachea*). As mentioned previously, many children with cerebral palsy have swallowing difficulties. This occasionally means that food is misrouted "down the wrong pipe" into the larynx and trachea and thereby into the lungs. This is called *aspiration*. Aspiration makes the small airways and lungs inflamed and can lead to lung infection, or *pneumonia*. You can often prevent aspiration by modifying food texture and by having your child positioned certain ways during feeding. If aspiration becomes a major issue, however, it may be necessary to stop oral feedings. In this case a feeding tube may be placed (see Chapter 7) through which liquid formula or food is given to your child.

Other Medical Problems

Children with cerebral palsy occasionally have trouble with urinary function and bladder infections due to a condition known as *spastic bladder*. Because of abnormal tightness in the special muscle tissue that composes the wall of the bladder, the bladder cannot fill properly, and your child's control of urination is impaired. Your child's doctor may consult with a urologist when this condition is suspected. It can usually be treated medically, without surgery.

Because of their decreased mobility, children with cerebral palsy are also at risk for skin sores. A sore begins with skin irritation followed by breakdown of tissue, especially at "pressure points" over a bony prominence such as the base of the spine. Severe skin breakdown results in *decubitus ulcers,* which may become infected and sometimes require hospitalization and surgery. Prevention is better than treatment. Encourage your child to move around. If your child is immobile, turn him or her at regular intervals, including at night. You can use a sheepskin or corrugated mattress to help reduce pressure on your child's body, and you should avoid having your child sit in a wheelchair for prolonged periods. The best treatment for such sores is relief of pressure and careful wound care. A daily check for small scrapes and cuts is also crucial (see the section called Skin Problems in Chapter 17).

ENSURING THE BEST QUALITY OF LIFE FOR YOUR CHILD WITH CEREBRAL PALSY

To enhance your child's quality of life, you can strive to help him or her gain independence in three areas: communication, daily living, and mobility.

Communication Skills

Communication skills are fundamental to all social interactions and are the basis for participation in society. Although some children with cerebral palsy are nonverbal because of severe cognitive impairment, many are nonverbal due to difficulties with the motor control required for speech. Other individuals may have specific problems with language development itself—such as understanding or using words—that impede communication. An array of technologies has been developed to promote nonverbal communication. These technologies and services are referred to collectively as *augmentative and alternative communication (AAC)* (see Chapter 21). Both traditional speech-language therapy and AAC techniques are best applied to achieve well-defined functional goals, and should be integrated into your child's individualized education program (see Chapter 12).

Daily Living Skills

Daily living skills (also known as *activities of daily living*) are the skills your child needs for independence in the areas of feeding, dressing, toileting, and personal hygiene (see Chapter 9). Both cognitive and motor processes are involved in these daily activities. The *occupational therapist (OT)* is the professional most likely to work on these skills with your child. Because most daily living skills require the use of arms and hands, the occupational therapist also works directly on improving your child's upper extremity function. Occupational therapists, as their name implies, also provide services aimed at improving competence and independence with work-related skills and activities.

Occupational therapists are often the ones who identify adaptive equipment that your child might use. *Adaptive equipment* includes a wide variety of devices such as specialized utensils, toys, and positioning devices that allow a person to perform a skill or carry out a task that he or she otherwise would not be capable of or would have great difficulty doing (see Figure 9.2 in Chapter 9). In recent years, *assistive technology* has grown dramatically, providing new methods (in addition to those offered by traditional adaptive equipment) for extending independence with daily living skills via the use of microcomputers and related electronic devices.

Mobility Skills

Because cerebral palsy is most directly associated with impairments of functional mobility, interventions aimed at improving mobility have received particular attention. The *physical therapist (PT)* is the professional most directly involved in this aspect of care. For some children, the primary goal of therapy is to walk (or *ambulate*) as independently as possible. But for many children, walking may not be the most effective means of locomotion, and alternative methods are provided.

Several types of devices are available to assist your child in gaining mobility. *Orthotics* represent a variety of splints and braces that provide structural and functional support to the limbs and trunk. The most commonly used brace for children with cerebral palsy is the *molded ankle-foot orthosis (MAFO)* (see Figure 9.2 in Chapter 9). The MAFO can be designed either to provide for proper positioning of the foot or to directly improve walking.

Crutches, walkers, and wheelchairs are types of adaptive equipment used to enhance functional mobility (see Figure 9.3 in Chapter 9). Many children with cerebral palsy may use a combination of these devices, either simultaneously or in sequence, at different times during their lives. The power wheelchair is especially helpful for children with severe motor impairments but who have relatively mild cognitive impairments.

Interventions for Etta

Etta's intervention plan emphasized helping her with walking. Following the initial diagnosis of cerebral palsy, Etta's pediatrician referred her to an early intervention program and to a pediatric orthopedic surgeon. Etta was assigned a physical therapist, who met twice weekly with Etta and her parents at home. Because Etta was already walking, a primary goal of therapy was to improve the quality and stability of her gait. The therapist believed that Etta would walk better if she could get her feet "down flat" more consistently (reducing her tendency to "toe walk"). The therapist suggested that Etta would benefit from MAFOs.

The pediatric orthopedic surgeon obtained X rays and found no sign of either a hip dislocation or spinal curvature (scoliosis). Etta was found to have moderately severe spasticity of the legs, especially at the ankles. The surgeon noted that it would be possible with some effort to stretch Etta's calf muscles so that her feet could move through their full range of motion. The surgeon explained that MAFOs could help keep Etta's feet in a neutral position, thereby encouraging walking. MAFOs could also help prevent or slow the development of contractures (permanent shortening of muscles so that they can no longer be stretched). The surgeon indicated that Etta might require other interventions if she began to develop contractures.

The surgeon also suggested that Etta might benefit from the use of forearm crutches during therapy. After some initial resistance, Etta adapted to her orthotics and crutches very nicely and was soon able to walk for short distances on her own. The family soon discovered that Etta became exhausted when using the crutches for long distances (such as going to the park or shopping at the mall), so the physical therapist measured Etta for a manual (self-propelled) wheelchair to be used for longer distances.

MEDICAL AND SURGICAL INTERVENTIONS THAT HELP IMPROVE CHILDREN'S FUNCTIONAL SKILLS

The medical and surgical interventions that exist to help counteract the motor impairments associated with cerebral palsy focus almost exclusively on the treatment of spasticity and its consequences. In general, therapies available to address the motor impairments associated with dyskinetic and ataxic cerebral palsy such as involuntary movements or problems with balance have been disappointing.

Physical Therapy

If your child has spasticity, he or she may undergo hands-on physical therapy, splinting, and casting to help stretch muscles to prevent contractures. These interventions, however, have only a temporary effect on the spasticity itself. Exercise of affected muscles also seems to reduce spasticity, but again the effects are temporary, not particularly dramatic, and have little effect on reducing spasticity.

Oral Medication

Several oral medications can reduce your child's spasticity. Valium (diazepam) is often used after orthopedic surgery to reduce spasticity and control muscle spasms. Its use on a long-term basis is limited due to problems with side effects—the medication tends to be sedating and to increase drooling.

Baclofen has similar effects to Valium, tends to be less sedating, but is more likely to cause vomiting. (If your child is taking baclofen, caution must be exercised in weaning your child from it because suddenly stopping baclofen can provoke seizures). Dantrium (dantrolene) acts directly on the muscle (as opposed to Valium and baclofen, which act on the central nervous system) to reduce spasticity but can in rare cases cause significant liver toxicity, so it must be used with great caution.

Other oral medications are becoming available for the treatment of spasticity but have not been well studied for use in children. In general, problems with the side effects of oral medications and a lack of clearly demonstrated improvements have limited their consistent use as a treatment for spasticity associated with cerebral palsy.

Intrathecal Medication

Special technologies have been developed to permit the direct administration of medication (usually baclofen) into the spinal fluid (*intrathecal* means *within the spinal canal*) (see Figure 19.2). Because the medication is administered directly to the spinal cord, much smaller doses are required than when the medication is taken by mouth and spread throughout the body. Spasticity may be reduced more dramatically, and there are usually fewer problems with sedation and other cognitive side effects. Because the pump that administers the baclofen is implanted inside the body, however, there is the risk of mechanical failure and infection. As of 2000, the use of intrathecal baclofen in children has not yet become widespread, although that could change as experience with the method increases and its safety in children is further documented.

Selective Dorsal Rhizotomy

Motor nerves emerging from the spinal cord carry impulses that cause muscle contraction and also regulate muscle tone. Sensory nerves move in the opposite direction, from muscles to spinal cord, completing a "feedback" loop that influences the output of impulses via the motor nerves. This feedback signal tends to cause an increase in muscle tone. The idea behind the surgical procedure known as *selective dorsal rhizotomy (SDR)* is that interrupting the feedback signal by carefully cutting selected sensory nerve roots can result in decreased spasticity. (*Selective* refers to the need to cut only the nerves that actually need to be cut, *dorsal* refers to technical name of the sensory nerves, *dorsal nerve roots*, and *rhizotomy* is the technical term for cutting a spinal nerve). A neurosurgeon performs the complex procedure. The advantage of SDR is that it permanently reduces spasticity in the legs (the arms are not usually affected by the procedure). It is difficult, however, to predict accurately which children will benefit most from the procedure, and there are

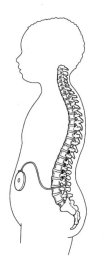

Figure 19.2.   Intrathecal baclofen. Baclofen is injected through the skin into a reservoir located within a pump placed surgically beneath the skin of the abdomen. The pump, which is about the size of a hockey puck, is programmable using a device placed against the skin and over the pump. Medication is continuously infused through a catheter that tunnels under the skin and into the spinal canal. Baclofen mixes with the spinal fluid that bathes the spinal cord, thus directly affecting the spinal cord and decreasing spasticity.

persistent controversies regarding whether the long-term benefits justify the surgery and the subsequent intensive physical therapy.

Botox Injections

It has been known for many years that injection of a nerve that goes to a spastic muscle with alcohol or phenol reduces the spasticity of that muscle for as long as 6 months. Because the procedure is difficult to perform and painful (sedation is usually required), however, its use has been limited in children.

Botox (Botulinum toxin type A) is a biological agent that binds directly to the microscopic junction of nerve on muscle. This binding prevents transmission of nerve impulses and decreasing spasticity in the injected muscle. The advantage of Botox over alcohol or phenol is that it is much easier to administer and is much less painful. Its effects last for 3–6 months (slightly less than with alcohol or phenol), and its main drawbacks are its expense and limitations on the total dose that can be used at any one time.

Botox is especially useful in situations in which a few individual spastic muscles are causing functional problems or in which temporary effects are needed. (By contrast, oral and intrathecal medications and selective dorsal rhizotomy affect multiple muscle groups.) For example, Botox is often used to help stretch a spastic muscle that cannot be stretched with physical therapy alone, thereby delaying the need for orthopedic surgery.

Orthopedic Surgery

If your child's muscles and tendons become permanently shortened due to long-term spasticity, interventions directed toward reducing spasticity alone are no longer adequate and your child may need surgery. The goals of orthopedic surgery can sometimes be accomplished by lengthening contracted muscles. In other cases, the point of insertion of muscle on the bone is changed to improve the movement of a limb. In still other instances, more extensive surgery is required to prevent degeneration of joints (as with hip dislocation) or to prevent impairment of heart/lung function (as with severe scoliosis).

SUMMARY

There is enormous variability in the degree of disability that may be associated with cerebral palsy. If your child has a mild form and mild cognitive impairments, he or she can function independently as an adult and will usually have a typical life span. If your child has a more severe form of cerebral palsy, he or she is likely to encounter more significant barriers to full independence and participation in society and may also face more complicated medical issues that can affect general health and longevity. There is hope in the fact that advances in medical care, improvements in educational and therapeutic interventions, and changes in societal attitudes toward people with disabilities are having a significant impact on improving outcomes for children with cerebral palsy.

Some Questions Answered

Is it possible to predict whether my child will eventually be able to walk?

Children with milder forms of cerebral palsy, such as spastic hemiplegia or spastic diplegia, are more likely to walk than are children with more severe forms of cerebral palsy, such as spastic quadriplegia. In general, children who sit without support by 2 years of age have a good prognosis for walking, whereas children who do not sit independently by 4 years of age have a poor prognosis for walking.

What is therapeutic electrical stimulation?

Low-intensity or therapeutic electrical stimulation (TES), administered at night while your child sleeps, is applied through an electrode placed on the skin surface over a weak muscle. Unlike the high-intensity electrical stimulation that has been used in adults with a variety of muscle disorders, TES does not cause muscles to contract. There is some evidence to suggest that TES may help some children with cerebral palsy improve motor skills (especially after SDR), but it is not known whether TES can help children in other situations. TES can cause a tingling sensation but is rarely uncomfortable; however, high-intensity electrical stimulation can be uncomfortable and is not recommended for children.

Do children with significant spasticity burn more calories than other children?

Many children with cerebral palsy have trouble gaining weight. Some have suggested that spastic muscles contribute to a higher metabolic rate; in other words, it has been suggested that children with cerebral palsy burn more calories than other children. This, however, does not appear to be the case. In fact, children with cerebral palsy actually tend to burn *fewer* calories than other children do probably because of diminished mobility. The most common reason for poor weight gain is insufficient calorie intake.

Hearing Loss

Annie Steinberg and Lisa J. Bain

One of the most amazing aspects of development during the first 3 years of life is your growing child's capacity to take in what he or she hears and, from that, develop a complex speech system. During this time, we use words to soothe, stimulate, and teach our children. If your child has a severe hearing loss, you may not have an intuitive sense of how to communicate with him or her, and the resulting barriers to communication can affect every aspect of your family's life. Yet, hearing loss is often hard to recognize in young children; it has been referred to as the "invisible disability." It cannot be seen and seldom causes physical pain. In addition, infants and young children cannot tell us that they are unable to hear. Further confusion results because babies who are born with a hearing impairment often startle normally at loud sounds and may even babble for a period.

In the United States, about 1 million children younger than age 18 have a permanent hearing loss. About one third of children with a hearing loss also have other disabilities, including attention-deficit/hyperactivity disorder, autism, or mental retardation. When hearing loss is combined with other disabilities, it further impairs the child's ability to function. And the presence of these associated disabilities requires special consideration in planning interventions.

This chapter provides information regarding hearing loss and the choices you need to consider as your child grows. This is likely only one of many sources you will explore. You should seek information not only from books, the internet, and professionals but also from other parents and individuals who have hearing impairments.

Sandra

Though at birth she appeared healthy, only an hour later Sandra turned blue and was whisked off to the neonatal intensive care unit, where she was found to have a congenital heart defect. Within days, she was found to have a spinal deformity and two fused ribs, suggesting a genetic syndrome. Although she passed a newborn hearing screen, her mother worried as Sandra did not react to loud noises such as the doorbell. When Sandra was 7 months old, after several bouts of ear infections, an auditory brainstem response hearing test, or ABR, was performed and revealed a profound hearing loss that could not be attributed to the infections. While trying to deal with their shock and grief, Sandra's parents also began to search for appropriate interventions. They learned about the benefits of hearing aids and the possibility of the surgical placement of a cochlear implant to restore a portion of Sandra's hearing. Two weeks later, a brain imaging study showed that Sandra lacked fully formed cochleas. Not only was an implant out of the question, but there also was no usable hearing to enhance. Sandra would not be able to use hearing aids.

After getting over this further shock, Sandra's parents focused on how she would learn to function in the world. Visiting a school for the deaf and talking to other parents relieved their concerns and gave them important information and support. They saw deaf children playing together, signing with teachers, and participating in a variety of activities. The family enrolled in the parent–infant program at the school and began to learn sign language.

At 28 months of age, Sandra already knows more than 80 signs and communicates with her parents at a level of a typical 2-year-old. Some neighbors and their children have also learned basic signing so that they can communicate with Sandra. She receives speech-language therapy twice per week at school and shows interest in learning to speak. Her heart condition has stabilized, and she has needed surgery only to remove her adenoids and to place tubes in her ears. She receives physical therapy for her low muscle tone, and her motor skills continue to improve.

HOW WE HEAR

The hearing system is complex, beginning at the ear and ending in the brain (see Figure 20.1). The peripheral auditory system is divided into the external, middle, and inner ear; the central hearing system includes the auditory nerve and the pathway to the brain where sound is ultimately interpreted and understood. In humans, the auricle (external ear) is the least important structure in hearing. The ear canal is a small tunnel about 1 inch long, with the eardrum located at the end. The ear canal protects the delicate structures of the middle and inner ear, and its walls contain glands that produce earwax, which helps keep dirt and other debris from reaching the eardrum. The ear canal also channels and increases the intensity of sound at the eardrum.

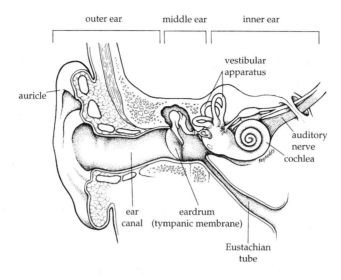

Figure 20.1.   The ear. The outer ear includes the auricle, the ear canal, and the eardrum. The middle ear contains three small bones that serve as a bridge between the eardrum, the inner ear, and the Eustachian tube, which connects the middle ear to the back of the throat. The inner ear includes the cochlea, the sensory organ for hearing, the auditory nerve, which carries hearing impulses to the brain, and the vestibular apparatus, which controls balance.

As sound waves move through the ear canal, they cause the eardrum, or tympanic membrane, to vibrate, setting the bones of the middle ear into motion. The sound is then transmitted into the inner ear, which contains the cochlea, the organ of hearing, and the vestibular system, the organ of balance. Within the cochlea are rows of more than 20,000 delicate hair cells that are connected to nerve fibers within the auditory nerve. These hair cells are thought to pick up mechanical vibrations from the middle ear bones, convert them into electrical energy via the release of chemical signals, and transfer them to the auditory nerve cells, which carry impulses to the brain. In the auditory cortex in the brain, these nerve impulses are combined with other sensory information and memory to allow perception and interpretation.

When we hear sound we are actually interpreting wavelike patterns of air molecules (see Figure 20.2). Frequency, measured in hertz (Hz), is perceived as sound pitch, whereas amplitude or intensity, measured in decibels (dB), represents the loudness of a sound. In speech, as in music, there are sounds with both high and low frequencies blended together. Although we can hear sounds with frequencies between 20 and 20,000 Hz, the most important sounds that occur in day-to-day listening have frequencies between 250 and 6,000 Hz. Vowel sounds such as "u" have a low frequency (250–1,000 Hz) and are usually easier to hear while consonants such as "f," "h," and "s" have higher frequencies (1,500–6,000 Hz) and are more difficult to detect.

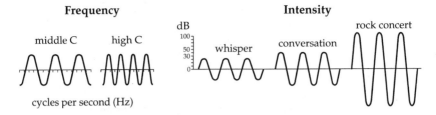

Figure 20.2. Frequency and intensity of sound waves. The pitch of a sound, or its frequency, is expressed as cycles per second, or hertz (Hz). Middle C is 256 Hz; one octave above is 512 Hz. Intensity of sound is expressed as decibels (dB) and varies from a whisper at 30 dB to a rock music concert at 100 dB or more.

Unfortunately, the consonant sounds convey more than 90% of the meaning in conventional speech. In addition, typical speech varies tremendously in intensity, so understanding speech can be challenging for an individual with a specific frequency loss. For example, a person with hearing loss that predominantly affects high-frequency sounds hears only the low-frequency (vowel) parts of words, so interpreting conversation is difficult.

A person with typical hearing can detect sounds ranging from 0 to 140 dB. The softest audible sounds are usually defined as 0 dB, whispers are 30 dB, a typical conversation is 45–50 dB, and a rock concert can be as loud as 110 dB (see Figure 20.2). Sound louder than 90 dB is uncomfortably loud, and by the time it reaches 120 dB (such as a chainsaw), it is painful and can lead to temporary hearing loss.

TYPES AND CAUSES OF HEARING LOSSES

A defect anywhere along the hearing pathway results in hearing loss. Hearing impairment caused by interference in the transmission of sound from the outer to the inner ear is called a *conductive hearing loss.* When hearing loss results from malfunction of the cochlea or auditory nerve, it is called a *sensorineural hearing loss.* A person can also have a mixed hearing loss with both conductive and sensorineural elements. *Central auditory dysfunction* results from an abnormality anywhere along the pathway from the inner ear to the auditory brain region. Hearing loss may affect one ear (unilateral loss) or both ears (bilateral loss). Sometimes hearing loss worsens over time, in which case it is called a *progressive hearing loss.*

The most common type of hearing loss is a mild conductive loss resulting from fluid accumulation in the middle ear during an infection. Most children have multiple bouts of middle-ear infections (otitis media) during their preschool years. Although these infections sometimes have no symptoms, many young children become irritable, develop fevers, pull at their outer ear, and sometimes stumble with impaired balance. A quick examination by your child's pediatrician can usually detect fluid collection or pus behind the eardrum. Treatment with antibiotics is often necessary and is generally successful. Your child may have a conductive hearing loss during the infection, but the loss usually improves within weeks. Your child's doctor may want to recheck the ear and do a follow-up hearing test. Recurrent infections may require the temporary surgical placement of tubes through your child's eardrum to permit drainage from the middle ear. Most conductive impairments are mild, temporary, and do not cause a substantial threat to your child's overall language development as long as the problem is identified early and prompt medical attention is obtained. Even if the conductive impairment cannot be completely corrected, hearing aids and special instruction often allow children to function typically.

Sensorineural hearing loss can be caused by infection during pregnancy. The classic example, now preventable by a vaccine, is German measles or rubella. A mother who contracts German measles during the first trimester of pregnancy has about a 30% risk of bearing an infant with a severe hearing loss. These infants also have congenital heart defects, visual impairment, and other developmental disabilities. The risk that rubella and certain other viral infections will cause hearing loss is highest when infection occurs during the first trimester of pregnancy, when the auditory system is developing in the fetus. Although rubella has been conquered by a vaccine, it has been replaced as a significant cause of a progressive sensorineural hearing loss by cytomegalovirus, a generally asymptomatic viral infection in women that can be passed from mother to fetus. A vaccine is under development for this infection as well.

An inner-ear hearing loss can also result from toxicity of medications including the antibiotic gentamicin and the chemotherapy agent cisplatin. Complications of premature birth, such as oxygen deprivation or hyperbilirubinemia (jaundice), and infections in infancy and childhood, such as bacterial meningitis, may also result in damage to the inner ear as well as brain damage (see Chapter 5 for more on the complications of prematurity). Mumps can result in unilateral hearing loss, whereas bilateral hearing loss can occur after measles and chickenpox. Finally, there are hereditary causes of hearing loss as in the case of Sandra. Genetic or hereditary causes of deafness occur in approximately 1 in 2,000 to 1 in 6,000 children, and more than 70 known inherited syndromes are associated with deafness. Even so, for approximately one third of children with sensorineural deafness, the cause is not known.

Finally, central auditory dysfunction, the least common form of functional hearing loss, may result from brain damage, such as from birth trauma. This can gradually improve over time as the brain "heals." The location and nature of the problem in the auditory pathway determines the degree and type of hearing loss. Yet, functional hearing among individuals with the same problem may be different.

Children with similar hearing losses may develop different receptive (receipt of) and expressive (production of) language capabilities. This results from many factors, most important of which is the age of the child when the hearing loss occurred. Losses occurring prior to 2 years of age, during the period of most rapid development of language, present the greatest challenge to the child in terms of developing speech.

TERMINOLOGY

Professionals have some disagreement regarding the basic terminology in describing hearing loss. Most audiologists use the term *deaf* to mean individuals whose hearing loss is in the profound range (hearing only sounds louder than 90 dB). By this definition, a person with less severe losses would be called *hearing impaired* or *hard of hearing*. Other professionals, however, use the term *deaf* to describe any individual with a hearing impairment who does not benefit from the use of hearing aids and/or who uses sign language or alternate forms of communication (regardless of the degree of hearing loss). In this chapter, the terms *hearing impaired* and *deaf* are used interchangeably to refer to all children with significant hearing loss. In addition, there is no consensus regarding the criteria for grading the severity of the loss. Because categories such as *mild* or *profound* may not actually reflect ultimate functional hearing, this chapter does not focus on these terms.

When a hearing loss is present at birth, it is described as *congenital*. As noted previously, this loss may be hereditary but could be environmental (such as due to a maternal infection). Similarly, many hearing losses occur as a result of a hereditary condition but are not evident until after the child is several years old. These can be considered congenital in nature, as the hereditary defect was present before birth. There can be significant confusion about the terminology.

IDENTIFICATION OF HEARING LOSS

You as a parent are usually the first to suspect a hearing loss, yet there may be a considerable delay between the first time you voice your concern and the diagnosis of the loss. This delay is in part because the hearing loss is "silent"; it is not accompanied by typical signs of disease such as fever, pain, or physical abnormalities. Furthermore, when children have other developmental disabilities, the delay in recognition of the hearing loss is often greater because there may be fewer expectations of and demands for verbal communication from the child. Early signs of hearing loss include not awakening to loud noises, delayed babbling, little experimentation with vocalization, and reduced response to parents' voices. Because it is difficult to rely on usual language milestones in a child with other developmental delays, a hearing screening is of even greater importance for such a child.

Hearing loss should be identified as early as possible. This may permit treatment of an underlying cause and early intervention, including amplification, speech-language therapy, parental counseling, and surgery, if appropriate. This gives your child the best opportunity to use residual hearing and stimulate brain pathways to develop speech and language skills during the critical early stages of brain development. The National Institutes of Health (NIH) has recommended that all infants be screened for hearing loss within the first 3 months of life. It is especially crucial that a child be tested for hearing loss if he or she has any risk factors, such as prematurity or other birth complications, congenital malformations of the head and neck, a family history of hearing loss, prenatal infection, or meningitis. Infant hearing screening is quick and inexpensive and does not cause discomfort. If the initial screen indicates a possible problem, your child will be referred for additional testing. Many children fail the initial screen but turn out to have typical hearing when given a more formal hearing test.

SIGNS OF HEARING LOSS

As your child grows, you can watch for signs that suggest a hearing loss. Between birth and 4 months of age, a hearing child will awaken momentarily when you talk loudly while the child is asleep, whereas a child with a hearing loss may not. As mentioned previously, however, even children with a significant hearing loss may startle momentarily to a loud noise.

The talking behavior of a baby may also reveal clues about hearing ability. Between 4 and 6 months of age, most children babble. A deaf child, however, stops babbling by around 9 months of age and may be silent thereafter. By 5–7 months of age a child with typical hearing should turn consistently toward a voice and begins imitating sounds made by adults and other children. The child with a hearing loss does neither. Children with mental retardation who have typical hearing also have delays in achieving these language milestones; however, all of their skills are similarly delayed, whereas children with hearing loss have much slower development in language than in other skills.

HEARING TESTING

A hearing assessment should address three questions: Is there a hearing loss? If yes, what is the severity of the hearing loss? Finally, what is the type of hearing loss—conductive, sensorineural, or mixed? The results of the assessment can also be used to compare the hearing of one ear with that of the other ear and can determine the "shape" of the hearing loss; that is, whether hearing is better at some sound frequencies. Infant hearing tests can determine if your child's hearing is impaired but cannot accurately predict the degree and type of hearing loss. In children older than 6 months of age, more precise information can be gathered about each ear and about the shape of the hearing loss.

The audiologist who tests your child's hearing may use one or more of several different methods. Two commonly used tests are the evoked otoacoustic emissions (EOAE) test and the more sensitive auditory brainstem response (ABR) test. These tests do not require active participation, and the infant must be still, such as while asleep or under sedation. The EOAE test assesses cochlear function by introducing a series of clicks or tones into your child's ear. A functioning cochlea generates a low-level sound in response to this stimulus; the absence of a cochlear response indicates the possibility of a hearing loss. The ABR test (also known as brainstem auditory evoked response, or BAER) assesses the cochlea as well as the pathway from the auditory nerve to the brain. In this test, EEG (electroencephalogram) electrodes are pasted to your child's forehead and tones or clicks of varying intensity are presented to each ear individually through headphones. The electrodes detect neural activity in the auditory brain-stem pathway. A computer displays a waveform that indicates where the hearing loss is and its severity (see Figure 20.3).

Although the EOAE and ABR tests have become valuable tools to test hearing in young infants, they have limitations. The most important is that the tests are not true tests of hearing; they provide information about the workings of the ear but do not tell what your baby actually hears.

When your child is 6 months to 2½ years of age, a method known as visual reinforcement audiometry (VRA) can more specifically identify the magnitude of the hearing loss at varying sound frequencies. This test takes advantage of children's natural tendency to turn toward a sound. A visual reward, such as watching a mechanical toy, is provided whenever your child responds correctly to a sound. The audiologist presents sounds of decreasing intensity and observes whether your child makes the appropriate head turn in response to the sound. When your child can no longer detect the sound, he or she ceases to respond appropriately.

The hearing of children between the ages of 2 and 4 years can be tested successfully using a procedure called *conditioned play audiometry*. Actually, this test does not differ much from the procedures used with older children and adults, except that children are asked to perform a task when an auditory stimulus is presented rather than directly indicating that they have heard the sound. For example, an adult might be instructed to push a button or raise a hand when a sound is heard. In play audiometry, your child is asked to perform a simple play task, such as placing a ring on a peg whenever a sound is heard. If the child performs the task, the audiologist knows that he or she has heard the sound. These behavioral tests generally provide the most accurate information about a child's hearing loss, that is, what he or she actually hears across a range of frequencies and intensities.

Whenever possible, the hearing test is performed using earphones so that the ears can be tested separately. Not all young children, however, are willing to wear earphones, although newer earphones that can be inserted in the outer part of the ear increase the likelihood of cooperation. Otherwise, sounds are presented by a loudspeaker, and the responses obtained are called *sound field responses* because the sounds were presented to both ears at the same time rather than to each ear separately. Thus, sound field thresholds

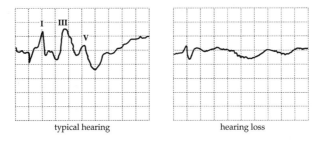

typical hearing   hearing loss

Figure 20.3. Results from auditory brainstem response (ABR) tests in an infant with typical hearing and in one with severe hearing loss. Note that the responses from the baby with typical hearing have three distinct waves that are labeled as waves I, III, and V. The response from the baby with hearing loss does not have this characteristic waveform.

represent a combination of the hearing in the better ear and in the more impaired ear.

The goal of all audiometry is to find the threshold, or the softest intensity, at which sound can be heard. It also permits the determination of threshold levels for low-frequency and high-frequency sounds. At the end of the hearing test, the results are usually graphed on an audiogram, which indicates the degree of hearing loss. Visit the Boys Town National Research Hospital's web site (http://www.boystown.org/Btnrh/Chlc/und_hl2.gif) for an audiogram that shows the frequencies of certain speech sounds.

Regardless of your child's age, the hearing assessment should also include a special test called *tympanometry*. This is not an actual hearing test but is designed to assess middle-ear function by measuring how well the eardrum transmits sound to the middle ear. The test is conducted by placing a small earphone in the outer part of your child's ear canal. During the test, your child hears a low-frequency tone and feels a slight pressure in the ear, much like the pressure sensation felt when riding up a fast elevator. The entire test takes about 5 seconds for each ear. The test most commonly detects middle-ear infections that alter the ability of the eardrum to transmit sound. Additional testing may be recommended to evaluate how the brain is interpreting incoming auditory signals if there is concern about a central hearing loss.

MAKING TREATMENT CHOICES

In the quiet of an office or an audiology suite, the moment following the report of a child's hearing loss is often magnified and frozen in time for parents. Although the diagnosis of deafness may seem far less dramatic than other chronic medical conditions, its impact on the life of your child and family is great. After receiving the diagnosis, you may feel pressured to make choices about amplification, surgery, communication modality, and educational approaches. Many parents describe a struggle to synthesize information and understand what is in the best interest of their child. To compound the problem of your initial lack of knowledge, you may encounter widely divergent and seemingly incompatible recommendations. At every point, passionate advocates for one specific option may leave you feeling more vulnerable and confused than ever. Take your time in making decisions, and remember that these are not life-or-death decisions. They can be reversed or adjusted if they don't work out. You will need to weigh the options, keeping in mind your child's strengths and needs in the context of your family and community. An interdisciplinary team including an otolaryngology (ear-nose-throat, or ENT) specialist, a speech-language pathologist, an audiologist, and an educator or an early intervention specialist is likely to help you make these decisions. Families have increasingly opted for making a plan in accordance with their child's developmental, cognitive, attentional, and sensory profile. In this approach, educational and communication methods are presented as a *series* of choices to be made based on the child's areas of strengths and continued needs at specific points in his or her development.

COMMUNICATING WITH YOUR BABY

Body language, gesture, facial expression, and touch are very important when communicating with a baby who is deaf. Sharing feelings such as happiness through frequent smiles, clapping, and exaggerated facial and eye movements all nurture your baby's visual attentiveness and communication. Think of yourself as an actor in a silent movie in which exaggerated body language can be very expressive of moods and give context to the surroundings. Babies and toddlers who are deaf also benefit from repetition as a way of both capturing their attention and reinforcing their communication efforts. It is interesting to note that deaf parents use a tremendous amount of movement when communicating with both their hearing and deaf children, exaggerating their facial expressions, moving their heads from side to side, touching their children, tapping, and waving their hands or objects. This may explain why deaf children of deaf parents tend to have excellent nonverbal communication skills.

Deaf infants are more likely to respond to visual cues than to auditory ones. Although many parents find it helpful to emphasize visual communication, others prefer to focus on stimulating and training their child's residual hearing. This mirrors the classic debate in education as to whether one should teach to a child's strengths or to his or her weaknesses. If one chooses to teach to weaknesses (the hearing loss), optimizing the learning environment is important. Although your child will respond consistently to visual stimuli, his or her response to auditory stimuli may vary according to weather conditions, the presence of colds or upper respiratory tract infections, and the acoustics in the environment. "Hearing" capacity in large, group settings with high ambient noise levels (such as in a shopping mall) is lower than in a quiet, well-lit, and more accessible environment (such as a classroom).

Once your infant moves out of the largely nonverbal or prelanguage phase around 1 year of age, you are both likely to become frustrated by the limits of what can be expressed and understood by body language alone. With spoken language not easily accessible, alternative modes of communication are needed. A wide range of options may be appropriate for your child. Many people choose to combine elements from several options.

COMMUNICATION OPTIONS

Oralism (also known as the auditory-oral or A/O method) emphasizes speech as the primary mode of communication and teaches listening skills and speechreading (lipreading). Auditory-verbal (A/V) therapy also emphasizes speech and the use of residual hearing, with a focus on hearing training and decoding of auditory information without the use of visual cuing such as speechreading. Cued speech, an alternate form of oral communication, uses spoken English and lipreading together with eight handshapes made in four different locations (cues) near the face to represent phonemes, or speech sounds.

A number of sign languages are used in English-speaking countries, the most common of which is American Sign Language (ASL). ASL is a visual, gestural language that combines specific hand shapes and movements with facial expressions and specific body postures to create a complete language with a grammatical structure and vocabulary distinct from English. Bilingual/bicultural educational systems teach ASL as the first language and English as a second language. This approach also incorporates teaching about Deaf culture. English-based sign systems combine ASL vocabulary with coined signs and fingerspelling to represent English sentence structure. Often, these systems are used simultaneously with spoken English, taking advantage of the additional visual cues presented through lipreading. Manually encoded English systems range from those that present exact English word order with special markers for word endings such as -ing (Signing Exact English, or SEE) to those that use less literal but more conceptually accurate signs (Pidgin Signed English, or PSE).

Regardless of the language used, deaf children of hearing parents typically miss out on much of the incidental learning that happens continually and without effort during a typical day at school and at home. For example, information transmitted at mealtimes may include the menu of foods served, the news of the day, news of the family, and so forth. Each subject has embedded critical information that adds to the development of social skills, interpersonal problem-solving, and world knowledge. The challenge for you as parents is to make this information available to your child with a hearing loss by other means, beginning in the earliest months of life, with ongoing and continual eye contact as a means of transmitting information. The importance of body contact and touch cannot be underestimated. Facial expressions and gestures are consistently cited by deaf adults as having been important when their parents were transmitting critical information to them as young children.

Many cultures minimize the use of facial movements, body gestures, and other forms of expressive communication and emphasize neutrality and subtle nonverbal communication. For you to communicate continually and understandably with your young child, you may wish to expand your own personal repertoire of gestural and facial expressive communication. Although your child is deaf, sound is an important part of life, and you should continue to talk to your child to support language development. Other language issues important for your young child are taking turns and engaging in dialogue. These can be emphasized through play and by engaging your child in a back-and-forth "conversation." You will need to have patience in awaiting your child's response, whatever form this may take.

In the preschool period, language activities such as making picture books or creating clocks with pictures of the events of the day allow your child to create a way to hold and describe experiences. When you are going on an excursion or even during daily activities, creating a story on paper, such as "My Day at the Zoo," that is illustrated with snapshots or drawings can be an enjoyable and important educational language tool. Hands-on activities and nonverbal play with puppets or other interesting tactile materials, particularly those that emphasize expressive and dramatic explorations, become increasingly important as a means for your child to take control of the immediate environment.

With school entry, reading becomes all-important in helping deaf children achieve full literacy potential. Brief practice periods at home should become routine. As your child grows older, descriptions of feelings, inner thoughts and inner experiences, such as daydreams, night dreams, imagined experiences, and fantasy should gradually replace more concrete and task-oriented conversation.

You should acknowledge your child's presence in all conversations. Deaf people often politely nod in agreement, even when they do not fully understand the conversation. Therefore, it is important that your child be an active responder so that you can be sure he or she is following the conversation. It is helpful to frame questions as a reporter does, using *wh-* questions (who, what, when, where, why, or which) rather than simple yes-or-no questions. Also, consider eliminating side conversations that are conducted as though your child were not present in the room. When family members say things about your child to others while your child is present, they erode much of the hard work you are doing to enhance your child's sense of individuality and importance. It is also important to remember, however, that the extra time you need to spend with your child who is deaf may place stress on your other children. You may want to develop special activities and devote time to each of your children to counterbalance this.

In terms of your child's behavior, you should expect appropriate social behaviors based on developmental level and apply the same rules and consequences for your child with a hearing impairment as for your other children. Although you will inevitably need to serve as an interpreter for your child with certain family members, establish the limits of this activity early on, and indicate your desire for all family members (including grandparents) to communicate directly with your child, even as a toddler. Your child should respond to your gestures, enjoy your company (most of the time), and relax in your presence. If this does not occur, consider consulting with a professional who is familiar with deaf children to explore possible psychological problems.

Amplification

Hearing aids amplify sound to take advantage of your child's residual hearing. Because only a small fraction of children with hearing loss lack usable hearing (like Sandra), hearing aids benefit the vast majority of children with hearing impairments. The degree of benefit an individual child receives, however, is variable and difficult to predict.

Children as young as a few months of age can be fitted with and may benefit from hearing aids. Even before children begin to produce words, at about 1 year of age, they learn the rudiments of language by hearing it spoken. For a child with a hearing impairment, boosting residual hearing is key to providing the fullest access to spoken language. If your child's hearing loss is severe to profound, hearing aids may not make speech intelligible but may still enhance your child's awareness of speech and environmental sounds and aid your child in interpreting visual cues.

Hearing aids consist of three components: a microphone that receives sound from the environment and converts it into an electrical impulse, one or more amplifiers that intensify the electrical signal, and a receiver that converts the signal back into sound and transmits it through an earmold into the ear canal. The hearing aid is powered by a battery, which should be protected with a tamper-resistant cover to prevent your child from removing and swallowing the battery, which may be toxic and a choking hazard.

Hearing aids come in a variety of styles; however, for most children, the behind-the-ear aids are recommended because they are safer and require fewer repairs than in-the-ear hearing aids do, especially with physically active and young children (see Figure 20.4). In addition, the casing size allows for more circuitry needed for assistive devices such as an FM receiver. With this system, a parent, teacher, or other person can wear a microphone that delivers their voice directly into the child's hearing aid. Some of the more sophisticated hearing aids are programmable, allowing the user to modify the settings to accommodate different listening environments such as a noisy classroom or the home.

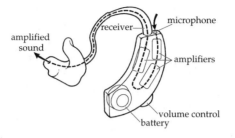

Figure 20.4. The components of a behind-the-ear hearing aid. The aid consists of a microphone, an amplifier power supply, and a receiver that projects the amplified sound through the earmold into the ear canal.

Your child's audiologist may be able to provide loaner hearing aids even before your child's hearing loss has been fully defined. During the evaluation, the audiologist will determine how your child responds to different frequencies so that the hearing aids can be tuned to amplify the frequencies that most need boosting. Because children with severe developmental disabilities may not be able to be tested by behavioral methods such as VRA, the hearing aid may be selected using only the information provided by an ABR test.

Surgical Interventions

The most common operation on the ear involves the placement of tubes through the eardrum. If your child has had multiple ear infections in a short time, your child's otolaryngologist may suggest placing pressure-equalizing (PE) tubes in the affected ear(s) to prevent or treat a conductive hearing loss. This is an outpatient procedure in which a slit is made in the eardrum and a small plastic tube is inserted into the middle ear. This equalizes the pressure, reduces pain, and allows ventilation of the middle ear. Once placed, these tubes remain for a few months and generally fall out spontaneously. The eardrum will heal after the tube comes out.

Recurrent ear infections may also be attributed to enlarged adenoids (lymphatic tissue in the back of the throat). This may block the Eustachian tube, placing your child at increased risk for middle-ear infections. Treatment involves removal of the adenoids (adenoidectomy) but not the tonsils. Sandra had PE tubes placed and an adenoidectomy with some benefit.

For many children with significant hearing loss, cochlear implantation (see Figure 20.5) may be an option. Sandra was not a candidate as she had a congenital absence of the cochlea. Cochlear implants are designed to restore partial hearing to individuals with sensorineural deafness. They were first approved by the U.S. Food and Drug Administration for use in children in 1990. At that time, the earliest a child could have the cochlear device implanted was at age 2. Earlier implantation has since been suggested as offering children significant benefits by providing earlier access to sound and speech. Many centers are now placing cochlear implants in children as young as 18 months of age. In addition, the technology used in cochlear implants is rapidly improving. Although the device does not restore hearing to normal, some children learn to speak and understand speech quite clearly.

Cochlear implant surgery is usually completed within a few hours. Your child generally would remain hospitalized overnight or as long as several days. Approximately 3–4 weeks later, after the surgical wound has healed, the stimulation process begins. Over a period of weeks or months, the device is gradually tuned, or "mapped," to optimize the input your child is receiving. Some children seem to perceive sound almost immediately after stimulation, whereas others progress more slowly. So, some parents may feel exhilarated soon after the implant, whereas others become frustrated with the slow progress. Some of the factors that influence outcome are the age at which hearing was lost, the age at which the device was implanted, the condition of the remaining nerve fibers in the inner ear, the individual characteristics of the child, and the amount of effort placed into rehabilitation of the child's hearing following cochlear stimulation. Your child must learn to interpret the sounds that are heard.

If you are considering cochlear implants for your child, he or she will need an otologic evaluation to ensure that there is not an active infection or anatomical problem that would interfere with implantation, a complete audiological assessment, a CT (computed tomography) or MRI (magnetic resonance imaging) scan, and possibly psychological testing. You should also receive information about the possible benefits and risks of the procedure and counseling to ensure that you have realistic expectations.

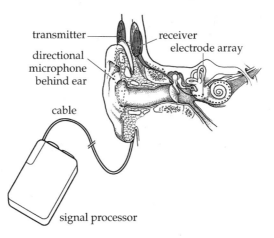

Figure 20.5. Cochlear implant. The cochlear implant consists of four components: a microphone that captures sound, a signal processor that converts the sound to electrical signals, a signal coupler (transmitter and receiver) that conveys the signal to the internal part of the device, and an electrode array threaded into the inner ear that stimulates auditory nerve fibers along the cochlea, thus relaying auditory information to the brain, resulting in sound perception. Magnets hold the transmitter over the implanted receiver.

There has been little research on the use of cochlear implants in children who have deafness in combination with mental retardation, autism, blindness, or other developmental disabilities. For some of these children, implants may offer significant benefits. For example, in children who are deaf and visually impaired, the additional auditory information they receive following the cochlear implant can be very helpful.

EDUCATION

As discussed in Chapter 12, all children with special needs are entitled by federal law to a free and appropriate education. Each state, however, carries out the mandates of this law somewhat differently. The audiologist who tested your child's hearing should be able to direct you to the agency that will work with you to oversee your child's education. The service coordinator, or case manager, who will integrate your child's services may or may not be familiar with the unique needs of a deaf child.

From birth until the age of 3 (see Chapter 6), your family is eligible for early intervention services. For a child who is deaf, these may include audiological services, a speech-language development program, and if you choose to pursue sign language as your child's mode of communication, sign language classes for the entire family. Early intervention services are generally provided in your home during your child's infancy and at a school or a private agency that provides services for children with hearing impairments by age 2. Many parents seek out and find early intervention services with a stronger focus on hearing impairment than those initially recommended by their service coordinator.

When your child reaches the age of 3, your local school district usually takes over responsibility for your child's education. Ideally, you will have a range of educational options available from which to choose. Your local public school system, however, may offer only one option, which you may feel is not appropriate for your child. Through advocacy, diligence, and persistence, some parents are able to convince the school district to support their preferred educational option for their child.

The type of educational environment you choose for your child depends in large part on the communication approach you have selected. Schools for the deaf usually take one of three general approaches: oral, bilingual/bicultural, or total communication. Total communication programs may incorporate ASL, manually encoded English, fingerspelling, gestures, speech, lipreading, and use of residual hearing.

Federal law also requires that a child with disabilities receive special education services in the least restrictive environment (see Chapter 12). There remains much controversy about what this means for a child with a hearing impairment. To some people, *least restrictive* means placement with hearing children in a general education classroom, often with an interpreter or other supportive services. Others maintain that the least restrictive environment would be one in which the child attends a special day or residential school for children who are deaf, in which all educational, social, and athletic activities are fully accessible and the child does not face a communication disadvantage.

Some parents and children, especially older children, feel that residential schools for the Deaf offer better opportunities for socialization and development of positive self-esteem. Others feel that those necessary components of a child's life are better addressed in the family's home. You need to consider your child's and family's strengths and needs in making this decision.

OUTCOMES

Your child's eventual skills depend on many factors, including intelligence, degree of hearing loss, age of diagnosis, and family environment. The higher your child's intelligence, the more adaptive he or she is likely to be and the faster he or she is likely learn. With a more severe hearing loss, however, you and your child will have to work harder to be successful. The age of diagnosis is important because earlier identification leads to more effective therapy, especially in your child's development of speech and language. Concerned, helpful parents and siblings can make a major difference in the outcomes for a child with a hearing loss.

Some Questions Answered

How can I find out about programs that are available where my family lives?

If your child's audiologist is unfamiliar with programs in the area, you should contact the department of education in your state. Your local school district or health department should also be able to provide some guidance. Many parents find that the most helpful information comes from other parents. Ask your child's audiologist or pediatrician for the names and telephone numbers of parents who would be willing to talk to you. You may also call national organizations or check their web sites (see the Suggested Readings and Resources at the end of the book) to ask if they have local chapters or contact people. As you begin your search, you are likely to encounter both professionals and parents who are ardent proponents of different communication methods, and you may find it difficult to get unbiased information. By considering divergent opinions, however, you should be able to get a balanced view of the options available.

Will using sign language inhibit my child's ability to talk?

Some people in the field of deaf education worry that because sign language is so much easier to learn than speech for a child with a serious hearing impairment, the child will not make the effort to learn speech during the critical years of language development (ages 1–5 years). The alternate view is that learning sign language in the early years is the best way for a deaf child to develop a solid language foundation. Despite several decades of research, no one has yet answered this question definitively. Many children who learn sign language first go on to develop excellent expressive and receptive speech, and many children who are taught oral methods go on to learn and communicate in sign language. No single approach is ideal for all children. You will need to consider your child's unique attributes and be flexible.

How can I learn more about what the future holds for my child?

Many parents find it helpful to meet adults who are deaf and learn more about the Deaf community and Deaf culture. Because deafness is a low-incidence condition and because 90% of children who are deaf are born to hearing parents, many parents have never met an adult who is deaf. They may find it difficult to imagine that deaf people live full and happy lives, go to school and college, have jobs, get married, and raise families. Meeting adults who have grown up deaf may relieve your anxiety and apprehension. In addition, young people and adults who are deaf may be able to give you practical guidance about the hurdles they faced and the strategies that worked for them. You may want to contact organizations such as those listed in the Suggested Readings and Resources at the end of this book or other organizations or schools for deaf children and tell them about your child and your desire to meet with and talk to an adult who is deaf.

21

Communication Disorders

Paul Wang and Ken Bleile

Speech and language seem like simple tasks for the majority of children and adults. Hardly a thought goes into the act of communication; you just open your mouth, and the thoughts come spilling out. But, in fact, communication is among the most complicated activities that human beings perform. Speech, the physical act of making word sounds, requires the coordinated activity of the diaphragm, chest, throat, palate, larynx, tongue, and lips. Then there is the truly complicated part of communication: language, which is having something to say and knowing when and how to say it. Using language requires a whole host of other skills, from understanding what someone else just said, to organizing what you want to say, to putting words together into phrases and sentences. In this light, it is not surprising that communication disorders are among the most frequent of the developmental disabilities.

For your child's communication abilities to develop typically, he or she must hear accurately what is being said, have the proper brain connections to understand what is being said, formulate thoughts into words, and possess the physical ability to speak. Impairment in any of these functions can cause communication problems. Communication disorders include speech, language, and auditory deficits. They range from relatively mild speech problems, such as pronouncing the word *rabbit* as "wabbit," to severe problems with understanding language or expressing oneself. Some children may have communication problems without other disabilities. In others, the communication disorder may be associated with developmental disabilities such as cerebral palsy, autism, or mental retardation.

Joon-Yi, Lia, Jane, and Billy

Joon-Yi is 3 years old and has been diagnosed with cerebral palsy. He does not walk, draw with a crayon, or feed himself with a spoon. He also does not say any recognizable words, although he does understand almost everything that is said to him. He reliably looks toward whatever he wants.

Lia is a 9-year-old with learning disabilities. Her motor development was always on target, but her language developed late. She now pronounces words clearly, but the words in her sentences seem to be in the wrong order, making it difficult to follow her conversation. Lia also says that she can't always think of the precise words that she wants to use. For example, when she was pretending to have a tea party, she asked her mother for cups and bowls instead of cups and saucers.

Jane is 6 years old and has mild mental retardation. She is functioning at a 4-year-old level in all areas except for her language skills. Her speech is difficult to understand because she has trouble pronouncing many sounds, such as "k," "s," and "l." Her mother feels that the length and complexity of Jane's sentences are the same as those of her 3-year-old brother. She recently told her aunt, "Mommy and Jane go to zoo today with you." Jane also seems to have trouble understanding what other people say to her.

Billy is 10 years old and has a severe hearing impairment. His speech is difficult for people who are not relatives to understand, and he seems to have trouble putting words together into phrases and sentences. He communicates very effectively, however, through sign language, and he enjoys baseball, bicycle-riding, and playing video games.

These four children's difficulties illustrate the wide range of potential communication problems. Joon-Yi is unable to perform the physical act of speaking and therefore has a speech disorder. Lia has no difficulty with speech itself but has trouble understanding and using language to express herself. In other words, she has a language disorder. Jane has both speech and language problems that are more severe than her other cognitive impairments. Finally, Billy has speech and language difficulties that are linked to his hearing impairment.

DEVELOPMENT OF COMMUNICATION SKILLS

The typical development of speech and language skills follows a similar sequence for most children, regardless of the language they are learning (such as English, Chinese, or even American Sign Language [ASL]). In the first year of life, children learn to make the sounds of their language; cooing (the production of vowel sounds) starts around 2 months, and babbling (consonant sounds) starts around 6 months. Children typically speak their first word when they are about 1 year old and have a vocabulary of 20–50 words by about 18 months. Children usually start speaking in two-word phrases around 2 years old, and they start forming complete sentences around age 3. By 5 years of age, most children use many verb tenses and can understand and tell short stories. It should be emphasized that these ages are averages and that there is considerable variability in the development of language skills. For example, typical children may say their first word anywhere from 9 to 18 months of age.

SPEECH DISORDERS

Speech disorders are the most common type of communication disorder for two reasons. First, speech occurs very rapidly. Even in casual conversation, we typically make 14 speech sounds per second that require the sequential coordination of many movements in the mouth. Second, a large number of body parts are involved in speech production. These include the lungs, voice box, throat, nose, mouth, tongue, lips, palate, certain parts of the brain, and various nerves coming out of the brain. Together, the parts of the body required for shaping the sounds in speech are called the *speech mechanism*. An impairment in any part of the machine will limit your child's effective production of speech sounds and overall communication.

Speech disorders and speech motor disorders (discussed later in this chapter) occur in 5%–10% of children who have no other developmental disability and occur more frequently in children with other disabilities. The prognosis for both types of speech disorders is good. With appropriate therapies, which may be required for a number of years, your child should be able to produce speech that most listeners can understand. A smaller percentage of children will learn to communicate through modalities other than speech, such as sign language or computer-assisted communication devices (also discussed later).

Speech disorders can be divided into those affecting voice, articulation, or resonance. Voice and articulation disorders involve problems of the mouth, nose, throat, and voice box. An extreme example of a voice disorder is found in premature infants who require prolonged placement of a tracheostomy tube (see Chapter 5). As long as the tube is in place, the child cannot speak because the tube bypasses the voice box (larynx). A valve can be inserted that will permit the child to have some speech by swallowing air and then expelling it. The result is a voice that sounds somewhat deeper than normal but with practice can be easily understood.

Resonance disorders are a type of voice disorder that occurs in children who have atypical oral or nasal tracts. The most common cause is a cleft palate (an incomplete closure of the roof of the mouth). If your child has a cleft palate or other atypical formation of the nose and mouth, he or she may be unable to make certain sounds, such as "b," "d," and "g" because air involuntarily flows through the nose. Some children have difficulty making any sounds except "m," "n," and "ng." Speech-language therapy involves helping your child learn to limit the amount of air that flows through the nose during speech. Surgery to repair the cleft palate usually improves the resonance disorder significantly. Your child, however, may still need therapy to overcome remaining impairments in the oral and nasal tracts and to extinguish incorrect speech patterns acquired prior to surgery.

Articulation disorders (sometimes called *phonological disorders*) are the most common type of speech disorder. The types of articulation errors that your child might make include substitutions (exchanging one sound for another, as in "wabbit" instead of "rabbit"), omissions (leaving out a sound as in "poon" instead of "spoon"), additions (adding a sound that should not be present, as in "joosa" instead of "juice"), and distortions (pronouncing a sound in an inaccurate way, such as an "r" sound that is halfway between an "r" and a "w"). Just because your child makes articulation errors, however, does not mean that he or she has a communication disorder. Young children with typical language development often make such errors at least until age 4. A specialist must make a careful speech evaluation to consider the type of articulation error and the frequency of these errors before determining that your child has an articulation disorder. If your child does have an articulation disorder, it is unlikely to result from a physical abnormality of the mouth or tongue. Marked damage to the mouth or tongue must occur before speech is affected. Unless your child has an obvious physical problem with his or her mouth, the speech disorder probably results from problems elsewhere in the speech mechanism.

SPEECH MOTOR DISORDERS

When the mouth, tongue, nose, throat, and voice box are structurally sound but the brain is unable to control them effectively, a speech motor problem results. The most common of these disorders are dysfluency (stuttering), dysarthria, and apraxia.

Dysfluency

The exact cause of dysfluency is unknown, but the disorder is thought to result from the brain's difficulty in controlling the timing of speech movements. Stuttering appears to be more common in children with mental retardation and children with learning disabilities than in other children. Some young typically developing children, however, have occasional dysfluencies as their speech develops. These dysfluencies may include repetitions of words or phrases, especially at the beginning of sentences, while the child is planning the next part of the sentence. Many of the grimaces, facial contortions, and tics often found in stutterers are the result of attempts to "force out the words" and are not actual neurological conditions. These behaviors also help clinicians to distinguish true stutterers from typically developing children who are just repeating themselves as they are learning to speak.

The best advice is to pay attention to what your child says, not how he or she says it. Avoid finishing your child's sentences, even during the longest stuttering block. Do not ask your child to repeat words that he or she stutters over. Stuttering often disappears on its own, especially during the preschool years. If it does not improve or if it causes significant impairment in your child's communication abilities, then you should seek speech-language therapy for your child. There is no known cure, however, for stuttering.

Dysarthria

Dysarthria arises from damage to the parts of the brain that direct the action of the muscles used in producing speech. If your child has dysarthria, he or she probably has difficulty with speech and other activities that involve coordinated movements of the mouth or throat. For example, your child may also have a problem moving the tongue both when speaking and eating. Some types of dysarthria make speech appear slurred. Other forms make speech sound monotone, hoarse, or strangled. This disorder is most commonly found in children with dyskinetic cerebral palsy (see Chapter 19). Speech-language therapy for dysarthria consists of helping your child to work around the problem or to find alternative ways to communicate. For example, if your child has a weak diaphragm (as in muscular dystrophy), he or she may be shown how to position the body to produce a louder voice. Alternative means of communication can also be considered for children who have more severe difficulties.

Speech Apraxia

Apraxia is the inability to carry out a purposeful movement. Speech apraxia therefore affects voluntary activities only, such as making complex patterns of movement with the mouth and throat during speech. Your child may be unable to touch his or her tongue to lip when asked to do so but may reflexively and unconsciously lick a crumb off while eating. Speech apraxia is often found in children who have brain injury, such as from a car accident or the removal of a brain tumor. Speech apraxia can also occur without any known cause and may result in delays in the development of speech and language skills. Treatment for speech apraxia often involves helping your child learn to gain voluntary control over the muscles that govern articulation. If your child has severe apraxia, he or she may not speak intelligibly. In this situation, your child's communication skills may be enhanced through the use of computers or other speech aids.

LANGUAGE DISORDERS

Although language is not the only way we communicate with other people, it is arguably the most important. Typically, children learn the rudiments of language by age 3 and master language almost completely by age 10. Children with disabilities, however, often need a longer time to acquire language, and a number of these children may never completely master it.

Language disorders are classified by the skills that are affected. *Receptive* (comprehension) language disorders are those that involve difficulty understanding or processing what other people say. Having a receptive language disorder does not mean that your child cannot hear, only that he or she has trouble understanding what is heard. *Expressive* language disorders are those that involve difficulty in expressing oneself. Having an expressive language disorder does not mean that your child cannot make speech sounds. Rather, it means that he or she has difficulty in formulating language to express thoughts to other people.

Children can have a receptive language disorder, an expressive language disorder, or both. Children with just an expressive language disorder generally have a better prognosis. With appropriate therapy, a child's expressive language abilities are more likely to "catch up" to the level of his or her receptive language abilities. For children with both receptive and expressive language delays, the prognosis is less predictable. With appropriate therapy, children's receptive and expressive language abilities can be enhanced.

In addition to the distinction between receptive and expressive disorders, language problems can be described by the areas of language that they affect: semantics, syntax, pragmatics, and discourse. These four types of problems are described next. Most children with language disorders have problems in more than one of these areas.

Semantic Difficulties

A child with semantic difficulties has trouble with the meanings of words and sentences. These problems can involve language comprehension, expressive language, or both. For example, your child might have trouble learning color words, the names of common objects, or adjective pairs such as *big/little* and *up/down*. Although everyone has occasional trouble finding the right word, a child with a semantic deficit has problems finding words so frequently that the ability to be understood is affected. Children usually learn the meaning of words through conversation. Children with semantic deficits, however, may require direct teaching of word meanings. If your child has word-finding problems, a speech-language therapist can work with you to teach your child techniques to find the right word.

Syntax Difficulties

To communicate effectively, we must understand more than the meaning of individual words; we must understand grammar, word order, pluralization, conjugation of verbs, and more as well. Knowledge of grammar tells us, for example, that the sentence *The cows were kicked by the horse* means that the horse did the kicking, that the cows got kicked, and that the kicking happened in the past. Similarly, we know that the phrase *the cows* refers to more than one cow. If your child has difficulties with syntax, he or she may be unable to understand many different aspects of grammar, such as the importance of word order in a sentence or the importance of suffixes that indicate tense or pluralization. Therapy for difficulties with syntax focuses on teaching grammar. For example, your child might be taught that the *-ed* at the end of the word *kicked* indicates past tense.

Pragmatics Difficulties

In addition to knowledge of word meaning and grammar, communication also requires us to know just how language should be used in social interactions. This aspect of language is called *pragmatics*. Pragmatics involves the use of terms such as *please* and *thank you*, the knowledge of how to take turns during a conversation, and the understanding of how to adjust our language depending on the person we are talking to and the situation that surrounds us. All children have difficulty using language in social settings now and then; however, a child who has difficulty with pragmatics has consistent troubles in this area. Such a child might not allow others to take turns in a conversation, may always say the wrong thing at the wrong time, or may not know how to start a conversation. Therapy for pragmatics disorders focuses on teaching the social rules of language. For example, an adolescent child with mental retardation might be taught how to interact appropriately with clerks in a grocery store or servers in a restaurant.

Discourse Difficulties

When people talk, they usually say more than one sentence at a time because telling a story, giving directions, or reporting an event requires more than a phrase. Therefore, good communication requires us to know how to organize sentences into discourse, or conversation. Learning such organization can pose significant problems to children with developmental disabilities. As with other language disorders, discourse problems can affect both comprehension and expression. For example, a 7-year-old with discourse comprehension problems may be unable to identify the basic plot in a simple story, even though he or she understands individual sentences. A 9-year-old who has an expressive discourse deficit cannot tell an organized story or retell a recent event. Therapy for these difficulties should focus on helping your child learn to organize a story into a beginning, middle, and end that make a cohesive whole.

EVALUATION OF COMMUNICATION DISORDERS

If your child has a communication disorder, your first step to developing a therapy plan is to set up a speech-language evaluation. The professional performing the evaluation should be a licensed speech-language pathologist, usually with a master's degree or a doctorate, and should be certified by the American Speech-Language-Hearing Association (ASHA; see the Suggested Readings and Resources for contact information).

You can expect your child's evaluation to begin with an interview during which the therapist will ask you basic questions about your child's development, medical problems that might affect communication skills, and the extent of the communication problem. If your child has had previous speech-language evaluations, the new evaluator may ask to see those reports. (You have the right to request such written reports from past specialists.) After the interview, the evaluator may ask you to leave the room so that he or she can see how well your child performs in a therapy or school-like environment. In other cases, especially if your child is very young, you may be asked to stay for the evaluation, which may last 1–2 hours. If other factors may affect the results—for example, if your child is sick, young, or easily distracted—the evaluation might be performed in shorter periods over a number of days. It can be helpful to observe some children's speech and language in natural environments, such as the home or classroom, in addition to evaluating them in a therapist's office.

A complete evaluation should cover all aspects of speech and language development. It should also include a hearing screening to determine whether a hearing impairment is contributing to your child's communication difficulties (see Chapter 20). If your child is school age, the evaluator will observe your child and give him or her a number of tests. In many of these, the evaluator will ask your child to point to pictures or to move objects. If your child is younger, the evaluation will be more play based and may involve your completing a report of your child's speech and language skills. During the speech evaluation, your child will be asked to name objects or pictures of objects and perhaps to tell some stories. The evaluator also will look in your child's mouth and ask him or her to move the tongue and lips around. Feeding or eating will be observed if your child has difficulty with those functions.

The speech-language therapist will determine your child's skills in a variety of areas and will report how your child compares with other children of the same age using a percentile score. For example, if a 6-year-old scores at the 12th percentile on a vocabulary test, this means that about 12% of children of the same age know fewer words (and about 87% know more words). When a child falls below the 10th percentile, there is reason for concern.

Another type of scoring, the age-equivalent score, indicates the age for which your child's skills are typical. For example, if a 6-year-old speaks in three- and four-word sentences, then the age-equivalent language score would be 2½–3 years, because that is the age at which most children speak in three- and four-word phrases.

Some aspects of speech and language skills are hard to measure in numbers. For this reason, some qualitative measures also are used. Qualitative tests depend on the educated opinion of the evaluator. Such tests are commonly used to evaluate oral-motor abilities and spontaneous language, especially in the areas of pragmatics and discourse. For example, an evaluator might observe your child during play and say that he or she "has difficulty following the content of a conversation." Such a description provides important insights into your child's communication problems. At the end of the evaluation, your child's therapist shares the results and creates a treatment plan with you.

The results of the speech-language evaluation should always be considered in the context of your child's medical history and other developmental skills. For example, medical conditions may influence where therapy can be performed, how long a session can last, and what type of therapy is more likely to be effective. If your child has a resonance disorder because of a cleft palate, for instance, he or she might need different therapies than another child with a resonance disorder having a different cause. Similarly, a child with autism might be expected to have particular difficulties with language pragmatics that should be given extra attention. It also is important to know the child's general developmental level to plan effectively, to identify strengths, to reach across various developmental areas, and to set appropriate expectations, because speech and language skills usually cannot exceed the child's general cognitive level. For these reasons, it is often helpful for your child to undergo a multidisciplinary evaluation instead of just a speech-language evaluation so that these other areas of development and important medical issues can be assessed.

After the evaluation, the evaluator should sit down with you to discuss the findings and to answer questions. Many times, the evaluator will also be your child's speech-language therapist. It is common, however, for different people to do the evaluation and the therapy, such as when the evaluation is scheduled through a hospital or school district. Regardless of whether the evaluator will be doing your child's therapy, you should obtain a report that lists suggested therapy goals.

THERAPY FOR COMMUNICATION DISORDERS

If your child has a communication disorder, he or she will need therapy. Factors to consider include where the therapy will take place (home, school, or the therapist's office), how frequent the therapy will be, and what treatment methods will be used. Speech-language therapy also should be coordinated with any other therapies and supports that your child receives. Most often, this would involve coordination with your child's teacher and occupational therapist, whose goals may overlap with the speech therapist's activities (see Chapter 12).

Approaches to Therapy

There are essentially three approaches to therapy: direct therapy, stimulation, and consultation with parents and teachers. In direct therapy, a therapist works with your child alone or in a group on some aspect of communication. The specific technique chosen by a therapist depends on your child's age and the nature of his or her difficulty. Drill—the repetition of specific sounds, words, or phrases—is only one tool among many therapy techniques. Other approaches can be almost as structured as drill but are more interesting, such

Home therapy is typically provided prior to age 3, or as a transition from an acute hospitalization, or when your family lives too far from a therapy center. For example, if your child has been receiving therapy during a hospital stay, home therapy can help your child make the transition between release from the hospital and enrollment in a community program. Infants and toddlers who are not yet enrolled in any center-based child care or preschool program may also receive home therapy.

Types of Therapy

Therapy can be individual or group. Some therapists recommend trying classroom therapy first and if not successful, trying individual sessions. In individual therapy, the therapist works one-to-one with your child. This approach is especially useful when your child is acquiring a new skill, such as learning to make a difficult speech sound. Individual therapy is usually performed in a treatment room. If a classroom is quiet enough, it can be a good alternative setting because your child may later find it easier to apply the skills in conversation with other children. If the classroom contains too many distractions, however, the benefits of individual attention most likely will be lost. At other times, the therapist may want to join your child during a classroom activity and assist him or her in participating by using the new skills they have been practicing in one-to-one sessions.

Group therapy typically is performed by a single therapist with two to five children and can be very useful in helping children learn to apply their new skills. Furthermore, in good therapy groups, the less advanced students benefit from being exposed to the more advanced students. Groups work best when they are small and when the children are at similar developmental levels. For groups with 1- to 3-year-olds, developmental levels should be within 6 months of each other, for groups with 3- to 6-year-olds, levels should be within 1 year of each other, and for groups with 6- to 18-year-olds, levels should be within 2 years of each other.

Because individual and group therapy offer different benefits, your child may receive both types of therapy at the same time. Such a balanced approach facilitates the learning of new skills and their application in real-life settings.

Amount of Therapy

The frequency of speech-language therapy varies from once every other week to five times per week. Once per week is appropriate if your child has relatively minor communication problems or is on a plateau. Parents sometimes ask, "Why not increase the amount of therapy in order to help move my child off the plateau?" Therapists typically will increase therapy on a trial basis to see if greater changes can be produced. This change needs to be done with caution. Especially if your child has severe communication problems, the rate of neurological development will determine his or her progress in speech-language therapy. If your child's neurological development is on a plateau, then pushing him or her too hard could result in frustration and a dislike of therapy. A history of failure may cause your child to become uncooperative. Allowing your child to remain at a plateau for a while works better in the long run.

Therapy two or three times per week is appropriate for most children with communication disorders, even for those whose problems are severe. Therapy at this level is often sufficient to produce major developmental changes, especially when reinforced by family activities, but is not so frequent that the child becomes bored or uncooperative. If your child is seen four or five times per week, he or she is receiving intensive therapy. Children with autism, for example, may need this level of therapy. Intensive therapy sometimes can produce quick changes in development. Children may also go through phases during which language development proceeds slower than at other times, even though intensive therapy is continuing.

Occasionally, a therapist will see a child either less than once per week or more than five times per week. If a child visits the therapist less than once per week, the therapist is probably not trying to improve communication abilities but is monitoring development, maintaining skills, and serving as a resource for the parents or teachers. At the other extreme, a therapist may see a child as often as twice a day, such as during recovery from neurological surgery to facilitate the return of communication skills.

All aspects of your child's therapy should be incorporated throughout daily life and the educational program. The speech-language therapist facilitates this goal by consulting with you, your child's teachers, and other therapists. In consultation with you and the other professionals, recommendations can be developed on how to encourage your child to practice newly acquired skills in natural environments throughout the day. This approach helps to maximize the benefit that your child can obtain from the therapy.

ALTERNATE MEANS OF COMMUNICATION

Some children's communication skills are severely limited by their speech impairments. For example, this may occur if your child has a severe hearing impairment, cerebral palsy that causes speech to be unintelligible, or autism spectrum disorder. In these instances, your child's oral communication may need to be supplemented with or replaced by other methods of communication. These other methods include sign language and augmentative and alternative communication.

Sign Language

Sign language is most commonly used by children and adults who are deaf (see Chapter 20). Sign language can also be helpful, however, for a child who does not have a hearing impairment but who has other communication difficulties or who may use signs to learn oral language. Signing has been found to reduce many children's frustration of being unable to communicate and can be a very effective tool if your child has not developed spoken language but has the physical and intellectual abilities needed for signing.

If your child's therapist suggests the use of sign language, you should ask whether the ultimate goal for your child is to use sign language exclusively or as a supplement to other forms of communication. If the goal is to use sign language as the primary method of communication, the therapist should be proficient in ASL, and your child must have the coordination and movement skills required to master ASL. If the therapist is not truly fluent in ASL, then your child probably is not being taught a real language. If the goal, however, is to use sign language in conjunction with speech, then any number of different sign systems can be used. Two other signing systems are Signing Exact English, or SEE, and Pidgin Signed English, or PSE. For some children, a combination of signing, lipreading, and hearing amplification may be used (this is referred to as total communication). Whatever the method, you should make a concerted effort to learn signing along with your child. Not only will this allow you to communicate more effectively with your child, but it also sends the message to your child that you accept him or her and are willing to work hard to communicate effectively.

Augmentative and Alternative Communication

Most children, including those with developmental disabilities, go on to become good verbal communicators. But a small number of children have such severe cognitive or physical disabilities that speech is impossible for them. The majority of these children have mental retardation, autism, or cerebral palsy. These children may be helped by augmentative and alternative communication (AAC)—special methods that provide an alternative to spoken language. For example, only 10% of the speech of a 4-year-old with cerebral palsy may be intelligible to others. For this child, pointing to images on a picture board or a computerized communication board may help communicate thoughts and feelings to other people.

Candidates for AAC generally should have at least the intellectual capability of a typical 18-month-old. Children who are developmentally younger than this age can often learn prerequisite skills for AAC, such as how to point to pictures or how to press buttons but generally do not become proficient in AAC.

An AAC evaluation generally consists of two parts. First, the evaluation team will determine your child's mental age or language age. After that, the evaluation is likely to focus on physical and sensory abilities. The evaluator will ask your child to manipulate switches, buttons, or toys similar to those needed to operate the AAC equipment. If your child has good arm movement but poor finger control, the evaluator will design an AAC system that maximizes the ability of your child to use arm movements but does not depend on precise finger movements. In many cases, the speech-language team will seek the help of an occupational and/or physical therapist for this motor assessment.

There are many types of AAC devices. The simplest are flat boards upon which squares are placed, with pictures or words on each square. The child points to a particular square to indicate meaning. With the advent of the computer age, such nonelectronic boards are typically used for temporary situations only, such as in a hospital when a child is unable to speak or when a child's computerized board is being repaired.

Electronic and/or computerized communication boards, called *voice output communication aids* (VOCAs), have many advantages over the older manual boards. They can be equipped with a voice synthesizer so that the board will "say" whatever your child points to. Electronic boards also permit much more rapid and varied communication. For example, a VOCA can be programmed so that your child only needs to touch one square to say a long sentence, such as "I want to go play in the park." Finally, VOCAs offer great flexibility. They can be easily reprogrammed as your child learns new words and sentences or as his or her interests change. The electronic flexibility also lends itself to alternate means of controlling the board. If your child has severe physical limitations, for example, he or she can use a beam of light attached to the forehead to activate the board.

VOCAs have greatly improved the quality of life for individuals with severe communication disorders. There are, however, still important limitations to these devices. Although faster than the manual boards, they remain a fairly slow way to communicate in comparison with spoken language. The speed of using VOCAs is influenced by your child's physical and intellectual abilities and the number of squares required to make a message. Speed of communication can be a particular hindrance for children with impaired cognitive and/or physical skills whose boards contain a large number of squares. If the communication becomes too slow, decreasing the number of squares on the board or simplifying the number of squares that your child must press to communicate a particular message may be wise.

Another problem with VOCAs is their expense. They typically cost thousands of dollars. Medical insurance companies and charitable organizations often help to defray the purchase price of AAC devices. The speech-language therapist who evaluates your child for AAC will often be able to assist you in acquiring the device and in identifying possible funding sources.

SUMMARY

Speech and language are complex abilities that have multiple facets: grammar, articulation, fluency, and more. Many biological and environmental factors can affect the development of these communication skills. Furthermore, these skills can be impaired independently of other abilities, such as general intelligence or gross motor skills. If you suspect that your child has a communication disorder, he or she should undergo a careful evaluation to determine exactly which facets of his or her abilities are impaired. Speech-language therapy should be tailored to address exactly those areas. Without appropriate therapy, a communication disorder can affect your child's performance in school and his or her relationships with others.

Some Questions Answered

Why does my child's ability to learn new communication skills seem so variable—excellent on one day, weak the next?

Parents and teachers sometimes come to believe that a child is lazy because he or she has variable communication abilities. It is common to hear frustrated parents say, "Sometimes she can make the 's' sound just fine. Other times she can't. She's just not trying." Your child's variable performance, however, is the hallmark of learning a new skill. Your child may also be confused when he or she is asked to perform slightly different tasks from one occasion to the next. For example, the first time your ask your child to say "s," you may be pointing to a picture of the sun, the second time to a picture of a star, and the third time to a picture of a bus. Although these words may seem to be equally difficult, in reality the single "s" at the beginning of a word (*sun*) is typically learned *much earlier* than the "s" in consonant clusters (*star*) is. So, your child's inability to say "s" consistently may be due to the varying difficulty of the tasks. Such subtle but important differences in task complexity are very common in many aspects of speech and language.

Will using baby talk slow down my daughter's communication development?

No. Baby talk is characterized by slow speed, clear articulation, and exaggerated intonation. All of these features usually help children to recognize the sounds that they are hearing and to understand their meanings. In general, you should talk in a way that helps your child have enjoyable interactions, and this often includes using baby talk. You may find it helpful to use word approximations when your baby is just beginning to learn words, such as "wawa" for water and "baba" for bottle. You can alternate the real word and the approximation.

My child has a developmental delay and does not speak yet. What is the latest age at which he might learn to talk?

The general rule of thumb is that if a child is to speak, he or she will start to speak words by about 5 years old. There are, however, exceptions to every rule, including this one. In fact, the vast majority of children with developmental disabilities do learn to speak, and many of the rest use speech in conjunction with sign language or other forms of AAC. Do not, however, wait until your child is 5 years old before seeking help. If your child is not producing voiced sounds and syllables by 12 months, words by 18 months, and word combinations by 28 months, it is important to seek help.

If my child learns sign language or uses augmentative or alternative communication, will it hold back the development of her spoken language abilities?

No. Careful studies have shown that teaching sign language to children with communication disorders does not delay the onset of their spoken language abilities. As long as your child continues to receive good verbal stimulation, he or she will start to speak when the brain and nervous system are ready. In the meantime, your child's ability to communicate in sign language will help him or her interact better with family, peers, and teachers and reduce frustration at being unable to share thoughts. Likewise, use of a VOCA is likely to encourage rather than prevent the development of verbal speech by allowing your child to practice positive and successful means of communication.

Do all children with language disorders have mental retardation?

No, most do not. Mental retardation means that both verbal and nonverbal skills are impaired. A language disorder is a problem with language but not necessarily with nonverbal reasoning abilities.

Eye Disorders
and Visual Impairments

Mohamad S. Jaafar and Mark L. Batshaw

Children can have a range of visual problems. Some are associated with conditions such as prematurity or developmental disorders such as cerebral palsy and mental retardation; others may be the child's only disability. In this chapter, the function of the visual system and various problems that can cause visual impairment in your child are discussed. How vision affects child development and approaches to treating and living with visual impairments are also addressed.

The eyes are your baby's windows on the world. While still in the delivery room, your child already has color vision and can see faces. Your infant's bonds to you are strengthened through vision, smell, and physical touch during the first days after birth. At this point, the shape of your face is most attractive, and bright colors catch your infant's fancy.

Vision is present at birth but is not very clear; it is only about 20/400 (that is, your infant is able to see 20 feet away what a person with typical vision can see 400 feet away). Usually, visual skills develop rapidly during infancy. By 1 month of age, your baby can visually fix on you, and by 2 months, your infant's eyes will follow a mobile as it rotates. Color vision develops more during the first 2–3 months of life. At 3 months, your infant will likely turn from one face to another, differentiating mother from father and parents from strangers. At 6 months, your child's vision improves to 20/40, and sometime between 12 and 24 months, it should reach the adult level of 20/20. Binocular vision (simultaneous visual perception from both eyes) and depth perception begin around 4 months and are usually well developed by 6 months.

Not only does vision permit your child to focus on the world, but it also is integral to the development of other skills. For example, learning to move is enhanced by having a goal to reach and seeing how others move. As a result, if your child has a severe visual impairment, he or she might learn to walk later than usual. Likewise, the development of speech involves imitation of mouth movements, so that language may be delayed in a child with visual impairment. Hence, vision disorders, even if not associated with other disabilities, can affect typical development. About 20% of children with developmental disabilities have a significant visual impairment. The risk is especially high in children with genetic syndromes, cerebral palsy, and mental retardation. Therefore, an eye exam should be an integral part of the medical evaluation of all children with developmental disabilities.

EYES AND THEIR FUNCTION

The eye works much like a camera. The lens of the eye brings an image into focus on the retina, the "photographic film" at the rear of the eye. The retina captures the image, which is then transported in the form of electrical signals to the brain. The brain integrates this visual information, leading to perception. An impairment anywhere along this pathway will interfere with vision.

The eyeball itself is a globe (see Figure 22.1). On the front, there is a central opening called the *pupil*, which appears black. Surrounding the pupil is the colored part of the eye (usually brown, green, or blue) called the *iris*. Like the shutter on a camera, the pupil opens and closes in response to light, dilating in dim light and constricting in bright sunshine. In front of the iris is a protective, clear window called the *cornea*. Behind the iris is the *lens*. Light rays hit the cornea first and are refracted, or bent, by the cornea and lens on their way to a focal point on the retina. Between the lens and the retina, the eyeball is filled with a jelly-like substance called the *vitreous*. Among the different cells of the retina are *rods* and *cones* that process the light and send the information via the *optic nerve* to the brain.

REFRACTIVE ERRORS

For a person to see clearly, light rays entering the eye must be focused by the cornea and lens to create a sharp image on the retina. Focusing problems, also called *refractive errors*, are usually not caused by a disease of the eye but by the relationship of the size of the eye to the strength of its cornea/lens system (see Figure 22.2). Children can have three different types of refractive errors that may require corrective lenses:

- *Myopia,* or nearsightedness, is often inherited. A myopic eyeball is often longer than normal, causing light rays to focus in front of the retina. This causes *near* objects to look clear, but distant objects appear blurred.

- *Hyperopia,* or farsightedness, is caused by light rays focusing behind the retina. A hyperopic eye may be shorter than typical, or the cornea/lens

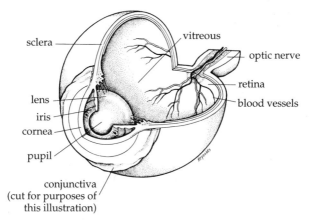

sclera

vitreous

optic nerve

retina

blood vessels

lens

iris

cornea

pupil

conjunctiva
(cut for purposes of
this illustration)

Figure 22.1.   The eye. The front of the eye consists of a clear window (the cornea), a central aperture (the pupil), and a colored surrounding area (the iris). Behind the iris is the lens, which helps the eye focus entering light rays. A transparent membrane (the conjunctiva) covers the white wall of the eye (the sclera). The vitreous is a translucent gelatinous substance that fills the inside of the eye and maintains its shape. At the back of the globe lies the film-like retina, blood vessels supplying nutrients to the eye, and the optic nerve carrying impulses to the brain.

system may be too weak. A person with hyperopia can see *far* objects but has difficulty seeing near objects clearly. Children, however, are often a little farsighted but have a large reserve of focusing power that allows the eyes to adjust and see well up close and at distances. In young people, only severe hyperopia needs to be corrected.

- *Astigmatism* distorts and blurs vision for both near and far objects. In an eye with astigmatism, light rays focus at different places on the retina, making a round object such as a basketball appear distorted, more like a football.

Identifying and correcting refractive errors early is important. Your baby's eyes can be checked for refractive errors even before he or she is able to participate actively with the testing. Using special eyedrops, instruments, and lenses, the ophthalmologist or optometrist can determine the correct lens power needed. Once the lens power has been determined, choosing eyeglasses that will fit your child's age, facial features, and activities is important. Flared and non-skid nose pads, cable temples, flexible hinges, and/or straps can be used to help the fit. Be positive about the glasses and your child's appearance in them. If your child is old enough, let him or her help pick out the frames. Prescription sunglasses can be purchased if your child needs to wear eyeglasses at all times. If your child refuses to wear the eyeglasses, always consider the possibility that the prescription might not have been filled correctly, and have the glasses checked or the frames adjusted. If the eye-

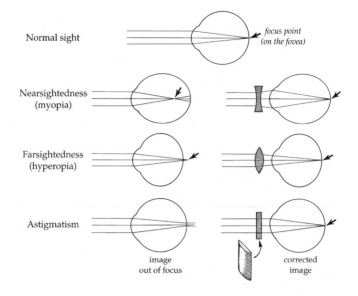

Figure 22.2.   The lenses in eyeglasses are curved to correct for the refractive error. Here are shown lenses for nearsightedness, farsightedness, and astigmatism.

glasses are correctly made but your child continues to refuse to wear them, you may find behavior management techniques helpful (see Chapter 11).

Contact lenses generally work as well as glasses, although children younger than 12 years often are unable to safely care for them. *Soft lenses* are the most commonly used type of contact lens except for people with astigmatism, who must wear *gas permeable hard lenses* or *toric soft lenses*. In general, contact lenses should not be worn overnight. Good hygiene is essential. Laser surgery to correct refractive errors is not approved for use in children.

LAZY EYE: AMBLYOPIA

For vision to develop fully, both eyes must be used throughout childhood. An eye that is not used well develops *amblyopia* (partial loss of sight) and is called a "lazy eye." The condition is common, affecting approximately 2 or 3 of every 100 children. The best time to correct amblyopia is during infancy or early childhood; earlier is easier and better. After about the first 9 years of life, the visual system is fully developed and cannot be changed. If amblyopia is not treated, several problems can occur: The weak eye may end up with a serious and permanent visual defect, depth perception (seeing in three dimensions) may be lost, and if the good eye becomes diseased or injured, a lifetime of decreased vision may result. Amblyopia has three major causes:

- *Strabismus* (misaligned eyes, which includes *esotropia,* or inturning, and *exotropia,* or outturning): When the eyes are not straight, the crossed or wandering eye conveys a second image to the brain. The brain rejects this double image, and soon the child unconsciously stops using the weak eye.

- *Unequal focus* (refractive error): When one eye is out of focus because it is more nearsighted, farsighted, or astigmatic than the other, the unfocused (blurred) eye can "turn off" and become amblyopic. This is the most difficult type of amblyopia to detect and requires careful assessment of vision.

- *Cloudiness:* An eye disease such as a cloudy cornea or lens opacity (*cataract*) may lead to amblyopia. This type of amblyopia is the most severe and can affect both eyes.

To correct amblyopia, your child must learn to use the weak eye. Eyeglasses may be prescribed to correct errors in focusing. In addition, covering the strong eye with a patch, often for weeks or months, may be necessary. Because the patch covers the good eye, your child will have trouble seeing at first and may try to take the patch off. This problem usually disappears as soon as your child gets used to wearing the patch and vision in the weaker eye improves. As a general rule, the younger your child and the shorter the time the eye has been "lazy," the less time it will take for treatment to be successful. As an alternative, amblyopia can be treated by temporarily blurring vision in the stronger eye with special eyedrops or with fogged lenses so that the weaker eye becomes stronger.

Michael

Michael was a healthy baby boy whose parents noted that his eyes started crossing shortly after birth. When his left eye looked at an object, the right eye tended to drift inward. The crossing persisted, and when Michael was 2 months old, his pediatrician referred him to an ophthalmologist who diagnosed him as having *esotropia*, or an inward crossing of the eye. The doctor started patching Michael's left eye for a few hours a day to improve vision in his right "lazy" eye and to prevent amblyopia. When vision became equal in both eyes, the doctor recommended eye muscle surgery to maximize Michael's likelihood of developing binocular vision.

EYE MUSCLE PROBLEMS: STRABISMUS

As Michael's story illustrates, the brain not only receives visual information from the eyes but also sends back signals that control eye movement, permitting us to look at an object, focus on it, and then follow (track) it as it moves. Six small muscles that surround each eye coordinate these movements (see Figure 22.3). If the brain cannot accurately control these muscles, however, the eyes will not move in synchrony and strabismus will result.

With normal eyes, both eyes aim at the same spot. The brain then fuses the two pictures into a single image, giving us depth perception. With strabismus,

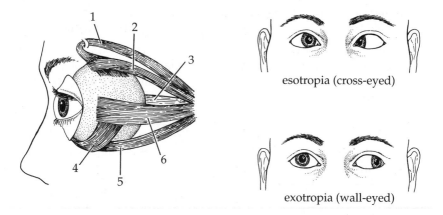

Figure 22.3.   The eye muscles. Six muscles move the eyeball. A weakness of one of these muscles causes strabismus. In esotropia, the eye turns in; in exotropia, the eye turns out. Esotropia and exotropia of the left eye are shown.

the eyes are misaligned, pointing in different directions and sending different pictures simultaneously to the brain. One eye may look straight ahead, whereas the other eye turns inward, outward, upward, or downward. The misalignment may or may not always be present. Strabismus occurs equally in males and females and affects about 4% of all children in the United States. Strabismus is especially common among children born prematurely or with disorders that affect the brain, such as cerebral palsy, mental retardation, hydrocephalus, and genetic disorders including Down syndrome. Cataracts or eye injuries can also cause strabismus. Strabismus may run in families and can also occur later in life. Adolescents and adults who develop strabismus often have double vision. A young child's brain, however, learns to suppress the image of the misaligned eye and loses depth perception. If the child always ignores images from the same eye, that eye becomes "lazy" and loses visual acuity.

A typical newborn baby's eyes may wander intermittently because the eye muscles are not well coordinated. Within a few weeks, however, the infant learns to move both eyes together. If the misalignment is constant or if it continues beyond the second month of life, prompt medical attention is required. Young children often have a wide, flat nose with a fold of skin at the inner eyelid that can make the eyes appear crossed (called *pseudostrabismus*). This condition will improve as the child grows. A child will *not*, however, outgrow true strabismus. An ophthalmologist can usually tell the difference between pseudostrabismus and true strabismus. Treatment of strabismus involves patching the stronger eye, wearing glasses, and/or undergoing surgery. Early surgery offers the best chance for the eyes to work well together. It is not, however, a substitute for using eyeglasses or wearing a patch, solutions that force the weak eye to "see." There is little evidence that eye exercises are helpful in most types of strabismus.

DISORDERS OF THE LENS: CATARACTS

A cataract is a clouding of the eye's normally clear lens. This inhibits light rays from reaching the retina and results in hazy or blurred vision. Although cataracts occur mostly in older adults, infants and children can also have cataracts. Infant cataracts may be inherited as part of a genetic syndrome or may occur as a result of a viral infection contracted during pregnancy. Childhood cataracts often result from an eye injury, chronic use of steroids such as prednisone, or certain chronic diseases such as diabetes.

Some childhood cataracts may only partially cloud the lens and do not interfere with vision. These small cataracts usually do not require treatment, but they should be checked periodically as they may become larger with time. Larger cataracts that interfere with vision require immediate surgery in which, using microscopic surgical techniques, an ophthalmologist removes the entire lens. Cataract removal, however, is only the first step in treatment. Your child will need a substitute lens (eyeglasses, contact lenses, or, for older children, intraocular lenses that are surgically placed in the eyes) to focus images onto the retina. Regardless of which method of visual correction is used, your child will need bifocals to see near objects clearly. The good eye may also need patching until vision improves in the eye that had the cataract. Children with cataracts often develop strabismus that may require eye muscle surgery.

DISORDER OF INTRAOCULAR PRESSURE: GLAUCOMA

Glaucoma is caused by increased pressure inside the eye due to inadequate drainage of the aqueous humor, a clear fluid filling the anterior chamber, or the space between the iris and the cornea. Like cataracts, the disorder usually occurs in older adults and tends to affect both eyes. Childhood glaucoma, however, usually appears in the first year of life. Children with glaucoma have severe sensitivity to light, excessive tearing of the eyes, and/or a large cloudy cornea. Any of these signs should prompt you to immediately consult an ophthalmologist for proper diagnosis and urgent treatment to prevent blindness. Treatment is primarily surgical to improve the intraocular drainage system.

Robin

Robin was born 3 months prematurely. Because of the risk of visual impairment as a complication of prematurity, an ophthalmologist examined Robin's eyes while she was still in the hospital. He found that new blood vessels were growing abnormally onto her retina, an early sign of retinopathy of prematurity. Using a special laser, he was able to halt the damage. Now 4 years old, Robin wears eyeglasses for her nearsightedness, the only residual sign of her retinopathy of prematurity.

DISORDERS OF THE RETINA: RETINOPATHY OF PREMATURITY AND COLOR/NIGHT BLINDNESS

If your baby is born significantly before term, as was Robin, the immature retinal blood vessels may start growing abnormally and begin to invade the gelatin-like vitreous humor that fills the interior of the eye. In this situation, called *retinopathy of prematurity (ROP)*, the blood vessels will eventually stop growing, leaving a fibrous scar that contracts and, in the most severe cases, pulls the retina away from the back of the eye. If enough retina is pulled away, your child will lose sight in that eye. As this process is likely to involve both eyes, in the most severe cases premature infants with ROP may become permanently blind.

To avoid visual impairment from ROP, ophthalmologists routinely check the retinas of premature infants while they are still in the hospital. In this way the abnormal blood vessel growth can be detected early and the retina treated with a laser that destroys the abnormal blood vessels and "tacks down" the retina. Although not always successful, this procedure has significantly reduced retinal detachment in premature infants. Children born prematurely may subsequently develop nearsightedness, crossed eyes, and amblyopia and need to be closely monitored throughout childhood.

Color vision impairment is often caused by a problem in the light-sensitive cells of the retina: the rods and cones. Rods are responsible for night and dim light vision. Cones are responsible for color and sharp vision. There are three types of cones, each having a different pigment, making it sensitive to a different color of light: blue, green, or red. By combining the signals of these different cones, the eye can see all of the colors of the rainbow.

The most common defect of the cones results in color blindness, a sex-linked trait that affects 6% of boys and 1% of girls. Color blindness prevents a person from discriminating certain colors, with telling red from green being the most common problem. This type of color blindness does not, however, cause a decrease in vision and is not associated with cognitive impairments. A colorblind person will just perceive the world differently.

Retinal disorders affecting the rods, such as *retinitis pigmentosa (RP)* and vitamin A deficiency, result in poor vision after dusk, are usually progressive, and may eventually result in blindness. Unlike color blindness, which appears in childhood, these disorders can appear anytime during a person's life. Early signs of cone retinal dystrophy are poor vision, light sensitivity, and possibly shaking of the eye (discussed next). With rod dystrophy, however, you may notice that your child stumbles or holds on to you tightly while walking outside at night. Any such symptoms or a family history of night blindness necessitates an early ophthalmological evaluation.

SHAKING EYES: NYSTAGMUS

Nystagmus (unintentional jittery movements of the eyes) usually involves both eyes, although sometimes one side is more affected than the other. It is often exaggerated when a person looks in one particular direction. There are many causes of nystagmus. Sometimes, the brain's control of eye movements is poor, resulting in an inability to look steadily at an object. Other times, nystagmus is a side effect of medications. The disorder can also run in families as an isolated problem (called *motor nystagmus*) or may accompany reduced vision, such as that resulting from *bilateral congenital cataract,* from albinism, from scars in the retina, from retinal dystrophy, or from an abnormal optic nerve. Occasionally, nystagmus can result from a brain tumor or other serious neurological disorder.

If nystagmus is present, a thorough evaluation by an ophthalmologist and perhaps by a neurologist is very important. Early surgery to remove a congenital cataract may allow better vision. Reduced vision also may be improved by eyeglasses and low vision aids (discussed later in this chapter). At times, a child with nystagmus may adopt a head turn to decrease the nystagmus and achieve better vision. Eye muscle surgery can help shift the child's optimal gaze position and alleviate this abnormal head position.

EYE TRAUMA

Trauma to the eye is quite common in children and most often involves something that gets stuck under the eyelid or an object that scratches the surface of the cornea. Small objects can usually be removed from the eye through the combined action of tears and by repeated lifting and sliding the upper eyelid over the lower lid. If your child complains of being hit in the eye, has pain, unexplained sensitivity to light, or watering of the eye that persists for an hour, you should take him or her to the pediatrician or the emergency room. Doctors can determine if there has been a corneal abrasion, bleeding inside the eye, severe inflammation, retinal injury, or other serious damage.

ASSESSING VISION

In the first 2 years of life, you are likely to be the one who has the best impression of your child's visual function. If you are concerned, arrange for a full evaluation by a pediatric ophthalmologist. The ophthalmologist can determine visual acuity through indirect ways such as watching how well your infant follows objects with one eye when the other eye is covered. There are also direct means of testing vision, even for nonverbal children ages 6 months to 3 years and for children with severe physical or cognitive disabilities. In addition to the clinical examination, ultrasound, CT (computed tomography), and MRI (magnetic resonance imaging) of the eyes and brain can help detect abnormalities that may interfere with vision. Using a combination of these techniques, the ophthalmologist can determine your child's vision and differentiate between a visual impairment resulting from retinal damage versus cortical blindness (discussed later).

In addition, *peripheral vision,* or *side vision,* which is very important for many daily activities, can best be measured by an ophthalmologist. Normal eyes can recognize objects over a field measuring at least 140 degrees (almost half of a circle). A child with a much narrower range of side vision (tunnel vision) may have trouble walking or recognizing people in a large room, even when central vision is excellent. This, however, is a rare problem in children.

VISUAL IMPAIRMENT AND BLINDNESS

When your child's best corrected central visual acuity is 20/200 or less in the better eye, or the side vision is narrowed to 20 degrees or less in the better eye, your child is considered legally blind even though he or she may have some useful vision. If neither eye can see better than 20/70, even with improvement from eyeglasses, your child is said to be visually impaired. Limited side vision, double vision, poor night vision, and loss of vision in one eye may also determine visual impairment. Within legal blindness are further degrees of severity: Vision can range from 20/200 in which your child can see the largest letter on an eye chart and read very large print, to vision sufficient to walk without assistance, to vision that allows your child to distinguish motion and shades, to perception of light, to absolute blindness with inability to perceive light.

Blindness is most commonly caused by abnormalities or damage to the optic nerve or retina. Blindness occurring when the eyes themselves are healthy is called *cortical* or *central blindness*. In this type of blindness, there is damage either to the nerve tracts leading from the back of the eyes to the visual centers of the brain (the occipital cortex) or to the occipital cortex itself, where the electrical signals sent through the nerves are interpreted (see Figure 22.4). Head trauma, brain infection, stroke, and lack of oxygen can all cause cortical blindness. Unlike peripheral blindness, which is irreversible, cortical blindness can spontaneously improve over time. It is difficult, however, to predict the ultimate visual ability of a young child with cortical blindness.

If your child has a visual impairment, good communication with the ophthalmologist will help you understand the cause of the vision impairment and learn whether it is temporary, stable, or likely to progress. You may also be able to learn if the condition is hereditary and presents a risk to other family members. Inquire about rehabilitation programs, devices, and supportive services. It is very important for your child to visit his or her ophthalmologist for regular checkups as the eye disorder may change over time, requiring a change in treatment. Because eyes can be affected by more than one disorder, detecting and promptly treating any new problem is important to preserve your child's sight.

LIVING WITH "ONE GOOD EYE"

Children growing up with vision in only one eye may never notice the difference and develop typically, although their depth perception may be impaired. Older children who suddenly lose vision in one eye will go through

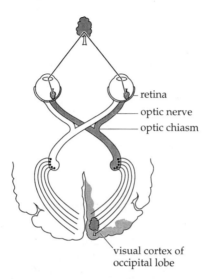

retina
optic nerve
optic chiasm

visual cortex of
occipital lobe

Figure 22.4.   The visual pathways. The image of a tree is imposed on the retina upside down and backwards, as is film in a camera. This is converted to electrical energy, which is conducted along the optic nerve, which emerges from behind each eye. A portion of the fibers of each optic nerve cross at the optic chiasm. Nerve tracts then lead to the back of the brain where the image is "seen."

a readjustment period, but they generally adjust well. In childhood, eye injuries are the leading cause of vision loss in one eye. Once vision is irreversibly impaired in one eye, taking care of the remaining eye becomes extremely important. Your child with vision in one eye should wear appropriate eye protection at all times during school, play, and sports or hobby activities. For everyday protection, impact-resistant eyeglasses with sturdy frames and polycarbonate lenses are sufficient. Your child should wear protective eyeglasses throughout life, even if no prescription is necessary for the correction of vision. Contact lenses alone should not be used, because they do not offer protection from trauma and may even increase the risk of infection to the good eye. It is important to emphasize that the better eye does not "wear out" or "work harder," even though it provides most or all of a person's vision. Nevertheless, regular eye examinations by an ophthalmologist are even more important for a child with vision in one eye because early detection of any disorder or disease is crucial.

LEARNING DISABILITIES AND THE EYES

There is little scientific evidence to suggest that poor vision, abnormal focusing, jerky eye movements, and/or misaligned eyes contribute to the development of learning disabilities (see Chapter 25). If your child has been diagnosed with a learning disability, however, he or she needs a thorough medical eye examination to detect any visual defect (such as eye muscle imbalance, astigmatism, or significant farsightedness) that may affect reading. There is no scientific evidence that visual training, special eyeglasses, or muscle, perceptual, or eye–hand coordination exercises can alleviate a child's learning disability.

DEVELOPMENT OF A CHILD WITH VISUAL IMPAIRMENT

Although most children with visual impairment have typical intelligence, many children with total blindness have developmental disabilities. These disabilities include most prominently cerebral palsy, mental retardation, and hearing impairment. Even children with typical intelligence who have severe visual impairment can have delays in the development of reasoning, language, social, and motor abilities. The child with sight learns many of these skills by following the comings and goings of parents and by imitating observed language and social skills. With the lack of visual input, your child's development will probably progress more slowly during early childhood (see Figure 22.5).

A child who is blind must learn to speak using auditory cues alone, without the aid of imitating mouth movements. As a result, your child may use echolalia, repeating words that have been said without necessarily understanding their meaning, or he or she may imitate environmental sounds, such as a car passing by, a dog barking, or a phone ringing. Your child may have difficulty differentiating *self* from *other* and refer to him- or herself in the third person. Although delayed in onset, the speech of most children with visual impairment is usually typical by school age. Your child may also have an unanimated facial expression. This does not mean, however, that he or she is sad or uninterested. You can learn to watch for subtle head and body movements that give hints of your child's mood. Because your child's communication is less likely to be accompanied by body and facial expression, you will want to work to develop age-appropriate conversation and social skills.

If you are concerned about your child's cognitive abilities, formal IQ testing can be performed. The results are most accurate when your child is old enough to be tested on language and verbal reasoning abilities rather than on the visual-perceptual skills that are prominently tested in preschoolers. The verbal section of the Wechsler Intelligence Scale for Children–Third Edition (WISC–III) is most often used (see Chapter 14).

Because muscle tone, which depends on visual perception, may be decreased in children with visual impairments, motor skills are also affected in early childhood, and sitting and walking may be delayed. Do not be surprised if your infant does not sit until after 8 months and starts walking only at about 2 years of age. Unless your child has a physical disability as well, he or she will catch up over time and motor impairments will not be a long-term concern.

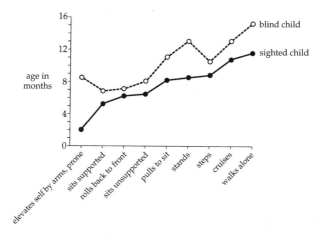

Figure 22.5.   The development of children with visual impairments who have typical intelligence is contrasted with the development of sighted children. The development of motor skills is delayed in blind children.

Fine motor skills, including self-feeding, may also be delayed or unusual. For example, your child may begin reaching out and grabbing for objects late, and instead of turning toward sounds, he or she may reach for them. In children with blindness and mental retardation, it may be difficult to distinguish what proportion of the developmental delay is due to vision loss and what is due to cognitive disability.

Individuals with visual impairment are often said to compensate by having other senses that are heightened. This may be true but does not occur automatically. For example, your child may not use his or her hands much, because he or she mostly ends up grabbing at air. Thus, you need to interest your child in different textures and shapes that can be explored manually or toys that make sounds when squeezed or turned. Crib gyms are also good for practicing motor skills.

Children with visual impairments can also become more sensitive to sounds. Your child can develop hearing for use in locating objects. For example, your child may be able to learn to navigate around rooms without bumping into things by memorizing the location of objects and by listening for the echoes bouncing off solid objects as he or she walks. This training to enhance the senses is frequently done by physical or occupational therapists.

BEHAVIORAL CHARACTERISTICS OF CHILDREN WITH VISUAL IMPAIRMENTS

Children with visual impairments may engage in a variety of self-stimulatory behaviors that are called *blindisms*. Your child may, for example, show repetitive behaviors such as twirling, rocking, waving fingers in front of the face, or head banging. In addition, there may be intermittent forceful blinking, gazing at lights, eye pressing, head rolling, or swaying back and forth. These behaviors usually become less evident after 4 years of age in children with typical intelligence but may persist throughout life in children with visual impairments and mental retardation.

The reason for the self-stimulatory behaviors is not known, but they may be attempts by your child to compensate for the sensory stimulation that he or she does not receive visually. The child with some dark/light vision may enjoy the changes of shading that can be produced by playing with his or her hands in front of the eyes. Another possible explanation is that a totally blind child may "see" light when rubbing the eyes. This is not the case, however, for children with cortical blindness, and they do not engage in eye pressing. If these behaviors become a significant problem, behavior management techniques can be used to decrease their frequency (see Chapter 11). Blindisms can be distinguished from the self-stimulatory behaviors of children with autism (see Chapter 23) because they are not accompanied by the social and language impairments typical of children with autism.

Your child may also have sleep problems. It is not unusual for a child with visual impairment to reverse day and night sleep patterns or maintain a prolonged (such as 27-hour instead of 24-hour) daily internal clock. Children who are blind also tend to sleep less. Treatment with melatonin at bedtime may help to establish a normal sleep–wake pattern and may be considered by your child's pediatrician.

TEACHING INFANTS AND YOUNG CHILDREN WITH VISUAL IMPAIRMENTS

Your child's formal education should begin as soon as a visual impairment is detected. Early intervention programs are available beginning in the first month of life for infants with visual impairments (see Chapter 6). Usually, this entails a once-per-week, home-based program in which an early childhood educator or therapist visits and works with you and your child. Along with language and exploration, the early childhood educator will work on motor skills and stimulating residual vision. The teacher will try to help your child develop protective reactions, such as extending the arms when losing balance. Your child needs these quick reactions in sitting and walking to have more confidence in exploring the environment. Your child may show little motivation and a lot of fear when learning to walk. Try using a desired object or destination (a favorite chair or toy) to motivate your child. Use your voice to guide your child in the right direction.

Different approaches to stimulating residual vision or other senses are required at different ages. For your infant, a mirror attached to the crib, brightly colored mobiles, or Christmas lights all stimulate the use of residual vision. Keep toys in the same part of the crib so that your child knows where to find them, or attach the toys by strings to a highchair so they can be thrown and then retrieved. Toys such as dolls and coloring books carry no interest for the child with severe visual impairment who has little idea of the shape of the human body or colors.

Encouraging fine motor skills is important because a sensitive touch can substitute for vision to some extent. Give your child finger foods that are unlikely to be crushed easily, such as celery, cookies, crackers, bacon, French fries, and M&Ms. Avoid giving your child soft, messy foods such as fruit slices; children with visual impairments generally do not like their hands being sticky, as they depend on a sensitive touch. Use a deep dish with straight sides to help your child learn to use a spoon and a "tippy" cup to teach drinking. Stacking blocks, nesting cubes, and colored rings may improve your child's eye–hand coordination. Other fine motor tasks can include using a toy work-bench, unscrewing bottle caps and lids to obtain desired objects, stringing large beads, and practicing buttoning. In teaching dressing skills, use Velcro straps when possible for shoes, pants, and shirts.

Touch and hearing should be particularly stimulated and encouraged. You must remember that if your child was born blind, then he or she will have no concept of the structure of the surrounding environment. If your child, however, had vision and then lost it, discovering the structure of the environment is less of a problem, especially if the visual impairment oc-curred after 2 years of age. Your child may learn by touching an object while you explain its name, its function, and its physical contours. Your child will explore by smelling, touching, tasting, turning over, and examining each ob-ject. Place your infant on his or her stomach rather than back to strengthen neck and trunk muscles and to make toys more attainable. Giving your child toys that have interesting surfaces to explore and that make noises will en-courage exploration and discrimination of shapes, orientation, and distance in space.

Safety and social considerations will demand close observation on your part, but you must allow your child as much freedom as possible to explore. This exploration can sometimes lead to uncomfortable situations. For exam-ple, your child may touch and smell objects or people as a learning tool that may not always be socially acceptable. Some compromises in propriety may be necessary in order for learning to occur, but your child must eventually respect personal space.

In terms of stimulating language, start talking to your child while you are at a distance to avoid startling him or her. When you are with your child, provide a running commentary on everything that is going on. In addition, give an explanation before, during, and after a task is performed. When mov-ing from one space to another, explain the purpose of the move and the ori-entation of the space. Talk as much as possible in a responsive way, and address your child by name frequently to include him or her in conversa-tions. Your child needs to react to your questions and take part in conversations, not just listen passively. Placing your child in front of a television set to learn words can lead to simple echoing of advertising jingles rather than the development of interactive language. A multisensory approach to learning will be most helpful. For example, as your child eats breakfast, allow him or her to smell and touch the cereal and to feel how it floats in the bowl, melts in the mouth, and tastes different from other foods. Have your child play outside in the grass, jump in the leaves, and dig in the dirt while you explain what these things represent. In your interactions with your child, use touch and physical affection. Remember that you cannot depend on using body language to convey your message.

By 3 years of age, children with visual impairments are usually ready for school-based programs. Over the next few years, listening, concept development, conversation, and daily living skills (dressing, eating, personal hygiene) are emphasized. The use of aids such as improved lighting devices, large-face clocks, and special kitchen tools is most helpful in promoting independence during this time.

AIDS FOR THE CHILD WITH VISUAL IMPAIRMENT

By school entry, the full extent of your child's visual impairment is usually clear. A child with better than 20/200 corrected vision who can read ¼-inch letters can and should be encouraged to read large-print books or use optical and electronic magnifiers to read regular print. Children with less than 20/200 corrected vision should learn to read braille, a symbolic language formed as a series of raised dots on a page and read from left to right. When your child is able to recognize small shapes, differentiate between rough and smooth, and follow a line of small figures across the page, he or she can begin learning braille.

Computers have opened an entire range of new possibilities for children with visual impairments. You should help your child learn to type on a computer by fourth grade. A great deal of other technology assistance is available. There are machines that can convert text to braille. Typed computer messages can also be converted into speech, and there are verbal note-taking devices and talking calculators. Computers can also connect the person with visual impairment to the Internet and libraries and can control various functions in the house, such as light switches, telephones, and door locks, thereby permitting greater independence. You can also encourage your child to use mobility aids for walking, such as a walking cane.

With these tools, children with severe visual impairments and typical intelligence often can follow the general education curriculum in school. They may need certain special services, however, such as classes on promoting listening skills, which range from auditory discrimination, to following complex directions, to using accelerated or compressed speech in recorded textbooks. Children with visual impairments and additional disabilities may be placed in an inclusive classroom.

WHAT THE FUTURE HOLDS

Outcomes for a child with visual impairment depend on the amount of residual vision, the child's intellectual abilities, the motivation of the child and family, and the skills of the involved teachers and therapists. In general, the less severe the visual impairment and the higher the IQ score, the better the outcomes. It is clear, however, that improved technology assistance and increased acceptance of individuals with disabilities in the workplace have increased the likelihood that children with severe visual impairments will function independently and successfully as adults.

Some Questions Answered

How old must my child be to wear eyeglasses?

Glasses can be worn as early as 6–9 months. In the case of a severe visual loss, correction with eyeglasses or contact lenses should be attempted immediately; however, a less severe refractive error of between 20/40 and 20/60 does not need to be corrected in a preschooler. Once your child has started elementary school, correction to 20/20 should be attempted.

Does wearing glasses or contact lenses make my daughter dependent on them? Do glasses change her condition?

Glasses are used to correct blurred vision. They neither make a child dependent on them nor improve the underlying condition. Keep in mind, however, that your daughter's eyeglass prescription will change with time. As the eyes grow, they usually become more nearsighted (or less farsighted), regardless of whether your child has been wearing glasses full time.

Can my child outgrow crossed or misaligned eyes?

Children do not outgrow crossed eyes, and without treatment, a child whose eyes are misaligned may lose depth perception and develop poor vision in one eye because the brain will "turn off" or ignore the image from the misaligned eye. In general, the earlier crossed or misaligned eyes are treated, the better. Treatment may include eyeglasses, patching, eye drops, or surgery.

Can using a computer or sitting close to the television damage my child's eyes?

Working on computers or playing video games will not harm your child's eyes. Often, when your child uses a computer for prolonged periods of time, just as when reading or doing other close work, he or she will blink less than usual. This makes the eyes dry, which may lead to eye strain or fatigue. Encourage your child to take regular breaks, to look up or across the room, or blink a couple of times. If the symptoms persist, however, you should consult an ophthalmologist.

Children often develop the habit of holding reading material close to their eyes or sitting right in front of the television. There is no evidence that this damages their eyes, and the habit usually disappears as children grow older. On the other hand, children with nearsightedness (myopia) frequently sit close to the television to see more clearly. If this behavior is consistent or if there is a family history of nearsightedness, your child's eyes need to be examined.

23

Autism Spectrum Disorders

Kenneth E. Towbin

If a doctor has said that your child has an *autism spectrum disorder,* you may be worried and puzzled. Or, possibly you have known all along that something wasn't right but couldn't quite put your finger on it. Since 1943, when autism was first described by Dr. Leo Kanner, a child psychiatrist at the Johns Hopkins University, a great deal has been learned about its causes, how children with autism grow and learn best, and how to help these children. But there is still much to be learned. These days we think of autism as a group of developmental disorders in which the give-and-take of ordinary social interaction and empathy do not develop in a typical fashion. These disorders are called *autism spectrum disorders (ASDS)* and reflect problems with being social and understanding the social behavior of others. Clinicians also sometimes use the term *pervasive developmental disorders (PDDs).* This chapter first defines these disabilities and discusses their causes and associated challenges. Then suggestions are offered for obtaining a complete evaluation and developing an effective intervention program. Finally, the chapter explores ways you can help support your child with special needs and your *whole* family and what you might expect for your child in the future.

WHAT ARE AUTISM SPECTRUM DISORDERS?

The three most common ASDs are autism, Asperger's disorder, and pervasive developmental disorder-not otherwise specified (PDD-NOS), each of which is described later. ASDs are relatively uncommon, affecting only about 1 in 1,000 people. It is important to know that autism and related conditions are developmental brain disorders resulting from a blending of genetic errors. The disorders are complex because so many genes are likely involved. Although ASDs run in families, your child is likely to be the only one on either parent's side to have this kind of disorder. ASDs are not a result of anything anyone has done or not done and are not produced by improper parenting or inexperience in playing with other children.

Amanda

Amanda was her parents' first child and was a quiet baby who ate vigorously and slept well. She sat and crawled on time but at 12 months had not yet said "mama" or "dada." Amanda also did not show much excitement in seeing her father when he came to pick her up from child care, and at 18 months he became worried because she was continuing to babble rather than developing a vocabulary. She didn't point or use other gestures, such as lifting her arms up to request "up," and she maintained only brief eye contact.

At age 2, Amanda seemed fascinated by ceiling fans and would watch them spin for 15–20 minutes at a time, frequently returning to this activity. Although she said a few single words, she did not put phrases together as is typical of 2-year-olds. At her child care center, staff members commented that Amanda kept to herself and became aggressive when other children approached her.

A speech-language evaluation and a hearing test at age 3 found that Amanda's hearing was fine but that she had significant delays in expressive language (using speech) and moderate delays in receptive language (understanding). In her play, Amanda focused on tiny beads and pieces of cloth, which she would carry around with her nearly all of the time. She did not request things of her parents but would cry or whine to get their attention. When injured, Amanda did not seek her mother for comfort and seemed to have a high tolerance for pain. She occasionally sat on her mother's lap for affection, but she did not like to be hugged.

By age 4, Amanda began to use some two-word phrases, but her voice was high pitched and singsong. As her language expanded, it seemed to be lifted verbatim from the videotapes or television programs that she insisted on watching over and over. She became proficient in naming different fabrics and colors and would spend 20–30 minutes at a time laying out different materials and stroking or stacking them. If other children tried to join in, Amanda would cry or walk away. She had no interest in pretend games (such as holding a tea party) or other imaginative play activities (such as outfitting a dollhouse).

This combination of language impairment, social skills deficits, and unusual behaviors led Amanda's parents to seek an evaluation by developmental specialists. The team diagnosed Amanda as having autism. With the family, the team helped design a comprehensive intervention program that included a special full-day preschool program and speech-language therapy three times per week. She has done well with this program, improving both in language and social interaction.

AUTISM

When health care or education professionals use the term *autism* or *autistic disorder* to describe your child's condition, they refer to a developmental disorder that affects three areas: social learning, language, and behaviors/interests (see Table 23.1). For the diagnosis to be accurate, your child should have had problems with one of these three areas before the age of 3 years. This does not mean that symptoms in all three areas need to be present before age 3.

Of course, every child develops in his or her own way, but in autism there is a pattern of immaturity or consistent delays in certain areas. In thinking back on your child's infancy, perhaps signs of impaired social communication were visible as early as 2–3 months of age, when your child did not begin to smile, or at 6 months, when he or she was not copying facial expressions. Perhaps your young toddler did not respond when you called or did not point to things or watch when you pointed. Later he or she probably did not bring things to show and tell at child care or did not play imagination games. As a preschooler, he or she may have had little interest in interacting with other children but may have been more responsive to certain individuals (especially to you). By the time your child entered school, problems with nonverbal communication (such as eye contact, gestures, and voice inflection) may have become prominent. Your child may have shunned or responded awkwardly to others who initiated social contact or perhaps initiated social contact awkwardly, without seeming to "read" or understand others' reactions.

Deficits in language skills may have affected your child's expressive language, receptive language, or both (see Chapter 21). As a toddler, your child may have shown less interest in language than in environmental sounds, turning toward a car horn but not reacting to your voice. Perhaps your child referred to him- or herself by the wrong pronoun ("You want juice" instead of "I want juice"). Some children with ASD have stereotyped speech that is mechanical or that has a repetitive singsong rhythm. Your child may have communicated only to make requests for specific needs. Your child may have responded better to brief phrases rather than to more complex language and may have learned better with visual rather than auditory cues. IQ scores are often below average, but about 40% of children with ASD have average (or even above average) IQ scores in nonverbal or verbal domains.

The repetitive patterns and narrow interests seen in children with ASD can be subtle or prominent. As a toddler, your child may develop self-stimulatory mannerisms or habits such as flapping the hands when excited or repeating the same sound many times. Examples of other repetitive behaviors include rocking, hand waving, spinning, toe walking, and head banging. Like Amanda, your child may also seek special sensory experiences by staring for long periods at ceiling fans, bright lights, mirrors, or things that sway. He or she may like to feel or hold certain fabrics or objects. Sometimes these are not typical cuddly, soft, furry toys but unusual objects such as sticks, a piece of string, or a detergent bottle. Some children become very attached to

Table 23.1.   Diagnostic criteria for autistic disorder

A.   A total of six (or more) items from the following groups:

Group 1[a]

1.   Marked impairment in the use of multiple nonverbal behaviors such as eye-to-eye gaze, facial expression, body postures, and gestures to regulate social interaction

2.   Failure to develop peer relationships appropriate to developmental level

3.   A lack of spontaneous seeking to share enjoyment, interests, or achievements with other people (such as by a lack of showing, bringing, or pointing out objects of interest)

4.   Lack of social or emotional reciprocity

Group 2[b]

1.   Delay in, or total lack of, the development of spoken language (not accompanied by an attempt to compensate through alternative modes of communication such as gesture or mime)

2.   In individuals with adequate speech, marked impairment in the ability to initiate or sustain a conversation with others

3.   Stereotyped and repetitive use of language or idiosyncratic language

4.   Lack of varied, spontaneous make-believe play or social imitative play appropriate to developmental level

Group 3[c]

1.   Encompassing preoccupation with one or more stereotyped and restricted patterns of interest that is abnormal either in intensity or focus

2.   Apparently inflexible adherence to specific, nonfunctional routines or rituals

3.   Stereotyped and repetitive motor mannerisms (such as hand or finger flapping or twisting or complex whole-body movements)

4.   Persistent preoccupation with parts of objects

B.   Delays or abnormal functioning in at least one of the following areas, with onset prior to 3 age years: 1) social interaction, 2) language as used in social communication, or 3) symbolic or imaginative play.

C.   The disturbance is not better accounted for by Rett's Disorder or Childhood Disintegrative Disorder.

[a]Qualitative impairments in social interaction, as manifested by at least two criteria from Group 1.

[b]Qualitative impairments in communication as manifested by at least one criterion from Group 2.

[c]Restricted, repetitive, and stereotyped patterns of behavior, interests, and activities, as manifested by at least one criterion from Group 3.

these objects and carry them wherever they go. They may also respond less than usual to pain or heat and overreact to environmental noises (such as from a vacuum cleaner), touch, or odors. When your child is preschool age, obsessive rituals and adherence to routines may be very important. For example, your child may insist that stories always be read in exactly the same order or that toys be lined up in a precise and unvarying formation. Your child may become distressed or have tantrums when there are minor changes in the environment, such as if a toy or piece of furniture has been moved from its normal place or if the bus route to school is altered. Sometimes restricted interests include food preferences; these may cause you to worry about your child's nutrition.

ASPERGER'S DISORDER

At about the same time that Dr. Kanner was collecting his series of patients with autism, Dr. Hans Asperger observed boys in Austria who displayed similar features of social impairment but had good expressive language skills, with an especially good vocabulary. Asperger's disorder, as the pattern of features came to be named, can be considered the high-functioning end of the autism spectrum. The core features are social learning problems and restricted patterns of behavior. Language is less affected, and understanding and use of grammar and syntax are good. Individuals with Asperger's disorder, however, commonly have significant problems with a flexible understanding of words (semantic problems) and cannot use their vocabulary and gestures in flexible, socially adaptive ways (pragmatic language deficits) (see Chapter 21). If your child has Asperger's disorder, he or she might seem aloof and indifferent to others and develop few friendships. Alternatively, he or she might make brief attempts to engage others socially, but the efforts are one-sided and he or she seems unresponsive to how others react. People with Asperger's disorder also often exhibit restricted interests such as memorizing train schedules, calendars, or patterns of numerical relationships. Your child may seem to think only about dinosaurs, insects, or airplanes and develop an extensive knowledge in that subject. He or she typically will have little interest in make-believe games or interactive activities. Delayed motor milestones and clumsiness are common, but intellectual ability usually falls within the average or above average range.

PERVASIVE DEVELOPMENTAL
DISORDER-NOT OTHERWISE SPECIFIED

The term *pervasive developmental disorder-not otherwise specified (PDD-NOS)* has been a source of confusion and ambiguity for clinicians and parents alike. Like all of the PDDs, PDD-NOS is a social learning disorder. It is probably the most common of the disorders on the autism spectrum but has been studied the least. Some professionals apply this term when the age of onset of symptoms cannot be firmly placed prior to age 3 years. Others use this diagnosis when a child's impairments seem too mild to be called autism. Still others have used this term for children who clearly exhibit a social learning disorder but do not meet all of the language or restricted pattern criteria for a diagnosis of autism.

CAUSES OF AUTISM SPECTRUM DISORDERS

It is most likely that ASDs are genetically caused developmental brain disorders. This implies that while the embryo was developing, your child's brain grew to be different from that of a typical child. There are no consistent findings in the brains of individuals with autism although the cortex is often large. Specialists do not yet understand how these findings specifically link to the abnormalities in communication, social skills, and behavior.

The evidence that the disorder has a genetic source is compelling. Twin studies and more extensive family studies suggest that the rate of autism is much greater among identical twins (70%–90%) than in fraternal twins (3%). The rates in identical twins, however, are not 100% as one would predict for a purely genetic disorder, so it is likely that there are some important nongenetic influences, too. If one child in a family has ASD, the risk of a second child having a disorder on the autism spectrum is about 5%–7%, versus 0.1% in the general population. This means that the risk is 50–100 times greater for such a family as compared with the general population. In addition, in families with a child who has autism, often some members have related but milder features such as rigid temperament, language delay, pragmatic language deficits, or stereotyped patterns of behavior. This has led some investigators to conclude that autism is probably the end result of 4–10 genes that act together. If only a few of these genes are affected, then partial or less severe impairment will result.

Considerable thought has been given to whether birth complications predispose a child to develop ASD. Although there seems to be an association, it appears that the disorder makes a fetus more likely to have complications at delivery rather than that problems in delivery lead to ASD. It is clear that ASDs are not caused by infections, adverse nutrition, maternal stress, or environmental circumstances. Data also do not support any effect of measles, mumps, or rubella immunization.

ASSOCIATED DISABILITIES

Certain medical conditions are often seen in individuals with ASD. The most common are mental retardation and epilepsy. Also, children with ASD may have certain genetic syndromes. It is important to identify these other problems early so that treatment can be started and your child can reach his or her full potential.

Mental Retardation

Approximately 60% of individuals with autism also have mental retardation (see Chapter 14). Typically, children with mental retardation have IQ scores that are similarly low across verbal and nonverbal functioning and have similar difficulty with adaptive functioning. This is not necessarily the case for children with ASD. Some people with ASD do have global impairments in functioning and IQ scores, but uneven scores also are common. An uneven pattern, sometimes called a *scatter,* may occur among a child's scores within domains on an IQ test or as a disparity among domains. This child does significantly better with some tasks than with others. For example, a child may perform better on tests of visuospatial skills and memory and poorer on tasks requiring symbolic or logical reasoning. Some children with autism may have higher functioning in musical skills, exceptional rote memory, an unusual capacity for jigsaw puzzles, or an ability to do rapid calculations.

It is also true that if your child has mental retardation (particularly a severe form) he or she is at a higher risk for autism than the general population. This close connection between these developmental disabilities creates difficulties in separating which features belong to which problem and complicates the diagnostic process. When social skills are on par with intellectual abilities, the primary diagnosis is mental retardation; when there are cognitive deficits but even greater impairments in social skills, your child is likely to have both ASD and mental retardation.

Epilepsy

Epilepsy is also more common in individuals with ASD (25%–30%), as compared with typical individuals (0.5%). In children with epilepsy who are otherwise developing typically, seizures usually begin in early childhood, but if your child has both ASD and epilepsy, the seizures are just as likely to begin in adolescence as in early childhood. There is no single type of epilepsy associated with ASDs. Among infants, major motor seizures are more common and tend to respond to antiepileptic medication (see Chapter 18).

Genetic Disorders

A few genetic syndromes appear to be more common among people with ASD: tuberous sclerosis, Tourette syndrome, and fragile X syndrome.

Tuberous Sclerosis   The genetic disorder tuberous sclerosis produces acne-like skin lesions and benign growths in the brain. It also is associated with a form of epilepsy of infancy known as infantile spasms (see Chapter 18). Nearly half of individuals with tuberous sclerosis have ASD. However, only about 1%–4% of people with autism also have tuberous sclerosis. Knowing that the two disorders are linked somehow is important because learning what it is about tuberous sclerosis that explains this high rate of autism may be a key to understanding the biological mechanisms of ASDs.

Tourette Syndrome   Tourette syndrome is a condition that produces sudden tics (often facial) accompanied by vocalizations that may be as simple as throat clearing or sniffing or as complex as whole words or phrases. Research strongly suggests that Tourette syndrome is a genetic disorder, but the precise genetic defect has yet to be discovered. There is growing evidence that Tourette syndrome may be more common among people with ASD than among typical individuals.

Fragile X Syndrome   At one point fragile X syndrome, the most common known cause of inherited mental retardation, was also believed to be a common cause of autism. Reported rates of autism among individuals with fragile X syndrome ranged as high as 60%. More rigorous investigations, however, have reported estimates closer to 4%–5%. Thus, it is now thought that fragile X syndrome is not a major cause of autism, although it is still more common in people with ASD than in typical individuals.

EVALUATING YOUR CHILD WITH AUTISM SPECTRUM DISORDER

The evaluation of your child requires time, collaboration between you and your child's health care and education professionals, and knowledge of ASDs. The following are necessary components of a comprehensive evaluation for ASD:

- A detailed developmental history with particular attention to social development
- Hearing and vision testing
- IQ testing
- Assessment of language development by a speech-language pathologist
- Neurological examination
- General medical evaluation
- An EEG (electroencephalogram, or brain wave test)
- Your family's medical history
- An understanding of your family's functioning and circumstances

Other than the EEG to look for seizures, there is no specific battery of medical tests required. Depending on the results of the initial evaluation, however, your child's physician may decide to perform an MRI (magnetic resonance imaging) scan, metabolic testing, and/or genetic studies. Depending on your child, additional assessments by an occupational therapist, physical therapist, and/or genetic specialist may be needed. An evaluation team might include a physician (a child psychiatrist, a developmental pediatrician, a child neurologist, or a pediatrician with expertise in autism), a clinical psychologist, a speech-language pathologist with experience in testing young children, and an occupational therapist.

It should be emphasized that the reliability of an evaluation of your child's strengths and areas of need hinges on there being multiple observers who assess your child over time and in a number of settings. A videotape illustrating your child's strengths and challenging behaviors can be very helpful. This is particularly true if your child feels intimidated by meeting strangers, being tested in novel settings, and/or being asked to do new things. With more familiarity and time, the anxiety of the experience declines and the testing results become more reliable. Rating scales are often used during the evaluations and can assist clinicians in organizing their observations. Rating scales used include the Autism Diagnostic Interview–Revised (ADI–R), the Autism Diagnostic Observation Schedule–General (ADOS–G), the Communication and Symbolic Behavior Scales (CSBS), the Child Autism Rating Scale (CARS), the Checklist for Autism in Toddlers (CHAT), the Gilliam Autism Rating Scale (GARS), the Parent Interview for Autism (PIA), and the Pervasive Developmental Disorders Screening Test–Stage 1 and 2 (PDDST).

APPROACHES TO TREATMENT

It can be confusing and overwhelming to hear about all of the different treatments for children with ASD. You will hear parents offer testimonials about any number of treatments that turned their children around. Unfortunately, the history of treating children with ASD also is riddled with eccentric, faddish, expensive care that is later shown to be needless or without merit. Relying on your best judgment is important. First, consider treatments that have sound supporting evidence and that will not be harmful to your child. Before moving forward with any novel or expensive treatment, investigate it carefully. If something is new or experimental, participate only as part of a study that takes steps to protect volunteers and that has specific consent forms telling about risks, benefits, and alternatives. The best starting point for good information is the team that evaluated your child. They should recommend specific services that are most likely to help your child and that relate to the strengths and weaknesses that surfaced in your child's evaluation.

Intervention in the Preschool Period

Currently, the mainstay of treatment for ASD is education starting as soon as your child is diagnosed. Autism is now classified as a special category of educational disability under the Individuals with Disabilities Education Act Amendments of 1997 (see Chapter 13).

There is no one best method for teaching all children with ASD. Two approaches that appear to help are the developmental approach (which focuses on engaging your child by reducing unpleasant sensory experiences and encouraging interactions with people), and the applied behavioral analysis (ABA) methods (which attempt to increase desired behaviors and decrease undesirable behaviors). Both rely on providing intensive services (20–25 hours per week) beginning in preschool. There are data to support both methods, but the methods are different in their objectives and philosophy. A combination of these approaches is also possible. The importance of your involvement as teachers/therapists and advocates for your child is critical.

Speech-language therapy is also essential treatment, particularly in the developmental approach. Language impairments interfere with your child's overall expressive and receptive communication. In addition to working on the development of speech, you may also consider focusing on alternative communication approaches (see Chapter 21) including signing, communication cards, picture symbols, and computer-generated speech. Improved communication skills can also benefit your child's behavior. Many children with ASD who have tantrums improve as they gain expressive language skills.

Intervention During the School Years

Your child's primary goals during the school years should be to gain academic, social, and social language skills. These goals can be achieved through a variety of approaches including inclusive classroom models (see Chapter 12), individual and small-group speech-language services, social skills training groups, "social stories," and supervised social group experiences. The particular techniques that are used will depend on your child's developmental level and skills. Your child may benefit from social skills training groups that teach greeting, taking turns in talking, staying on topic, and initiating conversations. Children with ASD have difficulty with unstructured settings such as lunch and recess. Having adult supervision can be critical for your child to learn how to interact successfully with classmates. Social stories target specific social situations that may create problems for your child, such as lining up at school or taking turns with equipment at recess. A social story offers information about how a person should behave in a certain situation. Children with ASD, however, are often unable to take what they have learned in one class to a new environment independently. Therefore, your child may need adults or other peers to help him or her apply skills in new situations. An integrated approach infuses language and social skills training into each classroom activity period rather than pulling your child out of class for special resource help.

Your Family's Role in Treatment

Although it can appear that your child has little interest, need, or ability to relate to you or others, this is not the case. Family members can have vital and trusting relationships with individuals with ASD. For almost all of these children, parents are the most important resource for learning about other people and for fostering social interactions. Beyond this, you are crucial for implementing treatment programs and for being advocates for your child's educational placement and other needs. Furthermore, you take on the role of interpreting the world and buffering your child from experiences that are too taxing or stimulating. Many parents report a loving yet different relationship with their child who has ASD.

Brothers and sisters are also influential because many children with ASD have their siblings as their primary peers. Your child's play with siblings can teach him or her to pretend, take turns, share, and become more flexible and interested in interactions with other children. In addition, an older sibling can be a guide when you are unavailable and a younger sibling can provide appropriate social opportunities. Siblings may also help you understand how a typical child develops and learns and can bring into sharper focus the difficulties and obstacles facing your child with ASD.

Medications

Medications play only a supporting role in the treatment of ASDs. No medication has been shown to be helpful to all children with disorders on the autism spectrum. Side effects are often a problem because these children can be very sensitive to seemingly insignificant changes in their world. Some medications pose few risks, but others have more serious risks or can make symptoms worse. Medication is most helpful when your child has symptoms that have not responded to a proper educational environment and adequate trials of behavior therapy. The safest way to think about medication is as a third line of defense. If symptoms severely hamper your child's participation in school, if behavior at home poses a risk to your family's safety, or if your child is distressed constantly, then you might consider medication.

Aggression, agitation, and self-injurious behaviors have been treated with psychiatric drugs such as haloperidol (Haldol) and risperidone (Risperdal). These drugs can calm your child without causing sedation, but they may cause weight gain and some unusual movements mimicking Parkinson's disease. Other drugs used for treating severe aggression are the antiepileptics carbamazepine (Carbatrol or Tegretol) and valproic acid (Depakene or Depakote), the anti-anxiety drug buspirone (BuSpar), and lithium. Ritualistic behaviors, stereotyped movements, anxiety, and difficulties in making transitions may decrease with serotonin reuptake inhibitors such as fluoxetine (Prozac), paroxetine (Paxil), sertraline (Zoloft), fluvoxamine (Luvox), and clomipramine (Anafranil). These drugs seem to decrease anxiety, lead to more socialization, and have some modest positive effect on language. Finally, symptoms of attention-deficit/hyperactivity disorder (see Chapter 24) can occur in children with ASD. Some children respond well to methylphenidate

(Ritalin) or dextroamphetamine (Dexedrine) but they may show increasing self-stimulatory behavior, irritability and social withdrawal. Clonidine (Catapres) has shown some short-term success in controlling hyperactivity and sleep problems but does little to improve attention. (See Chapter 10 for more on these medications and their side effects.)

LIVING WITH A CHILD WITH AUTISM SPECTRUM DISORDER

Your son or daughter influences your family as much as your family affects him or her. For some families, a child with special needs brings out everyone's best. The experience may make family members appreciate one another's positive attributes more. It can bring your family closer together and promote deep, mutually satisfying relationships. Family members may often feel more attuned to themselves, their family, and others in the community. They often can find support from their extended family, school and religious community, and neighborhoods.

But having a child with ASD also can be hard on you and your other children. Living with a child who does not give back much affection, empathy, or consideration can be draining. It can amplify disharmony that existed in your marriage prior to your child's birth. It can make it harder for your other children's needs to be met by the family and by their peers. Having a child with ASD increases your chances of becoming depressed and can make family members feel guilty because they believe that they are not doing enough, have failed, or are at fault for the problem. Living with your child can consume enormous energy and time; often you may worry about the future. The increased attention required by your child can reduce the time available for other relationships among family members and outside of the family, for community activities, for private time, and for work. When these burdens are heavy, you may find it helpful to speak to professionals who are knowledgeable about ASDs and their effect on a family. Sometimes family members benefit from family or individual therapy. The most important thing is for you and your children to speak about your fears, frustrations, and disappointments. This can help reduce personal barriers to resources available to you to meet your family's needs and provide the best environment for your child.

WHAT THE FUTURE HOLDS

The future for your child with ASD is closely linked to his or her verbal abilities, intelligence, family supports, and educational/behavioral programs. For example, some individuals with Asperger's disorder have successful professional careers although they still struggle with social interactions. This good outcome might not have been obvious when they were very young, so it is appropriate for you to be optimistic about your child's chances for significant improvements in cognitive, behavioral, and social skills. Developmental disorders such as ASDs, however, occur early and have a strong influence on later development. Your child will most likely continue to have some difficulty with social skills throughout his or her life. Depending on IQ and language abilities, he or she should be able to live independently or thrive in a supported or interdependent living environment and can be expected to have a typical life span. Early identification and good educational programs have significantly improved futures for children with ASD.

Some Questions Answered

Should we consider treating our child with alternative medicines and/or nutritional supplements?

Many parents and some professionals are paying considerable attention to the use of alternative therapy in autism as there is no "cure" using traditional medicine. The problem with alternative medicine and nutritional supplements is that they usually have not been tested in a careful manner. There are testimonials about the success of one treatment or another, but it can be hard to know whether the medication itself, a placebo effect, or something else was instrumental if the intervention was not studied in a controlled way. For this reason doctors generally do not *recommend* alternative medicine or nutritional therapy. However, people still use these approaches. If you decide to do so, remember that the treatment should not compromise your child's attendance at his or her school program or delay entry into a program and that it should be inexpensive and safe.

Should we tell people that our son has autism?

Whether you tell depends on who is asking and whether answering will be helpful to your son. What you decide to do may be different for family members, neighbors, close family friends, school or camp staff, and casual acquaintances. On the one hand, because there is so much outdated information around, your child may feel stigmatized if people have only a label and are operating in ignorance about the condition. On the other hand, it is in your son's best interests for those who work closely or spend a lot of time with him to know his strengths and needs and to know how his condition affects his language, behavior, and social interactions. The label is less important than a good description of his attributes and difficulties. For example, if your son exhibits unusual behaviors, others will be reassured to know in advance what the behaviors are and what they really signal.

You may find it helpful to meet people who will be working closely with your child to learn how open they are to exchanging ideas, their ability to respond flexibly, and their warmth and "empathy quotient." Their familiarity with terms such as *PDD-NOS, Asperger's disorder,* or *autism* is not as important as their ability to think positively about your son, consider his needs, and recognize that noncompliance does not equal disobedience. Above all, they must know they can turn to you when they have questions or when your son's progress seems slow. The most helpful approach is one that secures a successful line of communication.

24

Attention-Deficit/ Hyperactivity Disorder

Mark A. Stein and Mark L. Batshaw

Attention-deficit/hyperactivity disorder (ADHD) is one of the most common developmental disabilities, occurring in 2–9 of every 100 children. Symptoms of ADHD begin to appear in childhood, but the disorder can be diagnosed at any age. This disorder has had many different names over the years, such as *attention deficit disorder, ADD, hyperactivity, hyperkinesis,* and *minimal brain dysfunction.* ADHD can range in severity and can be an isolated disorder or can be combined with other problems. It affects children of all levels of intellectual functioning (including children with mental retardation) and predominantly occurs in boys.

If your child has ADHD, he or she may seem extremely inattentive given his or her level of development and may also be overactive and impulsive. He or she may appear to lack motivation, may become bored easily, and probably has difficulty anticipating the consequences of his or her behavior. Together, these attention and behavior problems often lead to impairments in functioning at home, at school, and in social situations. Parents report that having a child with ADHD is like having a child with perpetual "terrible twos" behavior.

For many individuals, ADHD is a chronic disability that stretches into adulthood; whereas for others it gradually disappears by adolescence. Mild ADHD is much more common than severe ADHD. Symptoms of the disorder are more evident when your child must devote sustained attention to a task and are less noticeable in novel or one-to-one settings or when your child receives frequent feedback and encouragement. Thus, the ability to play a video game, watch television, or construct with Legos for hours does not rule out a diagnosis of ADHD.

Lizzie and Jason

Lizzie is a 12-year-old sixth grader. She is well liked by her teachers and has several close friends. Lizzie did fairly well in primary school, but her grades have slipped since fourth grade. Except for art, her grades rarely rise above Cs, although she is thought to be quite bright and spends hours doing her homework. Despite her efforts, she seems unprepared for class and has difficulty keeping up with math and Spanish. She is described by her teacher as a daydreamer and by her parents as a "space cadet." Recently, her parents became concerned that her self-esteem is declining. She has made occasional but more frequent comments about being "stupid" and seems less motivated to achieve.

Jason has always been a "difficult" and "high maintenance" child according to his parents. He was a colicky baby with poor sleep patterns. As a preschooler, he was demanding and would exhaust his parents. His kindergarten teacher described him as "immature," and he was almost held back. Now that Jason is 7 years old and in the second grade, his teacher reports that he is having great difficulty with reading. He also is disruptive in class, frequently not listening to directions, getting out of his seat, making silly comments, and talking out of turn. Similar problems were reported by his first-grade teacher, but these difficulties were attributed to his adjusting to a new school. His parents, speech-language therapist, and soccer coach all have noticed his difficulty with following directions and paying attention.

DEFINING ADHD

There are two main clusters of ADHD symptoms: inattention and hyperactivity/impulsivity. These symptoms and the criteria used to diagnose the disorder are displayed in Table 24.1. Individuals who have six symptoms from each of the symptom clusters are said to have ADHD, Combined Type. For your child to be given this diagnosis, he or she must have had these symptoms before age 7 and they must have persisted for at least 6 months. ADHD, Combined Type, is the most common form of ADHD and the subtype about which the most is known from previous research.

The second most common subtype, ADHD, Predominantly Inattentive Type (ADHD-PI), refers to individuals who do not show significant levels of hyperactivity, although they have attention problems. In fact, these children may even be slow moving. Because of their subtle symptoms, their disorder is likely to go undiagnosed for many years. This subtype is more likely to be diagnosed in females than is the Combined Type. Lizzie is an example of someone with ADHD-PI. Children with this type of ADHD are less at a risk for disruptive behavior disorders, and the overall prognosis is usually more favorable, with educational impairments being the most prominent problem.

The third subtype, ADHD, Predominantly Hyperactive-Impulsive Type, describes young children who are believed to be at risk for ADHD, Combined

Table 24.1.   Diagnostic criteria for attention-deficit/hyperactivity disorder (ADHD)

Symptoms of inattention

Often fails to give attention to detail or makes careless mistakes

Often has difficulty sustaining attention

Often does not seem to listen

Often does not follow through on instructions and fails to finish tasks

Often has difficulty organizing tasks and activities

Often avoids or dislikes tasks that require sustained mental effort

Often loses things

Is often easily distracted

Is often forgetful

Symptoms of hyperactivity/impulsivity

Often fidgets or squirms

Often leaves seat when expected to remain seated

Often runs about or climbs excessively in inappropriate situations

Often has difficulty engaging in activities quietly

Is often "on the go" or "driven by a motor"

Often talks excessively

Often blurts out answers before questions have been completed

Often has difficulty waiting a turn

Often interrupts or intrudes on others

Type, but who have not yet reached the age at which attention problems are evident. Little is known about the course of this subtype and its response to treatment. An initial study suggests, however, that individuals with this type display impairments similar to those with ADHD, Combined Type.

HOW ADHD AFFECTS SCHOOL FUNCTION

In your child's first years of school, ADHD is likely to manifest as difficulty following classroom rules and teacher's instructions. Your child may have difficulty with circle time, the ritual of hanging up jackets on arrival, sitting at a desk, taking out books, and generally getting ready to follow directions and work. Instead, he or she may wander around the room touching other kids, may squirm or fall out of his or her seat, and may be distracted by every butterfly that flits past the windowpane. Information imparted by the teacher is invariably missed, and schoolwork assignments are done carelessly or are incomplete. Similarly, homework is not completed independently and eventually can become a major source of friction between you and your child. When ADHD is combined with a learning disability, school failure is a near certainty in the absence of intervention. ADHD, however, usually can be treated effectively if identified early.

HOW ADHD AFFECTS CHILDREN AND THEIR FAMILIES

Some children with ADHD are quite sociable and develop and maintain friendships that ultimately contribute to a healthy sense of self-esteem despite their attentional difficulties. Many more, however, are challenged in their interactions with peers and adults. They may have difficulty "reading" other people's body language or understanding their verbal responses. They also may not be able to inhibit behaviors that seem inappropriate, silly, and impulsive, and they often become the class clown. As a result, children with ADHD seem different to their peers and are often shunned and rejected. Children with ADHD-PI are more likely to be ignored. When combined with the physical clumsiness that often accompanies ADHD, children with the disorder may be seen as nuisances and are often excluded from sports and other group activities, resulting in increased frustration and demoralization.

In addition to difficulties with social functioning, children with ADHD often have marked impairments in their adaptive skills, which involve a variety of daily living, communication, and social skills necessary for self-sufficiency. The mother of an 11-year-old boy who was referred for evaluation of ADHD poignantly asked, "When do I get to stop being Nick's brain?" Even after Nick began effective treatment his mother reported, "I still have to check on him on an hourly basis, as he cannot or will not put his dirty clothes in the hamper, remember to turn in his homework, take his 4 P.M. dose of medication, or plan his Saturday mornings." This frustration often results in decreased parental expectations and reduced learning opportunities for these children. It also fosters dependency, increases parent–child conflicts, and leaves many adolescents with ADHD unprepared for independence in their young adulthood years. Consequently, it is important not to give up and to regularly readjust expectations.

In addition to these adaptive skills deficits, your child is likely to be noncompliant, and you may often have to repeat commands and shadow your child. Going to the market or the shopping mall can be an embarrassing and exhausting experience, complete with temper tantrums and a tendency to run off. Your child also probably tends not to respect the personal space of siblings, often entering siblings' bedrooms unannounced, taking their toys and clothes, and getting into verbal and physical fights with them. Neighborhood children may avoid your child because of his or her immaturity, erratic behavior, and lack of athletic skills and sportsmanship, thus putting more pressure on you to structure your child's environment and monitor behavior.

These problems can affect your entire family. Your other children may be made fun of in school, and they may be torn as to whether to agree with the tormentor or punch the kid in the nose. The behavior problems may also inhibit family activities or vacations and can lead you to feel chronically worn down. The end result is that your family may feel isolated and fatigued, which can lead to parental depression and/or lashing out against the child and/or siblings (verbally or physically). This puts stress on the marriage and often leads both parents to feel a sense of guilt and impotence.

These cumulative stresses point to the importance of early diagnosis and effective treatment of ADHD. A combination of medication, behavior management, parent support or respite care, and social skills training/counseling along with experience in structured socialization experiences (such as martial arts or summer camp) can be very helpful for your entire family. Parent and family education about ADHD and about being an advocate for your child is a must; national support organizations such as Children and Adults with Attention-Deficit/Hyperactivity Disorder (CHADD; see the Suggested Readings and Resources at the end of the book for contact information) are extremely helpful in this regard.

ORIGINS OF ADHD

The underlying cause of ADHD has much to do with how the brain works to control behavior. Although brain damage or dysfunction secondary to complications of labor and delivery or infection was previously thought to be the primary cause of ADHD, it is now recognized that the majority of children with ADHD do not display evidence of this. Instead, most often the disorder seems to have a large genetic component that affects the development of the brain prior to birth.

A genetic basis for ADHD has been suggested because of the high incidence of the disorder in parents, grandparents, and/or siblings of people with the disorder (10%–25%). Gene defects or mutations in the brain chemical dopamine have been implicated. This is not surprising because medications that are effective in treating ADHD, such as Ritalin (methylphenidate), act on dopamine. It is likely that more than one gene defect may increase the risk of ADHD.

The primary brain region affected in ADHD appears to be the frontal lobe, which serves as the "executive center" of the brain, selecting and implementing appropriate emotional and motor responses. This area is also rich in pathways, or "circuits," that use dopamine as the chemical messenger (neurotransmitter). Individuals with ADHD display impairments in several executive functions (working memory, internalization of speech, and self-regulation of motivation/arousal) that lead to problems in execution of goal-directed activities and behavioral flexibility and a poor sense of time. Advances in neuroimaging techniques such as functional magnetic resonance imaging (fMRI) are now being applied to the study of ADHD, and researchers have identified several areas of the brain that are smaller and presumably less active in individuals with ADHD. These areas of the brain include the frontal lobes and the caudate (in the center of the brain).

CONDITIONS THAT MIMIC ADHD

A number of medical and psychiatric problems can mimic ADHD (see Table 24.2). In addition, associated deficits (called *comorbid problems*) may complicate the diagnosis and treatment of ADHD. Identifying mimic and comorbid problems is crucial because many of these conditions require additional or different treatments.

As shown in Table 24.2, along with medical and psychiatric conditions that mimic ADHD, there are *social mimic* conditions. These are more subjective and therefore more difficult to evaluate. Social mimic conditions are usually the result of a poor fit between a child's abilities and the surrounding environment. One example is the child with typical abilities who is doing typical work yet whose parents and teachers expect much more. Some environmental situations also can conceal ADHD, such as when there are few expectations for independent work, when there is a chaotic environment, or when extra help is always available.

The three most common comorbid disorders associated with ADHD are behavior problems, learning disabilities, and psychiatric disorders. The most common behavior problems are oppositional defiant disorder and conduct disorder, occurring in approximately one third of children with ADHD. There is much debate as to the frequency of comorbid learning disorders with estimates ranging from 20% to 40%, depending on which tests and what criteria are used. Although many children have both ADHD and learning disabilities, ADHD is *not* a learning disability. Similarly, estimates given for comorbid psychiatric disorders, most commonly depression and anxiety disorders, vary considerably from study to study but average around 10%–20%. Other problems often associated with ADHD include sleep difficulties (especially getting to sleep), bedwetting, and family conflicts.

DIAGNOSING ADHD

Unfortunately, no single test clearly diagnoses ADHD. It is not like pneumonia, which can be diagnosed from an X ray. Instead, ADHD represents a syndrome, a group of clinical findings that together define the disorder. This group of findings has been developed by the American Psychiatric Association and published in the association's *Diagnostic and Statistical Manual of Mental Disorders, Fourth Edition.* The diagnosis depends on a comprehensive review of the child's behavioral, academic, developmental, medical, and family history. This information is obtained from you, your child's medical and school records, and from one or more standardized rating scales for ADHD,

Table 24.2.   Other problems that may resemble attention-deficit/hyperactivity disorder (ADHD)

Pediatric mimic conditions	*Test or procedure used in ruling out*
Vision, auditory problems	Vision or hearing screen
Fine or gross motor deficits	Neurological examination, Developmental Test of Visual-Motor Integration, occupational therapy evaluation
Poor nutrition	Physical exam, history, complete blood count
Sleep deprivation	Physical examination, history, sleep diary, actigraph (activity monitor)
Absence seizures	History, EEG (electroencephalogram)
Thyroid disease	History, physical examination, thyroid function tests
Medication side effects	List medication
Syndromes (such as fragile X, fetal alcohol, Williams)	Physical examination, history, genetic tests
Social mimic conditions	*Test or procedure used in ruling out*
Poor fit between child and parental expectations	Knowledge of child, family, and school
Chaotic home or school environment	Same, regular monitoring over time
Psychiatric mimic conditions	*Signs or symptoms*
Anxiety disorder	Worry, difficulty separating from parents
Mental retardation	Generalized intellectual deficits
Pervasive developmental disorders (autism spectrum disorders)	Little interest in peers, odd play, language deficits
Depression	Moodiness, poor sleep, eating disorder

such as the Conners' Rating Scales or the Child Behavior Checklist. The evaluation will also include a medical/neurological examination and psychoeducational testing. The latter should include an individually administered IQ test, such as the Wechsler Intelligence Scale for Children–Third Edition, and a measure of academic achievement, such as the Wechsler Individual Achievement Test or the Wide Range Achievement Test–Revised Edition. Don't be surprised if your child acts like an angel in the doctor's or psychologist's office. The combination of fear, a new and nondistracting environment, and one-to-one attention may help to keep the ADHD symptoms in check, at least briefly. Professionals expect this to be the case, so don't feel disappointed if your child doesn't demolish the doctor's office as he or she does your home. You may, in fact, want to bring a home videotape that typifies your child's behavior and reports from previous teachers or report cards.

The evaluation should be conducted by a professional who is familiar with your child and school and who has considerable knowledge and experience in ADHD as well as other related conditions. Often the pediatrician may conduct the evaluation in consultation with a child psychologist, developmental or behavioral pediatrician, child neurologist, and/or child psychiatrist. When your child is initially evaluated, the specialist will consider a number of possible diagnoses and will try to rule each one in or out. The objective is to determine whether there is a problem, whether the problem fits the pattern of ADHD, whether there are comorbid conditions and what the biological, psychological, and social roots of the problem are. It is also important to identify your child's academic, interpersonal, or other strengths. All of this information will lead to the development of an appropriate treatment plan for your child, including target behaviors to focus on and a plan for regularly evaluating your child's response to interventions.

CHOOSING A DOCTOR

With trends toward managed health care, there is concern that many children with ADHD are not receiving proper evaluations, increasing the likelihood of delayed or misdiagnosis and overlooked comorbid conditions. Often, families are put in the difficult position of not knowing how or where to find help. In looking for health care professionals, determining your child's primary care physician's practices with regard to ADHD is important (see Chapter 2). You will want to ask whether the doctors can and want to direct your child's care or instead wish to refer you to an expert in ADHD. Questions such as who, when, and what types of referrals are available, what their attitudes toward medication are, and what their previous training and experience with developmental disabilities and ADHD is may be helpful when you choose a physician.

TREATMENT APPROACHES

Once a diagnosis has been made, the next step is to design a treatment program. The most effective approach to treating ADHD and other problems that come along with it involves the combination of medication, behavior management therapy and parent training, and educational resources. These interventions, when individually tailored to a child's strengths and weaknesses, are called *multimodal therapy*. It is hoped that children who participate in such a treatment program will display better adjustment and fewer behavior problems than those who received medication alone. The following sections discuss aspects of multimodal therapy, beginning with medication.

Ritalin

Ritalin (methylphenidate) is by far the most commonly used medication to treat ADHD. Ritalin belongs to a group of medications called *stimulants*. These compounds lead to an increase in certain brain neurochemicals, most prominently dopamine, and likely norepinephrine and serotonin as well. These chemicals normally activate certain brain regions or circuits, especially in the frontal lobes, and children with ADHD presumably have lower levels or poor modulation of them. It is thought that deficient activity of these chemicals plays an important role in producing the symptoms of ADHD.

Since 1938, children with disruptive behavior problems and overactivity have been treated with stimulant medications, which increase neurochemical activity to more normal levels. The safety and benefits of these medications have been well established in hundreds of controlled studies. The core symptoms that Ritalin addresses are inattention, hyperactivity, and impulsive behavior. Your child can frequently describe the effects. One child told us, "In about half an hour I feel calmer, and people don't yell at me so much." Another said, "I don't act so crazy, and I can get my work done." The benefits are usually evident from the first days of its use. Overall, more than three quarters of children with ADHD will show significant improvement in behavior with Ritalin. The long-term effects on academic achievement are less clear.

Ritalin comes in both short-acting and long-acting forms. The short-acting form takes about 20 minutes to start working and lasts for close to 4 hours, although this can vary from child to child. The common practice is to give two or three doses per day. The first dose is given with breakfast, the second with lunch, and, if needed, a final dose is given around 4 P.M. The late afternoon dose of Ritalin is generally given to younger children who have significant behavioral issues at home or for older children who have prolonged homework assignments.

When Ritalin is first prescribed your child's doctor may suggest a "medication trial" to see whether the drug works. A low dosage is used initially, and the dosage is increased at 3- to 5-day intervals until it is found to be effective or is associated with significant side effects. Weight is not always a good predictor of effective dosage, so it is good practice for your child's doctor to evaluate several different dosages until significant improvement is seen. The medication trial involves having the teacher, who is most likely to see ADHD symptoms, fill out a questionnaire such as the Conners' Teacher Rating Scale concerning ADHD "behavior" while "blinded" to (not informed about) the treatment being used. For example, the teacher is asked whether the child "cannot remain still," "is easily distracted by extraneous stimuli," or "does not follow through on instructions." Usually the results are unequivocal and can be interpreted by parents and doctors. It is important to note, however, that this controlled trial of medication is not a diagnostic test because children without ADHD may also have improved attention on Ritalin. The trial should only be used once the diagnosis of ADHD has been established and specific symptoms have been identified as "targets" for stimulant medication.

The advantage of Ritalin is that your child does not need to take it every day to be effective. Therefore, its use can be restricted to weekdays or to the school year, and an afternoon dose can be given intermittently when your child has special work assignments. The point is that ADHD symptoms can be treated when the symptoms and impairments are most significant. For some children and adolescents with severe ADHD, this will be for most of their waking hours, although for most it will be primarily during academic tasks.

Ritalin also is available in a sustained-release form (Ritalin-SR), which lasts about 6 hours. It is only about two thirds as strong as the short-acting form, so higher doses must be given. The benefit, however, is that your child does not have to take a dose at school. This not only has logistical advantages but also helps your child avoid feeling stigmatized by visits to the nurse for medication. A new drug delivery system, Concerta (methylphenidate), is now available. One Concerta capsule has a similar effect to that of three doses of short-acting Ritalin.

Fortunately, Ritalin is a safe drug. In the short term, about 10% of children will get a stomachache, headache, or be moody/irritable when first put on the medication. Frequently these side effects disappear over a few weeks. Facial tics (twitches) or skin picking behaviors occur in less than 10% of children. In some children, however, these side effects may last longer and may be a reason to lower the dosage or switch to another medication. Some children also report that they feel less creative or social and more "blah" on the medication. If this happens to your child, this may be an indication that the dosage is too high. If this continues, you will need to weigh the advantages and disadvantages of your child's continuing on the medication. There is also the possibility of a "rebound" phenomenon when the dose of medication is wearing off (usually just after getting home from school). *Rebound* implies that your child actually gets more hyperactive than he or she is naturally. A small dose of Ritalin given around 4 P.M. can usually prevent rebound.

There are certain side effects that occur quite frequently. These include appetite suppression and insomnia. Although this appetite suppression does not affect breakfast or dinner in children receiving only two doses of regular Ritalin, it does affect lunch. Most children taking Ritalin are not hungry at noontime. You can get around this to some extent by using high carbohydrate/protein bars available in health food stores and some supermarkets or nutritional supplements such as Carnation Instant Breakfast bars. In some cases, changing the timing of the last dose of Ritalin can reduce insomnia. In other cases, behavioral treatment of insomnia or changing medications should be considered. Although stimulants can be abused, studies have shown that children on long-term Ritalin treatment do not have an increased risk of developing substance abuse as teenagers or adults.

It should be noted that medication response varies much more in preschoolers, and stimulants should be considered in children less than 5 years old only when the ADHD is severe. These medications should only be tried after environmental interventions (such as a structured preschool environment or parent training) have been provided and found to be insufficient. In all cases, a child's school achievement, behavior, mood, and growth should be monitored before starting the medication and at regular intervals thereafter to document effectiveness and side effects.

The duration of Ritalin treatment depends on the type and severity of your child's symptoms and the degree of impairment. Many children will benefit from it as long as they are in school (including college). Adolescents with ADHD who drive will benefit from treatment for longer periods of time to decrease the risk of accidents from inattention. One way of determining if the medication is still needed is for your child to have a "drug holiday." We recommend that for most children on Ritalin, a drug holiday be conducted every year during school. This is most commonly done in the late fall or spring, when there are few changes in the educational program and teachers are familiar with the child. This permits the child to be evaluated when he or she has settled into a routine. It can be carried out in the same way as the initial "blinded trial," with questionnaires used to determine continued effectiveness. Don't be too disappointed if the results show that the medication is still of benefit. Ritalin has not been associated with any long-term toxicity. Most children do not develop a tolerance to the medication over time, so they do not require repeated dosage increases just to maintain the same level of control. Dosage may be increased, however, to take into account your child's growth.

As your child gets older, he or she should be given increased responsibility both for taking the medication and for determining when and if a drug holiday should be tried. This gives him or her a level of control over the disorder that is part of growing up and accepting responsibility. When this should occur varies with each child but often coincides with adolescence. Yet, compliance with medication is a frequent problem in teenagers. Enlisting their active participation in treatment will increase the likelihood that they will follow through with treatment recommendations, especially when they report seeing benefits themselves.

Other Stimulants

There are a number of other medications that work in a similar way to Ritalin. These include Dexedrine (dextroamphetamine), Adderall (dextroamphetamine and amphetamine), and Cylert (pemoline). Dexedrine works about as well as Ritalin, but it may have a higher incidence of the side effects described previously. Pharmacies also are less likely to carry it because it is less popular. It also has the street drug name "speed," and some "entrepreneurial" adolescents with ADHD may try to resell it. It turns out, however, that the sustained-release form of Dexedrine (spansules) may work better than Ritalin-SR, so some doctors will recommend a Dexedrine spansule in the morning combined with a late afternoon dose of regular Ritalin, if needed. The dosage of Dexedrine is half of that used for Ritalin. Adderall is a recently developed drug that contains a mixture of two compounds related to Dexedrine and is formulated as a sustained-release compound. It appears to be a good but more expensive substitute for the sustained-release Dexedrine. Cylert is another medication that is long lasting. In very rare cases, however, it has been associated with life-threatening liver damage. As a result, a blood test to detect liver function needs to be done before a trial is initiated and at regular intervals. Because other effective drugs are available, Cylert is now used rarely in treating ADHD. Finally, a number of long-acting medications for ADHD are in clinical trials and are likely to come on the market in the next few years.

Caffeine is a weak stimulant that is associated with many of the same effects and side effects described previously. For most children with ADHD, however, the beneficial effects of caffeine are slight and not clinically significant. It is important to monitor caffeine intake, especially in adolescents, as it may increase the risk of stimulant side effects.

Treatment for Children Who Do Not Respond to Stimulants

When the overall effectiveness of stimulants is considered, approximately 90% of children with ADHD will benefit. For the few who do not respond, antidepressant medication and certain blood pressure medications may prove helpful. Compared with stimulants, antidepressants are less effective in controlling the core symptoms of ADHD but are clearly better than a placebo. In addition to being useful for people who do not benefit from stimulants, they are particularly helpful in children who have ADHD with comorbid depression, sleep disturbance, or anxiety. These children are slightly less likely to respond positively to stimulants. In contrast to stimulants, antidepressants have different side effects and need to be given continuously. Once effective, however, they last throughout the day. Unfortunately, antidepressants have more and potentially more serious side effects as compared with stimulants. For example, tricyclic antidepressants are potentially toxic to the heart, and an EKG (electrocardiogram) is obtained initially and later repeated when Norpramin (desipramine), Tofranil (imipramine), or Pamelor (nortriptyline) is used. These medications should not be stopped abruptly but need to be gradually weaned. It is also important to closely supervise where these medicines are stored as there is the potential for overdose.

Another alternative to stimulant medications is the chemically distinct antidepressant Wellbutrin (bupropion). The major concern with this medication is that it can induce seizures on rare occasions. The other major group of antidepressants are the selective serotonin reuptake inhibitors (SSRIs) of which Prozac (fluoxetine) is the best known. Other SSRIs include Zoloft (sertraline) and Paxil (paroxetine). Although the SSRI antidepressants have fewer and less severe side effects than the tricyclics do, they have not been shown to be effective in treating ADHD and in some cases can increase ADHD symptoms such as impulsivity.

There is also a group of blood pressure medications (called *alpha-2-noradrenergic agents*) that seem to be helpful in controlling hyperactivity, but they are less useful in improving attention in children with ADHD. These drugs include Tenex (guanfacine) and Catapres (clonidine). Their major side effect is sleepiness; less frequently they cause moodiness and irritability. They should not be abruptly discontinued because of the risk of transient high blood pressure developing. This may occur because of a "rebound" from low to high blood pressure if this medication is suddenly stopped. Some physicians will use Catapres at night and stimulants during the day. The night dose helps sleep problems as well as getting the child ready for school in the morning, whereas the stimulant works during the school day. There is controversy, however, as to whether Catapres in combination with stimulants can lead to cardiac arrhythmia. Until more studies have been conducted, these medications should be used in combination cautiously.

Behavioral Therapies

The second part of multimodal therapy is psychosocial treatment, often directed at comorbid behavior problems. This includes behavior management therapy and parent training. Behavior management therapy (such as contingency management, positive reinforcement or point systems, or time-out; see Chapter 11) is used to treat behavioral symptoms in the home and school. Parent training in such skills can be done individually or in groups. Many different parent training programs are available, and these programs have demonstrated their effectiveness. In contrast, there is little data to support individual psychotherapy or clinic-based treatment for children with ADHD, and the effectiveness of social skills training in clinic settings has been disappointing.

Meaningful behavior change is more likely to occur when intervention approaches are conducted in a naturalistic setting, such as in school or at home. A concern is that many children with ADHD are not given adequate intensity of treatment due to changes in the health care and educational system that restrict or limit evaluation and treatment services, especially psychosocial treatments.

Educational Resources

The third part of multimodal therapy involves providing educational resources. Academic underachievement is often the primary complaint reported by parents of children with ADHD. Identifying and highlighting your child's strengths both in and out of school are often keys to effective treatment. A good school for your child with ADHD is one that is aware of his or her difficulties and can make accommodations and provide supports so that he or she can succeed. Most children with ADHD do not require special education classes, although almost all benefit from extra assistance and accommodations. These issues are further discussed in Chapter 12.

NONCONVENTIONAL THERAPIES

As is true for many disorders for which cures have remained elusive, patent medicines and other unproven alternate therapies briefly sprout up and are often subsequently found to be ineffective. It is impossible to cover all of the alternate therapies that have been proposed for treating ADHD, so we present a few here. As of 2000, megavitamin therapy is quite popular for many disorders in addition to ADHD. For ADHD, at least, the few controlled studies show that there is no benefit and that there is even the chance of side effects from excessive doses of vitamins. EEG biofeedback is another untested approach in which your child is taught to control his or her brain wave patterns, with the assumption that this will also help control brain function. There is no evidence to support this approach either.

The situation is murkier with elimination diets. The classic diet for ADHD, named after its inventor, Dr. Feingold, eliminates artificial colors, preservatives, sugars, and artificial sweeteners. In controlled studies there have been no statistically significant effects, but in each group, one or two children do seem to respond. These children tend to be younger than most children with ADHD. As this represents only about 5% of all the children with ADHD, this does not support the widespread use of the diet. Moreover, following a restrictive diet is extremely difficult, even for adults who are highly motivated. Finally, because no one can predict who will respond, there is no way of knowing who should try the diet. There is no disagreement, however, that all children, including children with ADHD, benefit from a balanced diet. A good breakfast that includes some protein should be encouraged to get your child ready to learn.

In sum, you should be cautious of any treatment that has not been evaluated scientifically and should not assume such treatments are safe. These treatments can be contrasted with an approach that incorporates educational programs, behavior management, and medication, which has been proven to be effective in improving the core symptoms of ADHD in more than 95% of children. In addition, it is likely that scientifically valid approaches to treatment will emerge based on the explosion of knowledge about how the brain works and what can go wrong.

Lizzie and Jason: Results of Therapy

Lizzie was diagnosed with ADHD-PI and a mild learning disability. She responded very well to Ritalin given twice per day and some accommodations at school, such as a reduced amount of required written work. After making the honor roll for 2 years, Lizzie's medication was discontinued when she was 14, with no return of ADHD symptoms.

Jason started taking Ritalin after breakfast and with lunch. His behavior improved almost immediately, according to his teacher. It soon became clear, however, that he also had learning disabilities, and he started receiving resource help in school. Although he eventually learned to read, it still does not come easily. His behavior at home remained erratic, and he would often refuse to do his homework. To help him concentrate, a 3:30 P.M. dose of Ritalin was added with good results. He also started behavioral counseling with a private therapist. He continues to argue frequently with his mother and to struggle in school, but both he and his mother think that things are gradually getting better.

WHAT THE FUTURE HOLDS

Like Lizzie, about one third of children with ADHD gradually grow out of many or all of their symptoms by adolescence. About half still have some signs of ADHD into adulthood. It is clear that children who have developed comorbid conditions such as emotional, motivational, or conduct disorders have more challenges to face in the future. In general, the first ADHD feature to disappear is the hyperactivity. Common features that persist include deficits in organization, planning, and self-management required for longer-term projects in high school and especially college. Technological advances such as word processors, organizers, and planners obviously benefit individuals with ADHD. Planning for and restructuring schools and other social environments to allow individuals with ADHD to better employ their strengths are ultimately needed. Although most people with ADHD become well-adjusted, well-functioning adults, some have difficulty handling job stress, interacting with fellow workers, and juggling the demands of marriage, family, and work. Cumulative failure experiences and limited opportunities can cause adolescents with ADHD to develop depression and antisocial behavior, contributing to a poor outcome. Studies show that this occurs in 10%–15% of children with ADHD. The best predictors of a good outcome appear to be intellectual gifts, strong parental involvement, and early therapy that focuses on developing your child's strengths while also treating symptoms and areas of need.

Some Questions Answered

How common is ADHD?

Although diagnostic practices and frequency rates differ greatly across and within cultures, ADHD is detected everywhere when similar diagnostic criteria are utilized. For a variety of reasons that are still being clarified, there has been a dramatic increase worldwide in the number of individuals diagnosed and treated for ADHD. Depending on how the disorder is defined, the incidence of ADHD ranges from 2% to 9% of children. It is more common in boys, especially in clinical settings, in which the male–female ratio ranges from 9:1 to 3:1.

When does ADHD begin and how long does it last?

ADHD can be diagnosed at any age, but in retrospect the symptoms always begin in childhood. Most children are diagnosed between ages 6 and 10 years. Like most disorders, the more severe it is, the earlier it is diagnosed. Some children may show signs of ADHD in the preschool period. We are now identifying children as early as 3 years of age as likely to have ADHD. At the other extreme, extremely bright children with the inattentive form of ADHD may not be identified until adolescence, when the rigors of school and futures planning tax their compensatory skills. Symptoms may change over time, and generally the total number of ADHD symptoms decline over time. Yet, for many, ADHD is a chronic disability lasting into adulthood.

What about ADHD in girls?

In general, much less is known about ADHD in girls because more boys are referred for treatment. Girls do have ADHD, but as a group they are less likely to display comorbid behavior problems. Typically, they are older when they are first diagnosed and more likely to display the inattentive type along with mood and learning problems.

What is the best type of school for a child with ADHD?

There is no school that is "right" for all children with ADHD. Generally, however, children with ADHD do best in highly structured classrooms. Each child with ADHD needs a good teacher, one who challenges the child, recognizes strengths, and individualizes the curriculum and educational program to promote success. One goal of the psychoeducational evaluation for the child with ADHD is to identify cognitive strengths and weaknesses and to make educational recommendations based on your child. These are child-specific rather than diagnosis specific.

Is there a relationship between ADHD and adoption?

Yes, studies show that as many as 40% of adopted children in North America display ADHD. Because these studies include children adopted at birth, ADHD is not viewed as a psychological consequence of adoption. A more likely reason is that children who are placed for adoption are at greater risk to carry a genetic predisposition for ADHD. In addition, other risk factors for ADHD and learning problems in general, such as poor prenatal care, low birth weight, and exposure to fetal toxins such as alcohol and other drugs, are probably more likely to occur with children of unplanned and unwanted pregnancies.

Can someone with ADHD succeed in life?

Yes, although success is by all means easier when the individual receives the necessary supports, accommodations, and treatment. ADHD takes its toll both on those affected and on their families. Having a protective, consistent, and stable relationship with parents and friends, persevering through elementary and middle school, and finding opportunities and environments where one's strengths can be recognized are recommended strategies. Some individuals with ADHD can flourish in higher education or business, but they must recognize the situations in which they are vulnerable (such as classes in large lecture halls or instances when math is needed) and develop a realistic plan. Many colleges now have formal programs for students with ADHD.

Specific Learning Disabilities

Bruce K. Shapiro

Progress in school is the work of children. For your child to make good academic progress, his or her internal and external environment must work together properly. The internal environment includes your child's learning and emotional strengths, whereas the external environment encompasses the family and school. A problem in any one of these areas can result in school failure.

In terms of the internal environment, some children may underachieve in school because of developmental disabilities, including mental retardation, cerebral palsy, communication disorders, hearing or vision loss, or attention-deficit/hyperactivity disorder (ADHD). Others may have mental health disorders such as depression or anxiety that interfere with learning. In terms of the external environment, some children live in poverty, in a home in which education is not stressed or valued, or attend a school with inadequate instruction or resources. All of these children may also experience school failure, but a primary learning disability is not the reason for the failure.

Children who have typical intelligence and a supportive home, social, and school environment but are still not learning may have a specific learning disability. Children with specific learning disabilities can have co-existing developmental disabilities, but their learning disability is not the direct result of these conditions. Specific learning disabilities are one of the most common developmental disabilities of childhood, occurring in about 5% of school-age children. Half of all children receiving special education services are diagnosed with a specific learning disability.

The writing of this chapter was supported in part by the Maternal and Child Health Bureau of the Health Resources and Services Administration, U.S. Department of Health and Human Services, Grant No. MCJ 249149.

Specific learning disabilities are a group of disabilities that result in academic underachievement. They can be isolated to one learning area with reading, written expression, and mathematics being the areas most commonly affected, they can be a combination of difficulties in two or three of these areas, or they can affect all aspects of learning. Depending on the severity of the specific learning disability, its impact may extend well beyond the classroom to all aspects of your child's life.

TYPES OF SPECIFIC LEARNING DISABILITY

Reading is seen as the key to successful integration into our society and is a child's major academic accomplishment of early elementary school. Specific reading disability is by far the most common specific learning disability treated in special education and, therefore, has received the most attention. It may affect basic reading (decoding) or reading comprehension.

A second form of specific learning disability affects written expression. The terms *dysgraphia* and *graphomotor disorder* are frequently used to describe this form of learning disability. This difficulty with writing may be due to poor language abilities, fine motor dysfunction, or poor organizational abilities (also called *executive function*). Although children with a specific learning disability in written expression can write, they may do so slowly and imprecisely. Frequently this deficit goes unrecognized and may prove devastating to children whose trouble with written output results in declining grades and school failure. Specific learning disability in written expression is commonly associated with specific reading disability.

A specific learning disability in mathematics may affect computation or mathematical reasoning. This disorder, often called *dyscalculia,* commonly is seen in conjunction with other specific learning disabilities. Federal legislation also recognizes specific learning disabilities in oral expression and listening comprehension, although these are rarely isolated disabilities.

Scott, Julie, and Jim

Scott is a 6½-year-old who did well in preschool and kindergarten but is experiencing significant difficulties in learning to read in first grade. When asked to read a sentence, he will guess based on the first letter of the word. He reads *book* as *ball.* He attempts to sound out words but cannot master phonics (matching sounds to letters). In contrast, his 5-year-old sister, Sally, is beginning to read and will soon surpass him.

Julie is an 8½-year-old third grader. She did well in learning to read, but math remains a mystery to her. She has trouble with the concept of time and has difficulty carrying in addition and borrowing in subtraction.

Jim is a 12-year-old sixth grader who has struggled throughout school. Although he seems bright, he barely maintains a C average. Jim spends adequate time studying for tests but never seems to get the grades he deserves given the amount of time he studies. Jim, now entering adolescence, is getting frustrated. When he gets upset, he calls himself "stupid," and he is starting to "forget" to bring his homework home.

ORIGINS OF SPECIFIC LEARNING DISABILITIES

Specific learning disabilities do not start with school entry. It is now known that the brain dysfunction that results in a specific learning disability is, in most cases, present from birth and is often inherited. In some families, the disability is passed on from one generation to the next and may affect as many as half of the family members. Some children with genetic syndromes have specific learning disabilities. The genetic basis for specific learning disabilities is supported by the discovery of relationships between two particular chromosomes and reading or mathematics. It is also known that certain conditions in infancy, such as prematurity and delayed language development, place a child at increased risk for developing specific learning disabilities. Brain damage from birth trauma, traumatic brain injury, meningitis, lead poisoning, or near drowning may also be associated with specific learning disability. Despite increasing knowledge about learning disabilities, the origin of most children's learning disabilities remains unknown.

UNDERLYING MECHANISM OF
SPECIFIC LEARNING DISABILITY

The vast majority of children who receive treatment for a specific learning disability have specific reading disability, so it is not surprising that specialists know more about this disorder than other forms of learning disabilities and focus on it. Reading is very complex, and any problem in the processing or interpretation of written words can lead to a specific reading disability. Successful reading requires integration of the language, visual, spatial, memory, and motor functions of the brain. A problem anywhere along these pathways can lead to a problem in reading. Basic reading, called *decoding,* involves the translation of written language into its speech sound equivalents, called phonemes. If this decoding is not accomplished readily, reading will be labored and comprehension poor. Dyslexia can be viewed as a subset of specific reading disability. In contrast to specific reading disability, in which the impairment affects basic reading and or comprehension, the disorder known as dyslexia is marked by difficulties with basic reading alone. The International Dyslexia Association has proposed a biologically based definition of dyslexia as "a language-based disorder . . . characterized by difficulties in single word decoding."

It is suspected that most cases of specific reading disability result from a developmental brain abnormality that disrupts the network of nerve cells needed for reading. This theory suggests that the particular location of the problem determines the form of the specific learning disability. Unfortunately, the affected areas of the brain cannot routinely be detected. Certain experimental brain imaging techniques, however, are beginning to help define these abnormalities by showing areas of brain that have increased activity, marked by blood flow, while performing a task such as reading. Several studies have shown decreased brain activity in the left temporal lobe of the brain in adults with dyslexia. Other studies have shown decreased activity in the central auditory pathways and in brain regions involved in planning and attention. These findings show the diverse nature of reading disability, and other specific learning disabilities may have similar complexities. It is hoped that these techniques may ultimately lead to improved interventions for people with specific learning disabilities.

DIAGNOSING SPECIFIC LEARNING DISABILITY

The diagnosis of specific learning disability is often difficult to make, not only because there is currently no specific test for it but also because there is controversy about its definition. The Individuals with Disabilities Education Act (IDEA) Amendments of 1997, which provide federal funding for public school programs, define *specific learning disability* as "a disorder in one or more of the basic psychological processes involved in understanding or in using language, spoken or written, which . . . may manifest itself in an imperfect ability to listen, think, speak, read, write, spell, or do mathematical calculations." The most common method for making this diagnosis is by demonstrating a discrepancy between a child's academic potential and his or her academic achievement. Diagnosis using this "discrepancy" approach, however, has been criticized as being conceptually flawed, inflexible, and inadequate for classification. Another method of defining specific learning disability documents the child's failure to progress in an academic area. The problem with this approach, however, is that the child must show a prolonged period of lack of progress before a diagnosis can be established.

Identifying specific learning disabilities is often difficult and may delay the development of an intervention program for your child. The consequence of this is that your child may endure repeated failures until he or she "grows into" a diagnosis. And it means that you, as a parent, need to be an effective and assertive advocate for your child if you suspect a specific learning disability (see Chapter 12 for more on your child's educational rights).

TESTING A CHILD FOR SPECIFIC LEARNING DISABILITY: WHAT AN EVALUATION SHOULD INCLUDE

At minimum, the evaluation of your child for specific learning disability requires a measure of academic potential and a measure of academic achievement. Other evaluations may be warranted to document related conditions (such as ADHD), to further define the nature of your child's disability, or to develop a treatment program. Evaluations for specific learning disability should be based on individually administered rather than group tests.

Despite some concerns about IQ tests being an incomplete measure of academic potential, the Wechsler Intelligence Scale for Children–III (WISC–III) remains the most commonly used evaluation tool. The WISC–III yields a Verbal IQ, a Performance IQ, and a Full-Scale IQ (calculated from the first two scores). This test consists of increasingly difficult questions ranging from a 6- to 16-year-old level and is scored using age norms. In addition to measuring potential, the WISC–III is used to exclude intellectual limitation as a cause of your child's academic underachievement.

Academic achievement in written expression, reading, spelling, and math is typically measured by a standardized educational test. Among the most commonly used are the Woodcock Johnson–Revised: Tests of Achievement, the Wechsler Individual Achievement Test, the Peabody Individual Achievement Test–Revised, and the Kaufman Test of Educational Achievement. All are well accepted and provide an overview of your child's academic strengths and weaknesses. An educator or a psychologist can conduct educational testing.

It is difficult to detect academic underachievement using these tests in a child who is performing at less than a first-grade level. The tests may also fail to identify certain older children who will "pass" in the brief testing period but "fail" in a classroom environment in which prolonged attention and performance are required.

Other tests are available to measure speech and language abilities, quantify behavioral functions, and assess neurological (including motor and sensory function) and mental health aspects of your child. These tests provide additional information that may assist clinicians, but it must be realized that if enough tests are performed, some abnormality will be found in everyone. What is important is the presence of a consistent and significant pattern of abnormalities.

SUSPECTING SPECIFIC LEARNING DISABILITIES

You should suspect a learning disability when your child does not meet age-appropriate expectations. The more severe and complex the disorder, the more likely it is to be detected early. Thus, a child with global learning disabilities is likely to be identified soon after school entry. Similarly, a severe reading disability may be detected in first grade when a child fails to acquire basic reading decoding skills. Other reading problems, such as poor comprehension or chapter reading, may be identified later. The latter two forms of specific reading disability are generally *not* associated with difficulty in learning basic reading skills. Delayed diagnosis is also likely in the child with a high IQ score who develops strategies to circumvent the disability until high school or even college when it first becomes evident. Early diagnosis may occur when another family member has already experienced a specific learning disability and the family has an increased level of awareness.

Children with written language disabilities that are identified later in school often have poor coloring, painting, or pasting skills in preschool. Some of these children show poor pencil grasp, hand cramping, and/or excessive pencil pressure. Most written expression learning disabilities become evident in middle school when there are requirements for compositions, notebooks, and essay tests. In children with milder forms of the disorders and in brighter students, however, difficulties with written expression may not become evident until high school or college.

Math disabilities usually manifest as poor computation abilities. They are most often diagnosed in late elementary or early middle school, unless they co-exist with reading disability, in which case they may be diagnosed earlier. It is rare for a child to have mathematical comprehension problems without a computation disorder.

IDENTIFYING ASSOCIATED IMPAIRMENTS AND DISORDERS

Specific learning disabilities commonly are associated with other impairments and disorders. The most common reason for the lack of success of a treatment program is failure to address these co-existing problems. Somewhere between one quarter and two thirds of children with a specific learning disability have an additional developmental disability or mental health condition. The most common association is with ADHD (see Chapter 24).

In addition to these neurological impairments, children with specific learning disabilities may also have emotional and behavioral impairments. Children with specific learning disabilities may be socially clumsy and isolated, may not participate in extracurricular activities, and may have few close friends. The underlying problem may be an inability to take the perspective of others, poor conversational skills, and misinterpretation of body language. Your child may also have emotional disorders resulting from the experience of school failure. These may result in conduct disorders, withdrawal, poor self-esteem, anxiety, or depression.

It is important to identify these potentially complicating factors early because effective treatment of associated disabilities will increase the likelihood of a successful management program for your child and prevent the associated disorders from interfering with treatment. For example, if your child has ADHD, his or her inattention and hyperactivity will affect learning. Thus, when your child is being assessed for a specific learning disability, he or she should also be evaluated for other common impairments and conditions that may have an impact on learning and success at school.

GETTING THE DIAGNOSIS AND SETTING UP A PROGRAM

Testing for specific learning disabilities may be performed by a school psychologist at no cost to you. You may also choose to have your child tested privately. Reasons for choosing a private evaluation may be a backlog in testing at school or the desire for a second opinion. The cost of this psychoeducational evaluation may not be covered by your health insurance. If you are enrolled in an HMO (health maintenance organization), your child's primary care physician will need to make a referral to the psychologist for this service to be covered. Once the testing is completed, a school meeting will be set up to explain the results to you and to decide on a course of action (see Chapter 12).

ENVIRONMENTS FOR EDUCATIONAL INTERVENTIONS

The treatment environment for your child depends on a number of factors including the specific impairment(s), the degree of severity, and your child's age. Many children with specific learning disabilities, especially those with written expression problems, can be served in a general curriculum with some accommodations, such as being given more time to take written tests. Other children who require special instruction may be served in a pull-out or in an inclusive model. In pull-out services, your child is removed from the general education class for a single class period each day to attend a resource room with a few other students who have similar difficulties. In the inclusion model, a special educator works with your child within the general education classroom. There are advantages and disadvantages of both models. The resource room approach allows your child to have a controlled learning environment with a curriculum-based special education program. This approach, however, also identifies your child as being "different" and causes him or her to miss a regularly scheduled class. The inclusion model avoids these problems but replaces them with other issues. Remedial learning may be difficult in a large classroom that is moving at a faster pace or engaged in a different subject. The inclusion model also may afford less time for individualized attention from the special education teacher.

For only a minority of children with a specific learning disability is the traditional self-contained special education class the preferred option. Now, inclusion is the rule, and the use of self-contained classes is restricted to children whose learning disabilities are so severe or complex that they cannot be addressed in less restrictive environments. Children with specific learning disabilities most often requiring self-contained classes are children with global learning disabilities and those with co-occurring behavioral or emotional disturbances that are likely to be accentuated by the ebb and flow of the general classroom.

INTERVENTION: FOCUSING ON STRENGTHS OR NEEDS

There are two basic approaches to intervention for children with specific learning disabilities: remediation and accommodation. Remediation focuses on your child's needs and attempts to improve skills; most approaches to reading are remedial in nature. Accommodation approaches use your child's strengths and bypass weak areas; for example, your child might use a calculator if he or she has difficulty in math. Table 25.1 lists a number of accommodation strategies that are commonly employed for children who have specific learning disabilities in written expression. It should be emphasized that *accommodation* does not mean giving up on your child's progress in the problem area; it simply keeps a weak area from delaying your child's progress in other areas. In good educational programs, both remedial and accommodation approaches are used.

When should accommodation be used? In the area of written expression and mathematics, your child is not likely to experience a significant limitation in long-term function if an accommodation strategy is used following the failure of a remediation approach. For example, how many of us balance our checkbook manually as opposed to using a calculator or a software program? Many of us use computer programs to correct poor grammar and spelling as well. In the area of reading, when to use accommodation is a more difficult question to answer. Most educators resist accommodating a child with reading difficulties because illiteracy limits a person's options in life. Yet, in rare instances the teaching of reading will not be successful. For these children, other methods of information transfer have been used to bypass reading and maintain knowledge including volunteer readers, books on audiotape, videotapes, computers, and electronic readers/scanners.

HOMEWORK

Homework is usually difficult for children with specific learning disabilities and frustrating for their parents. For many children with specific learning disabilities, homework becomes the unwanted focus of their extracurricular lives. As a result, it can become a battleground between parent and child. To avoid this conflict, you should set up a routine for homework completion, develop homework aids to circumvent certain problems, and monitor the amount and type of homework given to your child.

In terms of developing a routine, your child will need to unwind after school, and you may not be home to supervise him or her until after your workday. So, your child may need to start homework in the hour prior to or after dinnertime. Whatever time you choose should be consistent from day to day. Ideally, your child should complete homework in a place with few distractions.

You can also help with accommodation techniques. For example, you can read the science material with your child who has dyslexia to ensure that his or her understanding of the information is not impeded by poor reading. Writing out your child's math problems may save a half-hour of homework time. Children as young as second or third grade may require secretaries (not editors!) and may need to use computers to compensate for their written language difficulties.

Homework assignments are also a sensitive measure of the appropriateness of your child's educational program. Adjustment of your child's program may be warranted if 1) the homework takes an excessive amount of time, 2) your child consistently does not understand or retain the homework information, or 3) you find yourself doing the work.

SOCIAL SKILLS TRAINING AND COUNSELING

Self-esteem and the development of social skills are important in preventing withdrawal from social contacts. You and your child's teachers can encourage the development of your child's self-esteem by finding activities that he or she does well and emphasizing them in school and extracurricular activities. Camp experiences are good summer opportunities for social skills training, and peer support groups are particularly helpful for adolescents who may be less likely to confide in adults. If your child requires increased support, social skills training can be provided in groups, using role-playing techniques, or in individual counseling sessions. Issues to discuss may include homework, discipline, parental expectations, and self-esteem.

EXTRACURRICULAR ACTIVITIES

Extracurricular activities should be an integral part of the treatment program and can include sports, scouting, music, drama, martial arts, and so forth. These activities provide opportunities for your child to socialize outside of school. Extracurricular activities also allow your child's nonacademic strengths to be demonstrated. The child who experiences success in an extracurricular area will often be more able to face problems in the classroom.

If your child cannot keep up with classroom demands, you should not stop his or her extracurricular activities in an effort to allow more time for academics. Some children show marked deterioration in their performance when extracurricular activities are curtailed. The tension between academic and extracurricular time requirements may be diminished by obtaining homework assignments in 1-week blocks and budgeting your child's time to meet both needs.

EFFECTS ON THE FAMILY

Learning that your child has a specific learning disability is likely to be very stressful. Many concerns arise: "Will he ever learn to read?" "Will she be able to attend college?" "Will I have to spend all my free time and money on tutoring?" "Whose side of the family did it come from?" However, a vast majority of children with specific learning disabilities eventually are able to read, write, do arithmetic, graduate from high school, and pursue higher education. In addition, few families are broken financially or emotionally by the experience.

Table 25.1.   Accommodations for specific learning disability in written expression (dysgraphia, graphomotor disorders)

Copying from the blackboard should be minimized. Teacher might hand homework and classwork to child.

Your child should avoid note taking. A peer note taker or a notebook buddy should be used to bypass note taking, or the teacher could provide lesson outlines.

Your child could use peer notes for studying (photocopying is helpful).

Designate a secretary to transcribe your child's dictation of book reports, essays, and other compositions.

Math problems may be copied by someone else, but your child should solve the problems.

Your child should be excused from showing his or her homework or classwork if the concepts are understood.

The teacher should note spelling and punctuation errors but not penalize the child for them.

Your child will benefit from modified testing procedures: multiple choice format, additional time, or oral testing to determine whether your child has mastered the material.

Your child could use a word processor or computer in the classroom.

Voice-activated software may be helpful to your child.

You may be able to assign blame for the inheritance, but it will help your child more to focus on treatment and support for his or her specific learning disability.

This does not mean, however, that success is simple, painless, or guaranteed. You will have many tasks to accomplish, including identifying the problem early, developing a treatment plan, monitoring the effectiveness of intervention, and keeping your child's spirits up. Siblings may pose particular challenges for the last of these tasks. It is difficult for siblings to understand specific learning disability. They may reason, "Jimmy looks the same as the rest of us. Why isn't he treated the same as the rest of us?" One answer is that each child gets the amount of time and attention that he or she needs and that this amount may not be equal. Be sure, however, that there are special times for each sibling to get individual parental attention, ideally on a daily basis.

ALTERNATIVE THERAPIES

There is currently no cure for specific learning disabilities, but many nonconventional therapies have been promoted. These have ranged from colored eyeglass lenses, to vision training, to special diets. None of these approaches have been tested scientifically and there is little in the scientific literature in support of using any of these approaches. Although alternative methods may seem innocuous, they are frequently costly in time and dollars, may place the blame for failure on the families that use them, and distract families from the main educational focus of therapy. Any new treatment approach should be tested in a scientifically valid manner before it is promoted for use in children with specific learning disabilities.

SEARCHING FOR INFORMATION ABOUT SPECIFIC LEARNING DISABILITIES

You will want to be kept up to date about new information about specific learning disabilities. The Internet is a powerful tool for obtaining this information, but the information is unfiltered. Some of it is current and correct and other information is outdated, presented in an unbalanced fashion, taken out of context, or inaccurate. It is best to rely on well-known specific learning disability web sites, such as those of the Learning Project of public television channel WETA (http://www.ldonline.org), the Learning Disabilities Association of America (http://www.ldanatl.org), and the National Center on Learning Disabilities (http://www.ncld.org), or to perform literature searches for peer-reviewed scientific articles through the free PubMed site maintained by the National Institutes of Health (http://www.ncbi.nlm.nih.gov/PubMed).

Parent groups can provide great support to your family. Local chapters may know the best schools, teachers, and programs in your area. Experienced members of the group are generally aware of available services within your community and how to gain access to them. These more experienced parents may also provide you with emotional support by sharing experiences and successes that will make you feel less alone and more hopeful. As you become more experienced, you may in turn be able to help others, which is both a giving and an empowering experience. In addition to local organizations, the national organizations of these groups provide up-to-date information about specific learning disabilities by sponsoring speakers and providing literature about a wide range of related subjects.

MONITORING YOUR CHILD'S TREATMENT PROGRAM

Your child's specific learning disability is not static. As a result, the treatment program will need to be modified as your child becomes older and academic demands change. Monitoring is a key part of an overall treatment program and can assume two forms. The first is close interaction between you and your child's teachers. The second is the periodic review of progress. The purposes of this periodic review are fourfold:

1. *To ensure that the program is still relevant:* Programs put into place in early elementary school are likely to need modification by middle school. Your

child may have met certain objectives and may no longer need remediation. Other objectives may not have been met, and alternate strategies should be tried. Some objectives may prove to have been inappropriate or unrealistic and should be changed.

2. *To provide anticipatory guidance:* Anticipatory guidance predicts the likely outcome of an event (for example, the need for multiple class changes when your child enters middle school) and the steps that should be taken to address it. Although each child is unique, certain events are predictable. Advance knowledge of potential problems may result in improved planning, less stress, and better outcomes.

3. *To address new or unresolved issues:* As your child gets older, new challenges emerge. Some of these events are the same for all children— adolescence, driving, dating—but the experiences may be colored by the specific learning disability. The normal testing of limits in adolescence may have an impact on dedication to schoolwork or homework.

   In addition to these new challenges, you may have unresolved issues or may need clarification of some information. For example, you may still wonder after all these years whether a cold you had during your pregnancy, a medication you took, or the forceps your obstetrician used caused your child's learning disability. Follow-up visits allow the opportunity for clarification and resolution of these issues. In this case, you would learn that there is no known relationship between any of these experiences and specific learning disabilities.

4. *To plan for the future:* Perhaps the most important part of the monitoring process is the ability to plan. Planning for the future is distinguished from anticipatory guidance because it focuses on your child rather than on the shared experiences of the group of children with specific learning disabilities. Planning is an insightful process that blends potential and achievement to revise goals and set new objectives. In effect, planning is a best guess about what will happen next with your child.

In the absence of problems, periodic review is best accomplished at times of transition: twice yearly in early elementary school, when moving from elementary to middle school, before entry to high school, and before entry to college. Past performance and measures of your child's current abilities should be reviewed. Reports of behavior and socialization and academic strengths and weaknesses should also be evaluated. Psychoeducational evaluations may require updating, and goals should be set for the next specified time period. When your child is in later elementary school or older, he or she should participate in the review process. If your child is involved in planning the future, he or she is more likely to support and follow through on the recommendations and make other important life decisions in the future. Finally, participation allows your child to "own" his or her disability.

AFTER HIGH SCHOOL: CAREER
EDUCATION, VOCATIONAL, AND COLLEGE TRAINING

Career education should be part of the program for your child from the primary grades. It involves teaching skills that are required for success in the workplace: cooperation, respect, responsibility, teamwork, organization, and how to seek information to solve one's problems. Your child should also have a transition plan, which is usually drafted in middle school (at age 14) and defines the goals of the management program (see Chapter 28). It is revised as your child progresses through school.

Vocational training starts as your child moves from middle to high school. Vocational education provides training in hands-on skills needed for future jobs but also stresses continuing education and encourages maximization of your child's abilities. Many of these programs are linked with community colleges on graduation from high school. Vocational rehabilitation services may be provided as part of your child's educational program if your child meets certain federally mandated criteria. They can lead to attendance at a technical school or on-the-job training after high school graduation.

Many children with specific learning disabilities will attend schools of higher education. Community colleges have long been committed to developing individualized programs for students with specific learning disabilities. Many colleges and universities also now recognize a responsibility to students with learning and other disabilities and provide accommodations for these individuals. Most colleges have a disability services office that helps students obtain support services. Some universities have developed extensive special needs programs. Because of the numerous options and the many individuals with disabilities, there are books devoted to assessing the suitability of colleges and universities for students with specific learning disabilities (for example, C.T. Mangrum's *Peterson's Colleges with Programs for Students with Learning Disabilities or Attention Deficit Disorders, Fifth Edition;* see the Suggested Readings and Resources at the end of this book for more information).

OUTCOMES FOR CHILDREN WITH
SPECIFIC LEARNING DISABILITIES

One key to a successful life outcome is preventing your child's disability from becoming a handicap. Most children with specific learning disabilities attain literacy and numeracy (basic math skills). Almost all attain these skills before the end of high school, although some learn to read as young adults. People with specific learning disabilities, however, often have persisting psychoeducational impairments. Adults with specific reading disability read more slowly, make more spelling errors, and acquire less information from texts. They tend to have difficulty in writing essays, completing heavy reading assignments, scoring well on timed tests, and learning foreign languages.

It is not possible to predict outcomes for individual children, and successful outcomes are not related to any one specific intervention. In fact, studies of large groups of individuals with specific learning disabilities have suggested that a number of factors influence outcomes. As expected, children whose disabilities are less severe and those with isolated rather than global learning disabilities tend to do better. Poorer life outcomes are associated with repeated school failure, poor family and/or school support, and co-occurring conditions, including mental health disorders. Good self-esteem, social skills, and ability to self-advocate seem to be related to good life outcomes.

Some Questions Answered

Should I delay my child's entry into first grade?

Delayed school entry is often recommended for children who lack academic readiness skills in kindergarten. Although this delay may be useful for the "late bloomer," it is of little value for the child with specific learning disabilities because delayed school entry will lead only to continuing academic difficulties. The preferred approach is to diagnose the specific learning disability and start appropriate intervention as early as possible.

Should I consider retaining my son in his current grade for another year?

Retention should be avoided for children with specific learning disabilities. These children do not close the gap with an extra year, and retention may lower self-esteem. If your child has an appropriate remediation program, there should be no need for retention. If your child is making insufficient progress, the goals of the educational program should be reviewed and modified.

My 5-year-old is writing his letters backward. Is this a sign of dyslexia?

Strephosymbolia, or twisted symbols (writing backward), was first associated with dyslexia by Dr. Samuel Orton, a pioneer in this field. It is now known that most children with dyslexia do not reverse their letters, and many children younger than 7 years of age who reverse their letters do not have dyslexia. Your 5-year-old's reversals probably indicate that the letters lack meaning rather than that he has a primary learning disability. There are, however, some early signs that do suggest an increased risk for dyslexia. It has been found that preschool children, ages 3–5 years old, who later develop reading disabilities have language delays including decreased length of utterances, receptive vocabulary, object naming, and pronunciation accuracy. If you notice that your son has any of these difficulties, then you should discuss the possibility of further evaluation with his pediatrician.

Will reading to my baby prevent specific learning disabilities?

Reading to your young child has many benefits. It is a chance to spend time together, perhaps as part of the ritual at bedtime. It provides you an opportunity to explain the world around your child, and he or she will come to love the sound of words and the images that written words can conjure up. Reading to your child, however, will not prevent a specific learning disability from developing as this is a developmental brain problem that likely predates birth.

Should my child undergo an EEG or an MRI scan as part of the evaluation for a specific learning disability?

Other than vision and hearing tests, there are no specific medical tests that need to be done for a child with specific learning disabilities. An EEG (electroencephalogram, or brain wave test) should only be done if your child might be having absence seizures that interfere with learning (see Chapter 18). Similarly, an MRI (magnetic resonance imaging) scan should be done only if some structural abnormality of the brain is suspected to be affecting learning. Both of these are extremely rare causes of learning problems. Eventually, functional MRI, an experimental technique that measures blood flow to various brain regions while a person is performing tasks such as reading, may be useful both in diagnosis and assessing effectiveness of treatment.

Are there medications that are helpful in treating specific learning disabilities?

Currently no licensed medications address the underlying problems in specific learning disabilities. Medication may be prescribed, however, for associated deficits. For example, if your child has ADHD as well as specific learning disabilities, the control of the attention disorder with stimulant medication such as Ritalin (methylphenidate) may help with the learning disabilities by improving your child's attention and frustration tolerance. Similarly, if your child has depression or severe anxiety, the use of antidepressants may improve the emotional environment and thereby improve learning.

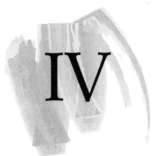

IV

What the Future Holds

26

What About Our Next Child?

Genetic Counseling

Cynthia J. Tifft

When you go to a genetics clinic you are likely seeking the answers to four questions: 1) What is wrong with my child (diagnosis), 2) why did it happen (cause), 3) what is going to happen to my child (prognosis), and 4) what is the chance it will happen again (recurrence risk)? Chapter 16 discusses the recognizable patterns of physical and developmental features of genetic syndromes that help geneticists and pediatricians answer the diagnosis and prognosis questions. This chapter discusses some of the causes of genetic syndromes by addressing the basic principles of genetic inheritance and some common genetic disorders. It also explains how a geneticist or genetic counselor can help guide you to clarify your own family's situation. The chapter then discusses how geneticists can help answer the question about the risk of recurrence and how prenatal diagnosis and a careful family history are useful. Last, the chapter mentions some therapies for the treatment of genetic diseases.

   In understanding genetic disorders, it is important to realize that nothing you did or did not do caused the genetic disorder to occur in your child. None of us has control over which genes we pass on to our children, and all of us have in our genetic background abnormally functioning genes that under certain circumstances or with a particular partner can give rise to a genetic disorder in a child.

ABOUT CHROMOSOMES AND GENES

Our body is made up of cells. All cells, with the exception of red blood cells, have a center, or nucleus, that contains the chromosomes. Chromosomes are tightly wound strands of DNA (deoxyribonucleic acid). The strands of DNA are made up of four chemical building blocks called *bases,* whose order determines the information contained in the genes, in much the same way as specific letters of the alphabet combine together to form words and sentences (see Figure 26.1). The four bases are called *adenine, thymine, cytosine,* and *guanine* and are often abbreviated A, T, C, and G, respectively. Genes are arranged along the chromosomes like beads on a necklace. The chromosomes are large enough to be seen under a microscope. The genes themselves are too small to be seen, but with special techniques, it is possible to "see" the genes and even determine the sequence or order of the bases that make up an individual gene.

Humans have 46 chromosomes arranged into 23 pairs. Normally, one chromosome in each pair is contributed by the mother, and the other by the father. A complete set of 46 chromosomes stores all of the instructions that the body needs to develop properly.

Each chromosome contains 500–2,000 genes, and according to estimates of the Human Genome Project, humans possess approximately 90,000 different genes. Every gene is made up of thousands, or even hundreds of thousands, of bases. Each gene occupies a specific position on one of the 23 pairs of chromosomes. The genes are the instructions for the development of the child from an embryo. They also determine physical traits such as hair or eye color, structural features such as bones and muscles, and enzymes necessary to control body metabolism.

Genetic disorders can be broadly classified as those that are caused by chromosomal abnormalities and involve large numbers of genes and those that are caused by abnormalities in individual or closely related genes.

CHROMOSOMAL ABNORMALITIES

To explain how some chromosomal abnormalities arise, the normal process of fertilization must first be described. Human cells contain 46 chromosomes, but sperm and egg cells are exceptions. The mature female egg and male sperm each contain only 23 chromosomes, one of each pair. At the time of fertilization, the egg and sperm come together to reestablish the 46 chromosomes that are needed to form the human embryo.

Among the 23 pairs of chromosomes is one pair that determines the sex of the baby. These two chromosomes are called the *sex chromosomes;* the other 22 pairs are called *autosomal chromosomes.* Sex chromosomes are referred to as the X and Y chromosomes. Boys have one X and one Y chromosome, whereas girls have two X chromosomes. The father's sperm can contain either an X or a Y chromosome, whereas the mother's egg can contribute only an X chromosome; therefore, the father's sperm determines the sex of the baby (see Figure 26.2).

Disorders Involving an Entire Chromosome

Chromosomal abnormalities can arise because of mistakes that occur when the egg and sperm cells are formed. At their earliest stages of development, the immature egg and sperm cells actually do contain 46 chromosomes, or 23 pairs. But as they mature, these cells undergo a division, called *meiosis*, that splits the paired chromosomes into separate cells, each with only one copy of each pair. Sometimes, however, the division proceeds unequally, resulting in cells with either 22 or 24 chromosomes. This phenomenon is called *nondisjunction* (see Figure 15.2 in Chapter 15). The cell with too few chromosomes almost always dies, because it lacks the necessary genetic information for development. But in some cases the cell with 24 chromosomes can go on to be fertilized, resulting in an embryo with 47 rather than 46 chromosomes; one of the chromosomes is present in triplicate.

This condition, called *trisomy*, most commonly occurs with chromosome #21, resulting in Down syndrome (see Chapter 15). Down syndrome is the most common genetic disorder and occurs in approximately 1 in every 650

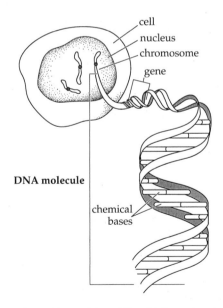

Figure 26.1. DNA (deoxyribonucleic acid), which carries the instructions that allow cells to make proteins, is made up of four chemical bases. Tightly coiled strands of DNA are packaged in units called *chromosomes*, housed in the cell's nucleus. Working subunits of DNA are known as *genes*.

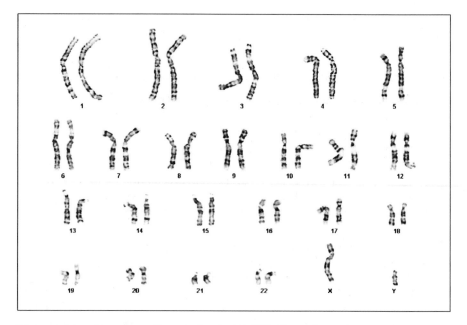

Figure 26.2.   Karyotype of a typical male (46, XY). To produce a karyotype, a teaspoon of blood and a chemical is added to stimulate growth of the white blood cells. After 3 days, the cells are harvested and placed on microscope slides. The slides are then stained to produce characteristic banding patterns for each chromosome. By analyzing the cells in a digital microscope, chromosomes from a representative cell can be electronically ordered from largest to smallest (chromosomes #1–22, X, and Y) to create a karyotype. Chromosomes are also checked for breaks or rearrangements.

births. You may have heard that children with Down syndrome are born only to older mothers, but in fact any woman can give birth to a child with Down syndrome. It is true that the risk of having a child with a chromosomal abnormality such as Down syndrome increases with a woman's advancing age. The higher birth rate among younger women, however, even when combined with the lower risk for Down syndrome, means that there is a higher total number of children with Down syndrome born to younger mothers. Once a young woman has had one child with a chromosomal disorder, her chance of having a second child with a chromosomal disorder is 1 in 100. Given this increased risk, she should be offered amniocentesis or chorionic villus sampling (CVS) during her next pregnancy to determine if a chromosomal abnormality is present (discussed later).

Chromosomal abnormalities often cause a child to be born with distinctive facial features and malformations in multiple organ systems such as the heart, brain, and kidneys. Many conceptions that result in chromosomal abnormalities end in spontaneous miscarriage in the first or second trimester. Indeed, 20% of all conceptions end in miscarriage, and half of these have chromosomal abnormalities. One reason for couples to experience recurrent miscarriages can be what is known as a *balanced chromosome rearrangement* in one of the partners. If this is suspected, both partners will be offered a blood test for chromosome analysis.

Microdeletion Syndromes

Scientists have discovered that some common genetic syndromes are caused by very small deletions of a particular portion of a chromosome. These disorders are called *microdeletion syndromes.* The microdeletions are too small to be detected on a standard chromosome analysis. If the physician suspects one of these microdeletion syndromes, a special test with the whimsical acronym FISH (fluorescent *in situ* hybridization) must be used to find them. Microdeletion syndromes include Williams syndrome, velocardiofacial syndrome (sometimes referred to as VCFS), Miller-Dieker syndrome (associated with a developmental brain malformation, short stature, seizures, and mental retardation), Smith-Magenis syndrome (associated with congenital heart disease, short stature, decreased muscle tone, and mental retardation), and some forms of Prader-Willi syndrome. The most common of these syndromes are discussed in Chapter 16.

SINGLE-GENE DISORDERS

The second type of genetic disorder arises when mistakes within individual genes are present. In this type of disorder, the message of a gene is scrambled or lost, and incorrect developmental or biochemical instructions are given. Profound changes in development may occur.

We inherit one copy of each gene from our mother and one copy from our father. Therefore, genetic *mutations* can also be inherited. When a baby is born with a single-gene disorder, he or she either inherited the mutation from one or both parents, or it occurred spontaneously as a new mutation early in development. Either way, the mutation is now a part of that baby's genetic blueprint. Inheritance of single-gene disorders is often called *Mendelian inheritance* after the Moravian monk Gregor Mendel, who first described certain inheritance patterns in his experiments with the garden pea in 1865.

To understand how genetic diseases are passed on from one generation to the next, it is necessary to understand certain basic concepts of heredity. The first two points have already been discussed: Chromosomes are composed of genes, and half of our genes come from our mothers and half from our fathers. The third important concept is that there are stronger, or dominant, genes that block the action of weaker, or recessive, genes.

Nearly 10,000 single-gene disorders have been described, and nearly 6,000 of these have been assigned to specific chromosomes. There are three major inheritance patterns for single-gene disorders: *autosomal dominant, autosomal recessive,* and *X-linked (or sex-linked) recessive.* The genetic change in an autosomal disorder occurs in a gene on one of the 22 pairs of nonsex chromosomes, whereas X-linked disorders involve mutations on the X chromosome.

Autosomal Dominant Disorders

Autosomal dominant disorders are caused by the presence of a single abnormal dominant gene that is inherited from either parent or that arises as a new mutation in a child who has two unaffected parents. In either case, the child has one abnormally functioning gene that is dominant over the normally functioning recessive gene. Individuals with autosomal dominant disorders have a 50% chance of passing the disorder to their sons or daughters, whereas unaffected individuals have no chance of transmitting the condition (see Figure 26.3). Just like tossing a coin, this means there is a 50% chance of passing the gene in *each* pregnancy regardless of the number of pregnancies. To pass a dominant condition to your children, you must have the condition yourself. Other autosomal dominant disorders include neurofibromatosis, osteogenesis imperfecta, Marfan syndrome, and achondroplasia.

Lena

Juan and Lucía's second daughter Lena was born with a large head and short arms and legs compared with her body. The family was puzzled because their first child and all of their extended family members were of average stature. They were worried that Lena might not grow typically. Lena's condition, called *achondroplasia*, is the most common form of dwarfism. Lena's achondroplasia is an example of a *new dominant mutation*, a spontaneous change in the DNA structure of a gene that started in that particular individual. This means that Juan and Lucía are not at an increased risk to have another child with achondroplasia, but Lena will have a 50% chance of passing the condition to her children. Lena's brothers and sisters are not at risk to pass the condition to their children.

Autosomal Recessive Disorders

Autosomal recessive disorders are inherited quite differently from autosomal dominant disorders. For your child to have a recessive disorder, he or she must have inherited two copies of the same abnormally functioning recessive gene, one from each parent. A double dose of the abnormally functioning gene is required for a person to have the disorder. In this situation, each parent has one normally functioning copy of the gene and one abnormally functioning copy; such an individual is called a *carrier* for that disorder. For autosomal recessive disorders only, carriers are healthy because one normal gene is sufficient. Most disorders involving the enzymes necessary for body metabolism are autosomal recessive (see Figure 26.4).

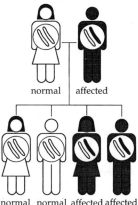

normal | affected

normal   normal   affected   affected

Figure 26.3. Inheritance of autosomal dominant disorders. Each time an affected person conceives a child with an unaffected person, there is a 50% risk that the child will be affected and a 50% chance that the child will be typical. About half of dominantly inherited disorders, however, represent new mutations in which neither parent is affected. In these cases, there is no increased risk of recurrence in subsequent children.

Tay-Sachs disease is an autosomal recessive disorder. The disorder results from a deficiency of one specific enzyme called *hexosaminidase A,* or *Hex A,* the production of which is controlled by a gene on chromosome #15. When Hex A is not present, the nerve cells in the brain are unable to break down a complex molecule in the brain called *ganglioside,* and it accumulates, eventually causing degeneration of nerve cells in the brain and death by age 5. There is no treatment for Tay-Sachs disease, although recent advances may make therapy possible in the future.

Jonah

Nancy and her husband Richard are both 28 years old. Last year, their 4-year-old son Jonah died of Tay-Sachs disease, a progressive and uniformly fatal disease of the brain. When Nancy and Richard went for genetic counseling, they were told that any baby they conceived had a one in four chance of inheriting Tay-Sachs disease. The counselor explained that Jonah had received two nonfunctioning genes for the Hex A enzyme and that this meant that both Nancy and Richard were carriers. Future children could inherit either two functioning genes, one functioning and one Tay-Sachs gene, or two Tay-Sachs genes. The baby would have Tay-Sachs disease only if he or she were to receive two Tay-Sachs genes.

The counselor told them that a test could be performed while Nancy was pregnant to determine whether the child did, indeed, have Tay-Sachs disease. During the fourth month of Nancy's second pregnancy, she underwent am-

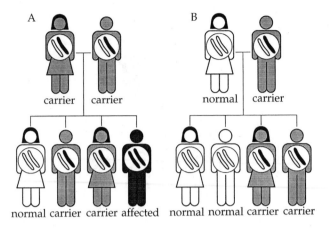

A   B

carrier   carrier   normal   carrier

normal carrier carrier affected   normal normal carrier carrier

Figure 26.4.   Inheritance of autosomal recessive disorders. A) Each time two unaffected carriers conceive a child, there is a one-in-four (25%) chance that the child will be unaffected, a one-in-two (50%) chance that the child will be an unaffected carrier, and a one-in-four risk that the child will be affected. B) If a carrier and an unaffected individual conceive a child, for each pregnancy there is a 50% chance the child will be unaffected and a 50% chance that the child will be an unaffected carrier; no children will be affected.

niocentesis (discussed later). The level of Hex A in Nancy's fetus was measured. Three weeks later, Nancy and Richard learned that their baby, a boy, had normal enzyme activity, meaning that he did not have Tay-Sachs disease. Steven is now a healthy 6-year-old.

It is important to remember that the one-in-four chance of inheriting the disease is a statistical risk. This does not mean that if a family already has one affected child, then the next three children will all be unaffected. Each new pregnancy carries the same one-in-four risk. It is as if you had a pair of dice and were throwing them over and over again. Two carrier parents could have four children, and by chance all four might be affected, all four might be unaffected, or there might be any other combination between these extremes.

A recessive disorder can only appear if two carrier parents have children. A carrier and a noncarrier will *always* have unaffected children, because all of their children will inherit a functional gene from the noncarrier parent. These children, however, will have a one-in-two chance of being carriers of the dysfunctional gene themselves. Siblings of affected children are not at a significant risk for having affected children themselves unless they carry the gene *and* they conceive children with another carrier of the disease. The chance of two carriers' marrying is rare, unless they are related by blood or unless the recessive disorder is more common in a particular ethnic group and both partners are from that same ethnic group (discussed later in this chapter).

Other examples of autosomal recessive disorders include sickle cell anemia, a disorder of the red blood cells common in African and African American people that causes blockage of blood vessels, resultant severe pain, and sometimes stroke; cystic fibrosis (CF), a disorder that affects multiple body organs, most prominently the lungs; and phenylketonuria (PKU), an inborn error of metabolism in which the amino acid phenylalanine, a breakdown product of protein, accumulates and causes brain damage if not treated.

X-Linked Disorders

Autosomal recessive and autosomal dominant disorders involve genes located on the 22 pairs of nonsex chromosomes. Diseases involving genes that are located on the sex chromosomes are called *sex-linked disorders*. Because no specific disease has been linked to the Y chromosome, these disorders are also referred to as *X-linked disorders*. Most sex-linked disorders are recessive. As with autosomal recessive disorders, a woman with one functioning and one nonfunctioning gene on her X chromosomes is a carrier. If a man, however, has a nonfunctioning gene on his X chromosome, he will be affected with the disorder because he has no second X chromosome to provide a functioning gene. Children of carrier women have a one-in-two chance of inheriting the nonfunctioning gene (see Figure 26.5). If the children are girls, they will inherit a functioning gene from their father (assuming he is unaffected) and be carriers like their mother. Boys who inherit the nonfunctioning gene from their mother, however, will have the disorder because they lack a functioning X chromosome. As a result, boys are much more frequently affected by X-linked disorders than are girls.

Color blindness and baldness are examples of mild X-linked disorders. But there are also more serious X-linked disorders such as Duchenne muscular dystrophy, the most common form of muscular dystrophy, a disorder

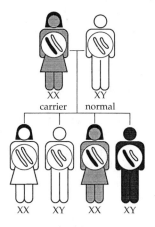

Figure 26.5. Inheritance of sex-linked disorders. Each time a carrier woman conceives a child with an unaffected man, with each pregnancy resulting in a male child, there is a 50% risk that he will be affected, and with each pregnancy resulting in a female child, there is a 50% risk that she will be a carrier (usually unaffected).

caused by mutations in the muscle protein gene dystrophin. A mother can carry the gene for muscular dystrophy on one of her X chromosomes and not be affected. Her male children, however, have a one-in-two chance of inheriting the abnormal X and developing muscular dystrophy. Her female children have the same one-in-two chance of inheriting the abnormal X and being carriers for the disorder.

Other examples of sex-linked disorders include hemophilia (Factor VIII deficiency), a disorder of impaired blood clotting, Menkes disease (a deficiency of copper metabolism leading to abnormal hair structure, seizures, and mental retardation), and some forms of mental retardation (see Chapter 14).

NONTRADITIONAL INHERITANCE

Geneticists have known for many years that some disorders do not follow the rules of Mendelian inheritance; that is, they are not strictly dominant, recessive, or X-linked. More recently, scientists have begun to provide explanations for these nontraditional inheritance patterns.

Imprinting

Not all genes in each cell are active all of the time. Some genes are active only in particular cell types; the genes for hemoglobin, for example, are only "turned on" in red blood cells. Other genes are active only at particular times during development, such as genes required for the migration of particular cells in the formation of the nervous system. In some cases, whether a gene or cluster of genes is active in the developing fetus depends on whether the cluster of genes came from the mother or the father. This phenomenon is called a parent-of-origin effect, and clusters of genes that behave in this way are said to be *imprinted*, or biologically "switched off."

Prader-Willi syndrome is the most well-studied example of imprinting. The syndrome, as described in Chapter 16, can be caused by the deletion of a small cluster of genes on the paternally acquired chromosome #15. The same cluster of genes on the maternal chromosome #15 is normally imprinted or switched off.

But Prader-Willi syndrome can also arise in a different way. As mentioned in the discussion about chromosomes, sometimes a nondisjunction of the chromosomes will cause an embryo to have three copies of a particular chromosome. In the case of Prader-Willi syndrome, the embryo may initially contain three copies of chromosome #15, one from the father and two from the mother. Fetuses with trisomy 15 are not born alive. Sometimes, however, during cell division in the early embryo, one of the trisomic cells may divide and one of the #15 chromosomes may be lost from the cell giving rise to a cell that now contains only two copies of chromosome #15 and the normal number of 46 chromosomes. If the chromosome #15 inherited from the father was lost, then the two remaining #15 chromosomes in the cell would both be of maternal origin. Because the maternal #15 chromosomes are imprinted (inactive), this child will have Prader-Willi syndrome. When both copies of a particular chromosome are derived from the same parent, it is called *uniparental disomy*. Deletions of chromosome #15 account for about 60% of occurrences of Prader-Willi syndrome; the remainder are a result of maternal uniparental disomy. Imprinted genes are also responsible for some occurrences of Angelman syndrome (see Chapter 16), Beckwith-Wiedemann syndrome (associated with a large tongue and other organs, umbilical cord hernia, accelerated growth, and low blood sugar in infancy), and Russell-Silver syndrome (associated with short stature beginning before birth, a triangular facial appearance, and sometimes developmental delay).

A couple's chance of having another child with Prader-Willi syndrome is very low. If your child has the syndrome, genetic testing is available to determine its cause. Prenatal diagnosis for Prader-Willi syndrome also is possible.

Anticipation and Triplet Repeats

Another principle of Mendel's laws is that genes are transmitted unchanged from parent to offspring. In an increasing number of disorders, however, the size of the gene is actually observed to change when passed on from parent to child. These genes have within them repeating sequences of the same three DNA bases. These sequences are called *trinucleotide repeats*. Expansion of the number of trinucleotide repeats within a gene beyond a critical number prevents normal functioning of the gene. The most well studied of the trinucleotide repeat disorders, fragile X syndrome, is the most common form of inherited mental retardation in males (see Figure 26.6). Boys with the syndrome have characteristic facial features, tall stature, a prominent jaw, and enlarged testes after puberty. They also typically have moderate mental retardation, communication disorders, and attention-deficit/hyperactivity disorder (see Chapter 16 for more on fragile X syndrome).

For many of the trinucleotide disorders, the number of triplet repeats in most individuals is variable (between 6 and 50 for the fragile X gene). Sometimes, however, when that gene is passed from parent to child, the number of repeats can increase to an intermediate size called a *pre-mutation* (50–200 repeats). Women with the pre-mutation are carriers for fragile X syndrome. They do not have mental retardation but may have excessive shyness or social anxiety. The risk for them is that the pre-mutation may expand again in their children, producing a full mutation (200 to more than 1,000 repeats). Boys who have 200 or more triplet repeats will have fragile X syndrome. Girls may also have a full mutation but are somewhat less affected than boys with a full mutation are. The greater the number of triplet repeats, the more likely the number of repeats will increase in the next generation. And generally speaking, the greater the number of triplet repeats beyond a critical threshold, the more severely an individual will be affected with the disorder. Geneticists call this phenomenon *anticipation*. Anticipation predicts an in-

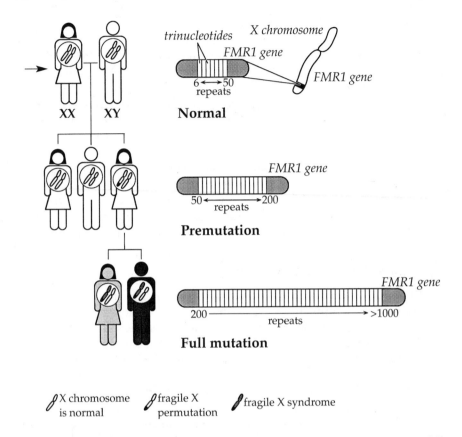

Figure 26.6. Representative family tree for fragile X syndrome. The grandparents of the affected child (indicated by an arrow) have a typical number of triplet repeats and are unaffected. The mother had an expansion of the triplet repeats and is a pre-mutation carrier. She has a daughter who received the expanded fragile X gene and is mildly affected and has a son whose triplet repeats expanded to greater than 200; hence he clinically has fragile X syndrome. The expansion, a full mutation, inactivates or turns off the FMR1 (fragile X mental retardation) gene, leading to abnormal brain development.

crease in severity of the features of a disorder when it is passed through subsequent generations.

MULTIFACTORIAL INHERITANCE

Some birth defects and genetic disorders are not determined by a single gene but rather by the interaction of several genes, often in combination with certain environmental influences. This is called *multifactorial inheritance* because more than one factor is involved. Many of the most common birth defects are multifactorial traits, including cleft lip and palate, club feet, and neural tube defects such as spina bifida (see Chapter 17). A fetus may inherit the tendency to develop a birth defect by inheriting some susceptibility genes from the father and some from the mother. When the number of susceptibility genes reaches a critical threshold, the birth defect occurs. Environmental factors, such as infections, drugs, or lack of proper nutrition, may further increase the chance for a particular birth defect to occur. This explains why even identical twins may differ in developing a particular birth defect; for example, one twin may have a cleft lip and the other may not.

Powerful statistical methods have been developed to uncover the susceptibility genes responsible for common genetically influenced disorders such as Alzheimer's disease, diabetes, autism, psychiatric illness, and some forms of cancer. By identifying susceptible genes in particular families, scientists hope to better understand at a molecular level how common diseases occur and how to prevent or identify them early.

Although geneticists do not completely understand all of the genes and environmental influences involved in common birth defects and multifactorial conditions, they can often determine recurrence risks for individual families by determining how many people in the extended family have the condition and how closely the affected individuals are related to the couple seeking the information.

GENETIC COUNSELING

The families described in this chapter all sought genetic counseling because they wanted to add to their families and knew that their future children might be at increased risk for a birth defect or genetic syndrome. You may be in a similar situation, or you may not have started your family yet because there is a history of a genetic disease in your family and you are concerned about the risks. Genetic counseling and genetic screening may be helpful to you. Whatever your particular situation, the first few steps are the same. First, contact a genetics clinic, which is usually found at a university hospital or another large medical center. Your obstetrician or your child's pediatrician can help you locate a clinic in your area, or your health plan may recommend a geneticist within your provider network.

You may initially meet with a genetic counselor who has a master's degree in genetic counseling and is very knowledgeable about genetic risks and prenatal diagnosis. He or she will take a thorough family history and construct a family tree, or *pedigree* (see Figure 26.7). The pedigree helps to identify family members who have the disorder in question and to clarify the inheritance pattern. From this information the counselor and the physician-geneticist are able to calculate if you have an increased risk of bearing a child with the disorder in the future. The pedigree also details the health history of extended family members and may identify other conditions such as high cholesterol, early heart attacks, or cancer for which your family may be at increased risk. The geneticist will review your reproductive history, and if your child or an immediate member of your family has the disorder in question, he or she may want to examine that individual. It is useful to obtain medical records for family members who have been tested or examined in the past. Even if your child was initially evaluated at birth or in early infancy and doctors were unsure as to the diagnosis, specific testing may now be available.

By putting together the information from the medical history, family history, examination, and diagnostic testing, the genetics team will be able to provide you with the most accurate estimate of your risk of having a child with the disorder in the future. A member of the team will also discuss which prenatal evaluations may be appropriate, and a letter summarizing all of the findings and specific recommendations will be provided to you.

GENETIC SCREENING

In the past it was only possible to test couples for a genetic disorder once it had appeared in their family. For a growing number of genetic disorders, however, specific carrier screening is now available. This is particularly important for disorders that are more common in particular ethnic groups. If you and your partner are of the same ethnic background, you may want to consider carrier screening for particular disorders more common in your ethnic background. For example, Tay-Sachs disease, Gaucher disease, and Canavan disease are more prevalent among Ashkenazic Jewish individuals. Sickle-cell anemia is more prevalent among African and African American

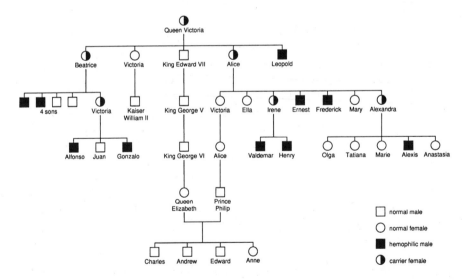

Figure 26.7. Family tree of Czarina Alexandra and Prince Alexis of Russia, illustrating the pattern of inheritance of the sex-linked disorder hemophilia. Approximately half of the women were carriers and half of the men had the disorder.

individuals, and cystic fibrosis occurs more commonly in Northern European Caucasians. Carrier screening is available for each of these disorders. The results of the screening tests will determine whether you, as a couple, are at an increased risk for having a child with a particular genetic disorder. Genetic screening, which usually involves a blood test, is available through genetic centers, where counselors can also help interpret the results of your studies.

There are a large number of rare genetic disorders for which screening or prenatal diagnosis is possible, but it is not practical to screen for all of them. Screening would be recommended if a particular disorder were known to be present in your extended family.

Screening tests for Down syndrome and neural tube abnormalities such as spina bifida are now routinely offered to all women during their pregnancies. The test, called a *triple screen*, measures the amounts of three substances (alpha-fetoprotein, unconjugated estriol, and human chorionic gonadotropin) in the mother's blood. Based on the levels of these substances and the gestational age of the fetus, an estimated risk for spina bifida and Down syndrome can be determined. If the screening test indicates an increased risk for either disorder, or for a rarer chromosomal disorder called *trisomy 18* (see Chapter 16), then more specific testing such as amniocentesis for chromosome analysis or high resolution ultrasound for neural tube defects can be performed to confirm the diagnosis. It is important to remember that many pregnancies initially identified through screening to be at increased risk will, after more specific testing, be found to be unaffected. A small number of affected pregnancies will be missed by maternal screening.

PRENATAL DIAGNOSIS

Several types of prenatal testing are currently available. Recommendations for testing should be tailored to your particular family situation and stage of pregnancy. If you are concerned about a specific genetic risk in your family, it is wise to seek the input from a geneticist as early in the pregnancy as possible to maximize the number of options available to you.

Before discussing the options, it is important to realize that in any pregnancy there is a 3%–4% chance of having a child with a birth defect or genetic disorder regardless of your family history. Likewise, there is no one prenatal test or combination of tests that, if results are normal, will guarantee a healthy baby.

Amniocentesis

Genetic amniocentesis has historically been the method of choice for obtaining fetal cells and amniotic fluid. It is usually performed at about 16 weeks' gestation. Under ultrasound guidance, a small amount of amniotic fluid (about 4 teaspoons) is removed by inserting a needle through the mother's

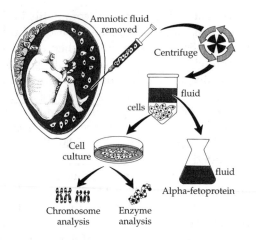

Figure 26.8. Amniocentesis. Approximately 4 teaspoons of amniotic fluid are removed at 14–18 weeks' gestation. The fluid is spun in a centrifuge to separate the fluid from the fetal cells. The fluid is used to test for neural tube defects. The cells are grown for a week, then karyotype, enzyme, or DNA (deoxyribonucleic acid) analyses can be performed. Results are available in 10–14 days.

abdominal wall and into the bag of amniotic fluid that surrounds the fetus (see Figure 26.8). The fluid is replaced naturally over the next 24 hours. The fluid contains cells from the fetus that can be grown for chromosome analysis, DNA testing for specific mutations, or biochemical analysis. In addition, the fluid itself can be analyzed. An increased level of alpha-fetoprotein (AFP) in the amniotic fluid is suggestive of a neural tube defect or abdominal wall abnormality in the fetus. Because amniocentesis is an invasive procedure, there are certain, relatively rare risks associated with it. The major concern is miscarriage, which occurs in about 1 in 200 procedures (0.5%).

Chorionic Villus Sampling

In the 1980s, prenatal centers across the United States began offering CVS. The procedure is usually performed near the end of the first trimester at 10–12 weeks' gestation. Using ultrasound guidance, a small catheter is passed through the cervix, and a tiny piece of tissue (chorionic villi) that will eventually become part of the placenta is obtained for analysis. The tissue can be used for chromosome analysis and DNA mutation testing. The results of a chromosome study are usually available within 2 weeks of the procedure. Other diagnostic tests may require slightly more time for the cells to grow in culture. The risk of pregnancy loss following CVS is higher than for amniocentesis, approximately 1%–2% at centers with physicians experienced in performing the procedure. You should contact the center where you are considering having the procedure in order to obtain complete information on which tests are offered and the experience of that particular center.

One advantage of CVS is that it is performed early in the pregnancy. If you receive abnormal results and you, as a couple, decide to terminate the pregnancy, the procedure can be performed at less risk to the mother. Because CVS does not sample amniotic fluid, however, alpha-fetoprotein testing for neural tube defects is not possible.

Ultrasound

With recent improvements in technology, ultrasound (or sonography) has become an increasingly valuable tool in evaluating fetal anatomy. It is a non-invasive test that uses sound waves that pose no danger to the fetus. At about 18 weeks' gestation, a detailed ultrasound, sometimes called a *fetal anatomy scan*, can identify many major malformations. These include cleft lip, some heart defects, brain and kidney malformations, defects in the abdominal wall or in the diaphragm that separates the abdomen from the fetal chest, club feet, and neural tube defects. The fetal sex can often be determined, and limb malformations or abnormalities in growth of the fetus can be identified. If necessary, several scans can be performed over a period of weeks to better define suspected malformations and to assess fetal growth.

Fetal Echocardiography

If there is concern about a congenital heart defect or if heart malformations can be associated with a suspected diagnosis (Down syndrome, for example), fetal echocardiography is available at some centers. This study, performed by a pediatric cardiologist at about 20 weeks' gestation, analyzes the structure and function of the fetal heart and can identify common malformations. Not all heart defects can be identified during pregnancy, however, because the circulation pattern during fetal life is somewhat different than the circulation in the newborn. Like ultrasound, echocardiography uses sound waves that pose no danger to the developing fetus.

Fetal MRI

Magnetic resonance imaging, or MRI, is an important technique that has been very useful in obtaining high-quality images of the brain and other body structures in children and adults. During pregnancy, it is sometimes used to clarify the presence of a specific malformation when an ultrasound has suggested an abnormality. MRI is particularly useful for identifying brain malformations or other structural abnormalities and may provide information useful in caring for the infant immediately after birth (see Figure 26.9). The procedure may also confirm the presence of normal anatomy when an abnormality has been suspected following ultrasound.

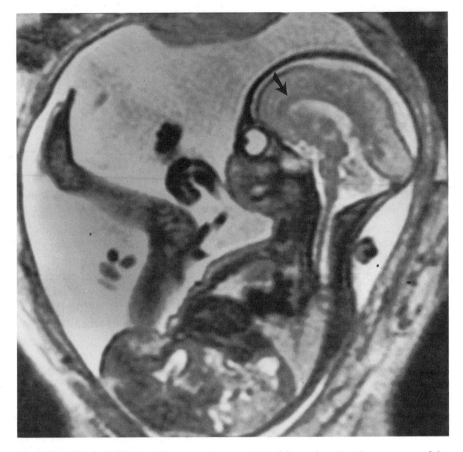

Figure 26.9.   MRI (magnetic resonance imaging) of fetus, showing the presence of the structure that divides the brain (the corpus callosum).

DECISION MAKING

During your consultation with the genetics team, you will probably be given a percentage of risk or likelihood that a specific condition may occur in a future pregnancy. Prenatal diagnosis for the condition may be available using one of the techniques just discussed. Your perception of the severity of the risk will depend on you and your particular family situation, and your decision about how to proceed will involve weighing the risk of having a child with the specific condition against the burden of that particular disorder. For example, the 25% risk for recurrence of a progressive neurodegenerative disorder such as Tay-Sachs disease, for which no therapy currently exists, will likely seem more significant than a 25% risk for PKU, for which effective treatment is possible. Likewise, a 50% recurrence risk may be acceptable to one family, whereas even a 10% risk for the same condition may seem too high to another.

The birth of a child with a disability is stressful for any family, and each has different coping strategies. Therefore, it is the couple involved who, when given accurate and timely information, are in the best position to decide what reproductive options are most appropriate in their particular circumstances. Advances in reproductive technology have increased the number of options for families who are at high risk for a genetic disorder. Some of the technologies include in vitro fertilization with pre-implantation genetic testing of the embryo, artificial insemination with donor sperm for disorders that are not sex linked, or the use of a donor egg for sex-linked disorders. Your obstetrician or geneticist will be in the best position to explain your options and guide you to an experienced center. Adoption is also an important consideration for many couples.

THERAPY

So far, this chapter has talked about genes, chromosomes, and different patterns of inheritance and has provided examples of a variety of genetic disorders. It has also discussed the concept of recurrence risk and mentioned some prenatal diagnostic tests that are currently available. This last section speaks briefly about therapies for genetic disorders.

Dietary Therapy

Some genetic disorders are caused by a deficiency of enzymes necessary to synthesize or break down compounds essential for normal body functioning. Like a dam across a river, the absence of a single enzyme in a pathway can lead to an accumulation of abnormally high levels of compounds upstream and/or a scarcity of the final product downstream. Either of these can lead to problems. PKU is one example. In the absence of the enzyme phenylalanine hydroxylase, phenylalanine (one of the building blocks of all proteins) accumulates to very high levels in the body. Abnormally high levels of phenylalanine are harmful to a child's developing brain, producing profound mental retardation. Early and lifelong dietary restriction of protein containing phenylalanine prevents this outcome, and children with PKU can develop typically and lead healthy and productive lives. Other disorders that can be treated with dietary management include galactosemia and maple syrup urine disease. All three of these disorders are part of the newborn screening test in most states.

Enzyme Replacement Therapy

Many genes provide the blueprint for enzymes that are important in body metabolism. Indeed, hundreds of these genes have been identified. In certain genetic disorders, the blueprint is flawed and a functioning enzyme cannot be produced. The goal of enzyme replacement therapy is to provide the missing enzyme to permit normal functioning. Because enzymes do their jobs in specific parts of the cell, the replacement enzymes must arrive at the correct place in an active form. Only one enzyme replacement therapy is currently available, alglucerase, for the treatment of a progressive neurological disorder called *type 1 Gaucher disease,* although others are currently being tested. Enzyme replacement therapy requires repeated intravenous infusions and is extremely costly.

For disorders whose missing enzyme is expressed in blood cells, bone marrow transplantation offers a potential therapy. Because bone marrow is self-renewing, repeated infusion is not required; however, there are still significant risks associated with the transplantation procedure. For this reason, bone marrow transplantation is performed only for life-threatening conditions.

Gene Therapy

Gene therapy involves the introduction of a known gene into specific body cells for the purpose of therapy. In gene therapy, multiple copies of the gene are packaged into carrier DNA called a *vector.* Multiple copies of the DNA-containing vector are then injected directly into the body or are added to specific body cells (such as bone marrow or liver cells) in culture, which are then reinjected into the body. Either way, the vector-containing gene must be taken into the cell and transferred to the nucleus, where it can serve as the blueprint for the desired protein. Although currently experimental, gene therapy is a new and powerful technology that will undoubtedly play a major role in the treatment of genetic disease in the 21st century.

SUMMARY

This chapter has discussed the basic principles of genetic inheritance, including chromosomal abnormalities, single-gene disorders, nontraditional inheritance, and multifactorial inheritance. This chapter has also presented examples of how a genetics team can be helpful in clarifying whether a genetic disorder is present in your family and what the risk would be of having a child with the disorder. This chapter has discussed some prenatal diagnostic tests that may help to determine if a fetus has a particular genetic disorder. Finally, therapies for genetic disorders have been discussed, ranging from dietary manipulation, to enzyme replacement, to gene therapy. This information may be helpful to your family by offering choices in treatment and in planning for future children.

Some Questions Answered

Our 2-year-old was born with a disability. Should we have prenatal diagnosis with our next child?

This decision depends on two issues. Is your child's disability likely to recur in future children, and can the disorder be diagnosed prenatally? For example, a woman who has had one child with trisomy 21 Down syndrome (see Chapter 15) has a 1 in 100 risk of recurrence. Disabilities inherited as autosomal recessive, autosomal dominant, or sex-linked disorders carry an even greater risk of recurrence—between 1 in 2 and 1 in 4. Thus, in each of these situations, prenatal diagnosis is of great value. If your child does not have a specific diagnosis or if the disorder cannot be detected prenatally but has a pattern of malformations that might be identified by ultrasound or fetal echocardiography, these may be other reasons to seek prenatal testing when expecting your next child.

Prenatal diagnosis should be offered to you regardless of whether you would be willing to terminate an affected pregnancy. Many families choose prenatal diagnosis to better plan for the birth of their child regardless of the diagnosis.

It is worth reemphasizing that doctors can only diagnose a condition that they are specifically looking for. Also, the absence of one abnormality does not ensure a healthy child, only one who does not have the specific disorder for which the test has been performed.

Are mistakes made in prenatal diagnosis?

The frequency of errors for most genetic tests is very low. You should ask about the specific error rates for the disorder that is being tested in your baby.

Should I consider terminating the pregnancy if the baby is affected?

At this time, there are very few diseases for which prenatal therapy is available. Therefore, if a child is prenatally diagnosed as being affected with a genetic disorder, the possibility of terminating a pregnancy may be discussed. Clearly this will not be acceptable to some families. Other families, however, would not want to risk the birth of a second affected child. In these instances, prenatal diagnosis can be viewed as giving the chance of life to children who would not otherwise have been conceived. Obviously, the ideal situation would be to identify affected fetuses and then treat them prenatally. For the vast majority of birth defects and genetic disorders, however, this simply is not possible, and for some diseases it may never be.

If you find out that your unborn child has a genetic disorder, the decision whether or not to terminate a pregnancy is for you and your partner to make, in consultation with your physician. In the event that you would not consider a therapeutic abortion but are at high risk for recurrence in future children, other reproductive alternatives may be consistent with your moral values.

Keeping Up with Changes in Health Care

Angelo P. Giardino

If your child has a disability, you are likely to have numerous relationships with a wide variety of medical professionals over time. In the coming years, these medical caregivers, described in Chapter 2, will almost inevitably be part of larger networks of health care providers working within tightly managed and monitored environments. This chapter paints a broad picture of the "system" issues that you will need to understand to make informed choices about health care for your child and to advocate for appropriate services.

Health care has undergone and continues to undergo tremendous changes in delivery and financing. The understanding of health and disease has advanced along with improvements in technology, allowing medical professionals to diagnose and treat illness and disabilities better. This advancement, however, has been accompanied by increased health care costs. These skyrocketing expenses, in turn, have led to the development of different models of delivering and paying for health care, the most popular of which is managed care.

Because children with disabilities, on average, use about twice as many health care services as typically developing children use, these changes in delivery and financing will have particular importance to you. As we look to the future in health care, the only certainty is that change will continue. Given that fact, you will need to make sure that your child's unique characteristics are not overlooked.

Shawn and Sherry

Shawn is a 2-year-old girl who was born 3 months prematurely and had many medical complications in the neonatal intensive care unit prior to her release from the hospital at 3 months of age. She still receives some of her meals through a feeding tube, and she takes two different antiepileptic medications. Shawn's mother, Della, has learned to manage the feeding tube and medications, so the home nurse has stopped her visits. Della's employer provides commercial insurance for most, but not all, of Shawn's health care needs. For example, her tube feeding equipment is not covered, nor is her nutritional supplement. To make up the difference, a social worker from the hospital's high-risk neonatal follow-up program helped enroll Shawn in her state's Medicaid program for back-up insurance. A patchwork of insurance coverage may be needed to ensure that a child such as Shawn can continue to receive all needed services.

Sherry is a 10-year-old with cerebral palsy; she has had seven orthopedic operations over the past several years to allow her to walk. She receives her health insurance from her state's Medicaid program and is enrolled in a multidisciplinary cerebral palsy program at a children's hospital. This clinic is funded by the state's Maternal and Child Health Block Grant program, which also provides case management services. Without the cerebral palsy program, Sherry would receive only the traditional types of health care services covered by Medicaid. Two months ago, Sherry's state implemented a mandatory Medicaid managed care program, and Sherry's parents had to pick one of three plans that were approved to participate in the program. In looking at each plan, her parents wanted to make sure that the orthopedic group practice that had been working with Sherry and had done each of her surgeries was listed as a provider. Fortunately, the orthopedists and the pediatrician whom Sherry and her family had been using were in all three plans, so Sherry's parents picked the plan that also had a special needs unit listed as one of the services. They had heard through their parent support group at the cerebral palsy program that the plan with the special needs unit was especially sensitive to the many unique needs of children such as Sherry. Sherry's story indicates the importance of choosing the right provider of health services and the need to research this before making a decision.

HEALTH CARE INSURANCE COVERAGE

The most common way for children to obtain health care insurance is through their parents' employer-based health insurance. The availability of commercial insurance, however, has been decreasing over time because of its high cost. More and more families are finding themselves with inadequate insurance coverage from the parents' employer(s). If this is your situation, your child may be eligible for public insurance under the Medicaid program. This is a combined federal–state program designed to provide health care coverage to individuals who have low incomes, are elderly, or who have visual impairments or other disabilities.

Medicaid, often referred to as *MA* or *medical assistance*, forms a safety net for children with disabilities who do not have commercial insurance coverage for a variety of reasons. These may include your not having insurance that covers your child, having exceeded the benefit maximum on your policy, or lacking coverage for a specific health care service. (It should be noted that the other form of public insurance, Medicare, rarely covers children.)

Medicaid is commonly subject to political cost-cutting efforts. As calls have come from the legislature to be more cost effective while maintaining benefits, Medicaid programs have started to incorporate the principles of managed care as a means of keeping costs in check. It is likely that if your child is covered by Medicaid (or even by private insurance), he or she will be cared for in a managed care system. How well this works depends on the plan design and its safeguards (discussed later).

OTHER GOVERNMENTAL PROGRAMS

A number of other governmental programs provide funding for services to children with disabilities. Among these are Supplemental Security Income (SSI) and components of the Individuals with Disabilities Education Act (IDEA). Supplemental Security Income is a program that provides both income support and access to Medicaid for individuals with disabilities. Even if children with significant disabilities do not qualify for income support, they can qualify for Medicaid coverage for health care services if they lack commercial insurance. Medicaid is always the payer of last resort, so if your child has commercial insurance, he or she would need to exhaust its coverage prior to using the Medicaid coverage. IDEA defines a wide range of education-related services such as physical therapy, speech-language therapy, and occupational therapy (see Chapter 12). In addition, states may have Title V Maternal and Child Health Block Grant programs that provide for a wide range of services for your child, often as an enhancement to Medicaid coverage. Finally, in an effort to assist states in expanding coverage to uninsured children, a combined state and federal initiative called the Children's Health Insurance Program (often called CHIP) now exists. This program gives states a lot of flexibility in designing and offering health insurance to children and families who are ineligible for Medicaid but whose incomes make it difficult to obtain health insurance. Each state operates its CHIP differently.

MANAGED CARE

As we look at the early part of the 21st century, ever-increasing numbers of people, including children with disabilities, will receive health care from managed care delivery and financing systems. The traditional fee-for-service system that essentially paid for health care after it was delivered (retrospective payment) has shifted toward a managed care approach that attempts to pay for health care services before they are provided (prospective payment). This move toward prospective payment is believed to shift the incentives toward the delivery of only appropriate services and hence keep costs as low as possible.

One of the more understandable definitions of managed care is offered by Family Voices, a group that advocates for children with disabilities and their families:

> Managed care is a way of providing pre-paid health care within a network that includes a specified group of health care providers and services. The network coordinates and refers patients to its health providers and hospitals, and monitors the amount and patterns of care delivered, the cost of care, and its quality. Managed care plans usually limit services that patients may receive by having physician visits, therapies, home care, pharmacies, specialists, clinics and hospitals available within their own system, and by using "gatekeepers" to make sure that services considered unnecessary or referrals outside the network are kept to a minimum.

There are a number of different types of plans in which the managed care concept unfolds, the three most common being HMOs (health maintenance organizations), PPOs (preferred provider organizations), and POSs (point-of-service plans). HMOs are the classic managed care design. In an HMO, you select a primary care provider (PCP) who is the "gatekeeper" for your family's health care usage. With some rare exceptions, all referrals to specialists, for laboratories and special studies, and to hospitals must involve this PCP, who for children is often a pediatrician. The primary care provider is capitated by the plan; in other words, he or she receives a monthly payment from the insurance company for each person assigned to the practice. The physician gets this payment regardless of how much or how little service is provided to the people assigned to the practice. The HMO is the most restrictive form of managed care in terms of your role in decision making because you can only use physicians approved by the HMO. A PPO is somewhat less restrictive and usually more expensive to enroll in. It comprises a network of providers who have negotiated a discounted rate that they will receive from the insurance company. You have more autonomy in a PPO than in an HMO, provided that you stay within the network of providers.

Finally, the POS plan combines elements of an HMO with those of a PPO, and the patient may exercise even more choice. On one hand, you can use it like an HMO and select a physician who provides referrals to network providers for various health care services. In doing so, you will have the least amount of out-of-pocket expenses because co-pays (the amount of money the family must pay out of their own pocket at the time of the visit) are at a minimum when a POS plan is used as an HMO. On the other hand, if you choose to use the plan more as a PPO, then you are able to choose which provider to go to. This avoids the need for referrals, but the costs are usually higher. Thus, the POS plan highlights one of the underlying principles of managed care: The more you are willing to restrict your own choices and, essentially, let the insurer have a role in these decisions, the lower the cost of the insurance.

MANAGED CARE AND CHILDREN WITH DISABILITIES

It is uncertain how well children with disabilities fare in a managed care environment. Research in the area is still at an early stage, and clear answers are not yet available. Potential positives of managed care include:

- Flexibility to design programs that meet your child's special needs, including therapies, home care, outpatient behavioral health services, and case management
- Coverage of well-child care, immunizations, and other preventive care that may have been excluded in traditional plans
- Less likelihood of lifetime maximums or benefit caps, unlike in traditional insurance plans
- Availability of POS plans that provide families with the benefits of an HMO but preserve the possibility of choice in providers if needed

Potential negatives of managed care for children with disabilities are:

- Coverage of specialty services only when significant improvement can be expected in a short period of time
- Lack of choice in and potentially limited access to specialty providers

A great deal of variability exists among plans, and the list created by Family Voices (see Table 27.1) includes a number of questions that you should ask when selecting a plan for your child.

PROVIDER ISSUES

In response to rising medical costs and the changes in health care brought on by managed care, health care professionals have had to change the way they function. In the last quarter of the 20th century, physicians began practicing more and more in groups; the solo practitioner has all but disappeared. In addition, the notion of an integrated delivery system has arisen in which provider organizations form large networks of professionals and institutions. These systems offer a wide range of services from primary care (rooted in individual communities) to tertiary care (often anchored to an academic medical center). To these ends of the spectrum are added home care, rehabilitation services, and residential facilities for older adults. The concept has emerged that a successful health care system needs to provide the full continuum of services that your family could possibly require. Such systems, integrated delivery networks (IDNs), are ideally suited to work with managed care organizations to cover an entire population from "cradle to grave" in a defined geographic area. As IDNs seek to be responsible for the health care needs of an entire population, some of the people requiring services will inevitably be children with disabilities. Because of the higher costs incurred by such children, these systems spend a great deal of time planning for their needs.

One way for the system to meet your child's needs is to incorporate a full set of pediatric services in the IDN that would be:

- Expert in meeting the continuum of your child's health care needs including preventive, primary, acute, subspecialty, post acute, rehabilitative, long-term care, and mental health
- Organized to work with managed care organizations and able to accept capitation for the services described
- Accountable to the public for the health of the population of children covered
- Appropriate for your child's immediate needs as well as for his or her long-term physical, psychological, social, educational, and spiritual development

Many children's hospitals are working to establish and maintain such systems of care on a regional basis.

With regard to the pediatrician and children with disabilities, the American Academy of Pediatrics (AAP) promotes the concept of a "medical home." This is not a place so much as a relationship between your child's pediatrician and your family. The relationship occurs in an atmosphere of mutual responsibility and trust. The medical home should promote care that is accessible, continuous, comprehensive, family centered, coordinated, and compassionate. Via this partnership, the AAP hopes to place your child's needs at the center of the discussion and sensitize government agencies, insurance companies, and a variety of other providers to the unique needs of children with disabilities.

PRACTICAL STEPS FOR FAMILIES
OF CHILDREN WITH DISABILITIES

With the preceding sections as background, how should you approach managed care? The answer is to do so cautiously and with as much information as possible. Preliminary information that you should have prior to choosing a managed care plan includes the following: promotional materials on the various plans, available options, time frame for making the selection, and

Table 27.1.   Questions to ask when selecting a health insurance plan

---

OBTAINING GOOD HEALTH CARE

Questions to ask

How are children with disabilities viewed by the plan? Is there a special department for children with special health care needs?

Do the primary care providers have any special qualifications for caring for children with disabilities?

How does a child gain access to pediatric specialists? What if they are not in the network?

How does a child receive coverage for therapies? Do the therapists have pediatric training?

What is the process for obtaining assistive technologies, durable medical equipment, medical supplies, nursing care, and support?

Do benefits include care coordination, transportation, home care, peer support, family counseling, genetic services, and respite care?

How does the plan handle requests for experimental procedures, alternative medical therapies, nonroutine treatments, and medications?

Is there a benefit cap on the amount of services a child can receive in one year? Is there a lifetime cap?

How are emergencies handled? Are there alternatives to the emergency room? What about out-of-town emergencies?

Can health care services be delivered in alternative environments such as child care and school?

What to look for

A plan that is responsive to the needs of children with disabilities typically has a case management approach toward meeting a child's and family's needs and makes clear that they understand that the managed care principles that apply to routine populations may need to be altered to meet the unique needs of children with disabilities.

ENSURING CONTINUITY

Questions to ask

What commitment exists for keeping the pediatricians, specialists, and therapists who now care for your child?

Are specialty hospitals part of the network? Do they provide primary care?

What happens if the child's provider leaves the network?

How long has the plan been serving children with disabilities?

(continued)

Table 27.1.   *(continued)*

What to look for

Plans interested in serving children with disabilities have policies that value continuity of care over strict adherence to network rules. Because most pediatric specialists work out of children's hospitals, it is essential that these be included in the plan.

HAVING CHOICES AND MAKING DECISIONS

Questions to ask

Can families choose primary care providers, specialists, therapists, home care providers, durable medical equipment vendors, and counselors?

By what process are services determined to be "medically necessary?" What is the appeal mechanism?

Who are the "gatekeepers," and what are their qualifications? How are they monitored?

How are second opinions handled? Are there policies about who pays and timeliness?

What to look for

Responsive plans allow families to play an active role in choosing the health care providers to serve their child and have clearly defined appeal mechanisms regarding medical necessity determinations.

QUALITY ASSURANCE AND FAMILY-CENTERED CARE

Questions to ask

Is consumer satisfaction measured? If so, how often, and are results available to consumers? How do consumers get involved in quality assurance?

Are there internal quality standards? Are there external standards? Is the plan accredited by an outside body? Who is responsible for reporting on these and communicating with consumers?

How is care monitored for children with disabilities? How is data collected about how children with disabilities are faring? How does this information affect the way care is delivered?

Does the plan use the principles of family-centered care? Is this part of the quality assurance program? Is training in family-centered care offered to network providers?

Is there a family advisory board?

How does the plan address family, cultural, and language characteristics?

What to look for

Family-centered care is based on an approach to health care that respects each family's values, cultures, resources, and strengths. Care and services provided are perceived by the family as flexible, accessible, responsive, and sensitive. The family is seen as a constant source of support for the child.

COSTS

Questions to ask

What are the costs to the family, including premiums, co-pays, and deductibles?

How does the plan address the expenses associated with caring for children with disabilities?

Are physicians penalized for the high costs associated with treating children with disabilities?

Are premiums raised based on high utilization?

What to look for

Ideally, the plan is structured so that costs to the individual/family and the physician's practice are kept to a minimum. Cost control should be based on effective case management and coordination, *not* on limitation of services provided.

COORDINATING CARE WITH OTHER CAREGIVERS

Questions to ask

How are services coordinated with Title V and schools? How are financial and delivery responsibilities dealt with between the plan and other providers, such as a school?

Is there a relationship between the managed care organization and the regional children's hospital?

How is the health care for the family coordinated with the care for the child with special needs?

What to look for

Responsive plans identify a service coordinator or case manager who works with the family to facilitate the flow of information about the child to the various programs and support services. Ideally, the case manager is the child's advocate in navigating through the various systems through which the child receives services.

SOLVING PROBLEMS

Questions to ask

How are problems with the child's health care resolved, including billing problems? Who is the contact person? What is the typical time frame?

What are the grievance procedures? Does a state agency monitor these and distribute the results? Is there a relationship between the managed care organization and the regional children's hospital?

What to look for

The plan's appeal and grievance procedures should be readily available in the member handbook. If not, the state's insurance commissioner's office should be able to provide either the grievance procedure or the manner by which to obtain it.

information on other, related programs to which your child may be entitled, such as SSI. After reviewing the background materials and information, you may want to use the list of questions in Table 27.1 to assist you in learning more about your options.

SUMMARY

Interaction with the health care system and health care insurance providers (both public and private) will be inevitable as you work to get your child all that he or she needs to grow and develop to the fullest potential. Although this may appear a daunting task, keep in mind that there are many resources to help you and your family make sense of all the pieces. In addition, other families and your child's health care providers (doctors, nurses, and social workers, to name a few) can help you pull all of these pieces together. Ultimately, you will need to ask a lot of questions, gather information, and discuss it with friends, family, and the professionals with whom you work to decide what makes the most sense for you and your child with special health care needs.

Some Questions Answered

Is managed care good for my child with special needs?

The answer depends on the particular plan and how it approaches the unique needs of your child. Some aspects of managed care can be ideal for a child with special needs (such as a focus on prevention and care at home), whereas other parts could be detrimental (such as complicated precertification processes and limited within-network providers). The answer for your child depends, however, on what is covered by the plan and on your child's specific needs.

Are all children on Medicaid enrolled in a managed care plan?

The provisions of Medicaid vary from state to state. States are, however, increasingly turning to managed care plans as a way to control costs and in some cases to expand coverage to more children. Some state Medicaid plans have moved toward mandatory Medicaid managed care in which everyone enrolled in the program must join a managed care plan. Other states have chosen a voluntary approach in which the family can choose to stay in the traditional fee-for-service plan or can opt to join a managed care plan. In these voluntary situations, the managed care plan may offer added benefits that serve as an incentive to join the plan.

If I join a managed care plan, how do I make sure that my daughter will be able to continue to see the same health care providers who have been treating her?

You will need to look at the plan's provider directory and check to see that your child's doctors are participating providers. Check for both primary care and specialty care. If you do not see your child's physicians listed, call the plan (and your child's doctors) and ask if the doctors are participating because the directory may not be current.

28

Success on the Road to Adulthood

Patience H. White,
Andrea Edelman, and Vincent Schuyler

Transition into adulthood is a process, not an event. It evolves over many years and involves the entire family and possibly other caregivers and support personnel. For young people with disabilities, transition hinges on their ability to become self-advocates and to actively determine what actions they need to take to become independent and self-sufficient adults. Appropriate parental expectations; clear, caring, and consistent roles; the belief that a disability is not a handicap; and letting go so that your young adult can take personal responsibility for his or her future all facilitate successful transition. Thinking about this transition process should begin at the time of identification of a disability. Careful planning is the key to success. For those who are identified as having a disability within the special education system, federal law (the Individuals with Disabilities Education Act [IDEA] Amendments of 1997) requires that an individualized transition plan (ITP) be in place at age 14 (see Chapter 12). Goals for independence and self-determination, delineated on a schedule that is constantly reevaluated according to the child's abilities, interests, and preferences, are important parts of the transition planning.

The four major transitions discussed in this chapter are moving from dependence to independence, changing from secondary to postsecondary education, making the transition from pediatric to adult medical care, and moving from a school to a work environment. Each transition is based on the premise that your child has acquired the necessary knowledge, skills, and abilities and has access to supports to be successful at the next step.

As a parent, you play a crucial role in ensuring that your child has the opportunity to accomplish these transitions. To help your child become independent, you must have an expectation that he or she can and will make these transitions.

Kenisha, Greg, and Shana

Kenisha is a 21-year-old with cerebral palsy. She always received special education services in school. Kenisha's dream in high school was to have a job. She has never worked, requires many trials to learn a task, and needs constant support and direction. Her parents believed her to be unemployable. They were not aware that transition planning, which includes transition to the world of work, was a required part of her individualized education program (IEP) and that her school was required to help her with her dream of becoming employed (see Chapter 12). Her parents were not informed of the resources available, such as their state's Department of Rehabilitation Services, to help her with employment efforts after graduation. As a result, Kenisha, who graduated last spring, spends her days watching television.

Greg is a 19-year-old with epilepsy. He developed seizures in early adolescence, experiencing both complex partial and major motor episodes (see Chapter 18). While Greg was in school, his parents worked with the school and service agency staff to ensure that accommodations were in place to allow him to succeed. Through his IEP and ITP, he participated in a time-limited paid internship. His teachers worked with his employer to educate his co-workers about epilepsy and how to accommodate him in the workplace. He excelled at his internship. Following graduation, Greg found employment on his own. Greg, however, did not disclose his disability, did not ask for any accommodations, and did not educate his co-workers or boss about epilepsy and how it could affect him at work. As a result, Greg was laid off when his seizures became difficult to control and affected his work performance.

Shana is a 22-year-old with spina bifida and associated learning disabilities. Through the provisions of her IEP, she was able to receive excellent accommodations in high school and graduated with honors. Through her active participation in IEP meetings, she learned how to identify her needs and developed excellent advocacy skills. She worked with her teachers and parents to develop a comprehensive ITP that focused on identifying and developing strategies to provide for her anticipated needs after high school. She identified herself to the Office of Services for Students with Disabilities at her community college and worked with them to develop accommodations. She has since graduated and is employed full time as a computer specialist. She is very successful in her work and believes that her success is due to her knowledge of her rights as a person with a disability and her ability to advocate on her own behalf so that her identified needs are met.

FROM DEPENDENCE TO INDEPENDENCE

The transition from dependence to independence occurs gradually. We marvel as our children master a first word, take a step, or learn to spell their name. We expect them to grow from an infant, to a child, to an adolescent, and finally to a young adult. It is important that parents of a child with disabilities recognize that although their child's development may not follow the same route as that of a typically developing child, he or she is still capable of participating in a full and fulfilling life. We must encourage children with disabilities to become as self-reliant and independent as possible so that one day they will be capable of taking care of themselves and addressing their own needs to the best of their abilities.

A child begins to gain intellectual and social skills early in life. As the child matures into an adolescent, a sense of self and identity develops. At this time, the adolescent starts to separate from the parents, and friendships and peer relations take on primary importance. Adolescence is a time when self-concept is formed and reshaped, and young adults strive for autonomy. For individuals with disabilities, successfully negotiating this stage of development is just as important as it is for typically developing teenagers. Individuals with disabilities, however, may require more support than is needed by their counterparts without disabilities.

Your own beliefs play an important role in your son's or daughter's capacity to become independent. If you believe that the disability will prevent your child from becoming independent, you may find that you do not actively encourage the activities necessary for independence. Your child may start to believe in his or her own limitations. Conversely, if you believe your child is capable of becoming independent in spite of the disability, you will probably foster participation in activities that build your child's confidence and skills that will ensure later success.

There are many things you can do to encourage activities that foster your child's positive self-image and feelings of self-worth and that ultimately promote independence. Most important, you must recognize that your son or daughter is a person first and is not solely defined by the disability. This is the subtle difference between referring to "a child with cerebral palsy" rather than "a cerebral-palsied child." Although your child may have a disability that requires special attention or accommodation, you should encourage age-appropriate activities and promote new challenges and responsibilities as he or she demonstrates the ability to learn and accomplish them. In other words, you should define your child by his or her abilities, not by the disabilities.

At home, you should have certain expectations for your child with a disability just as you have for your typically developing children. You may ask your child to clean his or her room, to care for the family pet, or to set and clear the table. As your child matures and becomes more capable, encourage greater responsibilities, such as grocery shopping, preparing and cooking meals, doing the laundry, and learning to balance a checkbook. Countless tasks at home provide children with the opportunity to acquire the skills and abilities they need to function as independent adults. Through your expectation that your child can perform these tasks, your child will learn that he or she is capable. This fosters a positive self-image and a sense of worth.

At school, you should expect your child to learn about the impact of the disability on his or her education. You can model advocacy skills and encourage your son or daughter to self-advocate. You can encourage your child to be an active participant in identifying educational needs and preferences and developing necessary accommodations. You can teach your child to investigate community resources and how to take advantage of them and to be an active participant in the development of the ITP at school. The knowledge, skills, and abilities your child develops in attaining educational goals can be easily transferred to the postsecondary environment and the world of work, in which parental involvement is curtailed.

You should also encourage your son or daughter to participate in age-appropriate activities. Though often overlooked, it is important to recognize and foster the development of social and sexual identity. You can encourage involvement in school-sponsored clubs, community-based recreational activities, social outings, and dating. As your child approaches the age to drive, you can explore driving (adapted driving, if needed) or teach him or her how to use public transportation. You can help your child seek volunteer or paid work experiences. It is important that adolescents and young adults with disabilities have experiences that are similar to those of their peers so that they can develop friendships, learn social and interpersonal skills, experience the world of work, and learn to resolve conflicts independent of their parents.

Because your goal is for your child to achieve the maximum level of independence as a young adult, you should explore community resources and establish necessary support systems while he or she is still living at home. If an IEP exists, it must include an ITP (see Chapter 12), which focuses on future employment, housing, and social needs and identifies appropriate community resources to facilitate transition. In addition, the Center for Independent Living in your state can assist you in identifying independent living options, programs to foster independent living skills, and other resources, if needed. Your state vocational rehabilitation agency, which provides vocational rehabilitation services for adults with disabilities, may have a counselor specializing in independent living. You should contact both to determine how they can best assist your child.

Part of achieving independence involves your child's taking "ownership" of his or her disability. This requires learning about and becoming responsible for its medical management and understanding the impact of the disability on activities of daily living and education. This includes learning how to gain access to medical care and being aware of the resources, services, laws, accommodations, and technology that will assist your son or daughter to be independent. Your child also needs to know his or her rights in the workplace as defined by the Americans with Disabilities Act (ADA) of 1990 (PL 101-336).

FROM SECONDARY TO POSTSECONDARY EDUCATION

Planning for effective transition to postsecondary (college or work) environments greatly influences future success. A student is entitled to receive special education services or any other accommodations in the secondary school system. When this same student leaves the K–12 school system (or reaches age 21, whichever comes first), and moves into the postsecondary education environment or the world of work, he or she is no longer entitled to services. Instead, your son or daughter must prove eligibility for services or accommodations, identify his or her needs, and initiate action on his or her own behalf. Too often, students and their parents moving into the postsecondary environment are unaware of this change and how it affects them. And, too frequently, students with disabilities or other special health care needs do not take into consideration how their disability-related needs will change in this new environment. The IDEA legislation requires that a student's IEP provide a statement of transition services that will be needed, including a statement of the interagency responsibilities and links (see Chapter 12).

The American Council on Education listed four essential elements (see Table 28.1) that should be addressed as part of a transition plan for the postsecondary school environment for an individual with disabilities: education, environmental considerations, medical needs, and activities of daily living. Assessing how the disability has an impact on the student in these four areas, developing strategies to minimize or alleviate those impacts, and anticipating how needs might change in a postsecondary environment form the core of the transition plan. In addition, the student must have the maturity to successfully implement the transition plan. To help plan for this transition to postsecondary education, Table 28.1 lists questions that should be addressed in these four areas.

Knowledge, skills, and abilities needed to successfully implement the transition plan include 1) the ability to take responsibility for oneself, including assessing needed supports, 2) an understanding of one's civil rights, 3) an awareness of why, when, to whom, how, and what to disclose about a disability, and 4) the knowledge to manage medical needs. It is also important to fully assess the college's or vocational school's ability to address disability-related educational needs, the surrounding community's resources available to meet the student's personal and disability-related requirements (such as transportation), and the health care coverage provided to meet any significant medical needs.

By the time individuals move into the postsecondary environment, they must have the skills needed to act independently on their own behalf. As stated throughout this chapter, you will have many opportunities to foster your child's development of these skills. This is crucial to success in the post-

Table 28.1.   Essential questions to be addressed as part of a transition plan to post-secondary education

---

Education

Did the disability necessitate any special accommodations in high school?

Was a class that met at a certain time of day missed because of the student's need to perform a health care routine?

Did the disability affect the student's overall attendance?

Did medication affect the student's ability to concentrate or participate in school?

Did the student require extra time to complete classwork, tests, or homework?

Was technology used in the classroom or at home to fulfill academic requirements?

Was in-class assistance required, such as a person to take notes?

Environmental considerations

Do certain environmental factors affect the student's health and well-being?

Does the student need to limit exposure to noise and distractions?

Does the student require a special (controlled) living environment?

Are certain activities (walking long distances, climbing stairs) difficult?

Medical needs

Is the student restricted from participating in any activities?

Does the student require specialized medical care facilities?

Does the student require the coordinated care of many health care providers?

Does the student have a care routine that must be performed at specific times of day?

Does the student have a care routine that can be performed only by a specially trained individual, such as a physical therapist, respiratory therapist, or nurse?

Is there a medication schedule that must be adhered to strictly?

Are required medications difficult to locate?

Is the care of a medical specialist required? If so, how frequently?

How does the student plan to cover medical expenses?

Activities of daily living

Is assistance required in getting out of bed?

Is assistance with food preparation/eating needed?

Does the student require a special diet?

Does the student need assistance in bathing or using the bathroom?

Is assistance with dressing necessary?

Is assistance with mobility required?

---

secondary environment and to your child's ability to lead a productive, independent life as an adult.

FROM PEDIATRIC TO ADULT MEDICAL CARE

Medical transition is the planned movement of young adults with disabilities from pediatric care to adult-oriented care. When your child went to a pediatrician, you had primary responsibility for communicating with the physician and ensuring health maintenance. In adult medical care, these responsibilities fall to your son or daughter. The goal of medical transition is for health care to be uninterrupted, coordinated, developmentally appropriate, psychologically sound, and comprehensive (including primary and subspecialty care). You may question why this transition is needed when everyone feels so comfortable with the pediatric providers. The reason is that adults in our society obtain their care from physicians trained in adult health issues. Setting the expectation that your teenager with a disability will, like all teens, seek physicians knowledgeable about adult health issues will make him or her feel that he or she is entering adulthood. Remaining in the pediatric system of care may reinforce the teen's dependence, feeling of being different, and fear of being incapable of becoming an adult. In most states, adolescents reach the age of majority at 18 and are legally expected to make decisions about their own medical care. This is a good time for your son or daughter to make the transition to the adult health care system.

In planning for this transition, make it a collaborative process that involves you, your teenager, and the health care provider. Help your teenager identify the components of adult health care he or she will need, including medical and rehabilitation specialists. Identify the skills your teenager will need to manage the disability. Plan to slowly transfer responsibility for health issues to your teen. Break down this process into achievable steps such as your child's arranging for appointments, communicating needs to the physician, and making some of the medical decisions as soon as appropriate.

In anticipation of your child's becoming an adult, review your health insurance policy to determine age limits. You can retain coverage to age 23 if your son or daughter is a full-time student and indefinitely if your child has severe disabilities (see Chapter 27 for more on health insurance). If your child is not eligible for either, he or she may be covered for 3 years by using the federally mandated Consolidated Omnibus Budget Reconciliation Act self-pay provision of your policy. This can serve as a bridging policy until your child can obtain health insurance through his or her job. Check with your employer to be sure that you are aware of all of the options available through your insurance program. If your teenager is pursuing postsecondary education, carefully review the offered school health coverage policy. Many postsecondary educational institutions do not cover students while they are on summer break or are taking a leave of absence. In summary, carefully plan to transfer the responsibility for health care from you to your teenager. Accomplish this while your child is still under your watchful eye so that if he or she falters, you are around to guide him or her toward healthy adult choices.

FROM SCHOOL TO WORK

Having a job provides financial security, engages a person in society, and builds positive self-esteem. Yet, in a 1998 Harris poll, two thirds of Americans with disabilities ages 16–64 were unemployed. When adolescents with disabilities were asked in the survey what they wanted from transition services, they all identified job training as their most important need, with independent living skills, college, and vocational guidance close behind. Research has shown that the essential developmental milestones needed in identifying a career and finding a job are the expectation that there will be future employment, development of communication and social skills, exploration of vocational challenges, and early work experiences. All of these milestones must be met if your son or daughter is to move successfully into the competitive work force.

The future technology-driven economy will require constant reviewing and upgrading of skills. Work force data for individuals with disabilities show that the more education one obtains, the more likely one is to be employed and have a higher salary. Therefore, postsecondary education or training is key to success in the competitive work-place. If your son or daughter, however, is unable to work in a competitive environment, there may be other appropriate opportunities, such as supported employment. The transition plan that is part of your son's or daughter's IEP should address employment goals (see Chapter 12). The teacher and vocational counselor will be able to assist your child in identifying the type of employment that is most appropriate. They may also be able to link him or her with community resources that can help in seeking employment after high school.

The parent's role in this vocational planning process is central. You should be actively involved by doing the following:

- Setting the expectation that your child can and will work in some capacity
- Learning the basic components of vocational development and ensuring the attainment of basic career development (in conjunction with your child's IEP process)
- Enabling your child to explore career options and have work experiences as early as elementary and middle school
- Assisting your child in obtaining the best education possible
- Gaining an awareness of resources such as your state's vocational rehabilitation agency and relevant laws such as IDEA (see Chapters 12 and 13), Section 504 of the Rehabilitation Act Amendments of 1992 (PL 102-569), and the ADA (see Chapter 13)

SUMMARY

Assisting your child to become a successful adult is a rewarding experience. It is never too early to develop a plan. Take one step at a time, do not underestimate your child's capacity for independence, and let go. At the same time, identify "safety nets" so your son or daughter can take risks, falter, and recover. Most of all, enjoy the challenges, laugh, and take care of yourself, too.

Some Questions Answered

Why is it important to understand the difference between *entitlements* **and** *eligibility?*

By law (IDEA and the Rehabilitation Act Amendments of 1992, especially Section 504), elementary and secondary schools are required to identify students with disabilities and provide accommodations when the disability affects their education (see Chapter 12). The burden of identification generally falls on the parents of the child with a disability. Students are entitled to accommodations under these laws when disability-related issues interfere with their educational success. When students leave the public school system, however, these *entitlements* end, and they must enter the world of adult-based services that are provided based on *eligibility.* It is important that you understand how these systems differ, because the change will have a great impact on your son or daughter in postsecondary education and/or at work.

In postsecondary education, there are no entitlements. The responsibility for identifying needs and developing appropriate accommodations shifts from the school to the individual with the disability. Students with disabilities must identify themselves to be eligible for services, must provide documentation of their disability, and must request necessary accommodations. In college, the student must disclose the disability to the school's office of services for students with disabilities, which is responsible for assisting students with disabilities on campus. If the student does not disclose a disability and initiate the accommodation process, the school is under no obligation to provide accommodations to the student. Some examples of accommodations that may be found in postsecondary education include priority registration, seating, parking, extended time for assignments and exams, provision of note takers, relocation of classes, and distance (home-based) learning.

In the workplace, many laws cover individuals with disabilities, including the ADA (see Chapter 13). The ADA gives civil rights protections to individuals with disabilities. According to the ADA, the person must be qualified to perform the essential functions or duties of a job, with or without reasonable accommodations, to be protected from job discrimination. Some examples of reasonable accommodations in the workplace include 1) making existing facilities readily accessible to and usable by an individual in a wheelchair,

2) offering part-time or modified work schedules, 3) acquiring assistive technology (such as TTY device for a deaf individual), 4) modification of equipment or devices (such as larger computer screens for an individual with visual impairment), or 5) modifying employment exams (such as extended time).

How can my son find a college or university that can accommodate his disability?

Although a college's ability to accommodate disability-related needs greatly affects postsecondary experience and success, selecting a school on this basis alone is not recommended. The academic program desired should be the first consideration in the college selection process. Your son should identify his educational goals, assess the school's academic programs, admission requirements, cost, size, location, activities/programs of interest, housing, student–teacher ratio, and any other factors that are important to him. Once he has found a school that meets these criteria, it is important for him to consider how the disability will have an impact on his educational experience and activities of daily life (see Table 28.1). His final decision should be based on how well the school and surrounding community can meet his goals and needs. Staff who provide services to students with disabilities on the campus can help him assess the capacity of the school and surrounding community to meet his disability-related needs. In the final analysis, both academic goals and disability-related needs must be considered.

Suggested Readings and Resources

CHAPTER 1: FINDING OUT YOUR CHILD HAS A DISABILITY

Brazelton, T.B. (1996). *New visions for the developmental assessment of infants and young children.* Washington, DC: ZERO TO THREE: National Center for Infants, Toddlers and Families.

Israeloff, R. (1998, September). Detecting disabilities early. *Parents Magazine, 73*(9), 223–226.

Miller, N.B. (with "The Moms": Burmester, S., Callahan, D.G., Dieterle, J., & Niedermeyer, S.). (1994). *Nobody's perfect: Living and growing with children who have special needs.* Baltimore: Paul H. Brookes Publishing Co.

Nagler, M., & Nagler, A. (1997). *Yes you can!: A guide for parents of children with disabilities.* North York, Ontario, Canada: Stoddart Publishing.

Pueschel, S.M., Scola, P.S., Weidenman, L.E., & Bernier, J.C. (1995). *The special child: A source book for parents of children with developmental disabilities* (2nd ed.). Baltimore: Paul H. Brookes Publishing Co.

Wexler, K., & Wexler, L. (1994). *The ABC's of prenatal diagnosis.* Denver, CO: Genassist.

Wodrich, D.L. (1997). *Children's psychological testing: A guide for nonpsychologists* (3rd ed.). Baltimore: Paul H. Brookes Publishing Co.

The Family Village, Waisman Village, University of Wisconsin–Madison, 1500 Highland Avenue, Madison, WI 53705 (http://www.familyvillage.wisc.edu)

National Information Center for Children and Youth with Disabilities (NICHCY), Post Office Box 1492, Washington, DC 20013 (800-695-0285; http://www.nichcy.org)

National Parent-to-Parent Support and Information System, Post Office Box 907, Blue Ridge, GA 30513 (for parents: 800-651-1151; 706-374-3822; http://www.nppsis .org/index.htm)

Parent's Guide Unlimited, 2200 West Chester Pike, Broomall, PA 19008 (610-325-7704; http://www.parents-guide.net; parentsguide@yahoo.com)

Parents Helping Parents, 3041 Olcott Street, Santa Clara, CA 95054 (408-727-5775; http://www.php.com)

CHAPTER 2: MAKING THE MOST OF DOCTOR VISITS

Jones, M.L. (1985). *Home care for the chronically ill or disabled child.* New York: Harper-Collins.

Nelson, K.B., & Leviton, A. (1991). How much of neonatal encephalopathy is due to birth asphyxia? American Journal of Diseases of Childhood, 145, 1325–1331.

American Academy for Cerebral Palsy and Developmental Medicine (AACPDM), 6300 North River Road, Suite 727, Rosemont, IL 60018 (847-698-1635; http://www.aacpdm.org)

American Academy of Pediatrics (AAP), 141 Northwest Point Road, Elk Grove Village, IL 60007 (847-434-4000; http://www.aap.org)

American Association of University Affiliated Programs for Persons with Developmental Disabilities (AAUAP), 8630 Fenton Street, Suite 410, Silver Spring, MD 20910 (http://www.aauap.org)

Beach Center on Families and Disability, 3111 Haworth Hall, University of Kansas, Lawrence, KS 66045 (919-864-7600; http://www.lsi.ukans.edu/BEACH/html/d11.htm)

Children's Seashore House of The Children's Hospital of Philadelphia, 3405 Civic Center Boulevard, Philadelphia, PA 19104 (http://www.childrens-seashore.org)

National Easter Seals Society, 230 W. Monroe Street, Suite 1800, Chicago, IL 60606 (312-726-6200; http://www.easter-seals.org)

PEDINFO (http://www.pedinfo.org)

Society for Developmental and Behavioral Pediatrics, 19 Station Lane, Philadelphia, PA 19118 (http://www.dbpeds.org)

Society for Developmental Pediatrics, Kennedy Krieger Institute, 707 N. Broadway, Baltimore, MD 21205 (410-502-9400; http://www.kennedykrieger.org)

CHAPTER 3: WHY MY CHILD?

Batshaw, M.L. (Ed.). (1997). *Children with disabilities* (4th ed.). Baltimore: Paul H. Brookes Publishing Co.

Creasy, R.K., & Resnik, R. (Eds.). (1994). *Maternal–fetal medicine: Principles and practice.* Philadelphia: W.B. Saunders.

Moore, K.L., & Persaud, T.V.N. (1998). *Before we are born: Essentials of embryology and birth defects* (5th ed.). Philadelphia: W.B. Saunders.

Moore, K.L., & Persaud, T.V.N. (1998). *The developing human: Clinically oriented embryology.* Philadelphia: W.B. Saunders.

Pasquariello, P.S., Jr. (Ed.). (1999). *The Children's Hospital of Philadelphia book of pregnancy and child care.* New York: John Wiley & Sons.

CHAPTER 4: HOW A YOUNG CHILD DEVELOPS

Accardo, P.J., & Whitman, B.Y. (with Laszewski, C., Haake, C.A., & Morrow, J.D.). (1996). *Dictionary of developmental disabilities terminology.* Baltimore: Paul H. Brookes Publishing Co.

Einon, D. (1999). *Learning early.* New York: Checkmark Books.

Frankenburg, W.K., Dodds, J., Archer, P., Shapiro, H., & Bresnick, B. (1992). The Denver II: A major revision and restandardization of the Denver Developmental Screening Test. *Pediatrics, 89,* 91–97.

Golinkoff, R.M., & Hirsh-Pasek, K. (1999). *How babies talk: The magic and mystery of language in the first three years of life.* New York: E.P. Dutton.

Gopnik, A., Meltzoff, A.N., & Kuhl, P.K. (1999). *The scientist in the crib: Minds, brains, and how children learn.* New York: William Morrow & Co.

Greenspan, S.I., Weider, S., & Simon, R. (1998). *The child with special needs: Encouraging intellectual and emotional growth.* Reading, MA: Addison Wesley Longman.

Hodapp, R.M. (1998). *Development and disabilities: Intellectual, sensory and motor impairments.* New York: Cambridge University Press.

Leach, P., & Matthews, J. (1997). *Your baby and child: From birth to age five.* New York: Alfred A. Knopf.

Let's play and learn: Over 160 fun and easy activities. (1999). Grand Rapids, MI: Instructional Fair. (Available from the publisher, Post Office Box 250, Grand Rapids, MI 49502; 800-443-2976; http://www.instructionalfair.com)

Reitzes, F., Teitelman, B., & Martle, L.A. (1995). *Wonderplay: Interactive and developmental games, crafts, and creative activities for infants, toddlers and preschoolers.* New York: 92nd Street YMCA Parents Center.

Singer, D.G., & Revenson, T.A. (1998). *A Piaget primer: How a child thinks.* Madison, WI: International Universities Press.

Umansky, W., Hooper, S.R., & Fallen, N.H. (1997). *Young children with special needs.* Upper Saddle River, NJ: Prentice-Hall.

Widerstrom, A.H., Mowder, B.A., & Sandall, S.R. (1997). *Infant development and risk: An introduction* (2nd ed.). Baltimore: Paul H. Brookes Publishing Co.

CHAPTER 5: YOUR BABY WAS BORN PREMATURELY

Ahmann, E. (Ed.). (1996). *Home care for the high-risk infant: A family centered approach* (2nd ed.). Gaithersburg, MD: Aspen Publishers.

Harrison, H., & Kositsky, A. (1993). *The premature baby book.* New York: St. Martin's Press.

Klein, A.H., & Ganon, J.A. (1998). *Caring for your premature baby: A complete resource for parents.* New York: HarperCollins.

Madden, S.L. (1999). *The preemie parents' companion.* Boston: Harvard Common Press.

Manginello, F.P., & Digeronimo, T.F. (1998). *Your premature baby: Everything you need to know about childbirth, treatment, and parenting.* New York: John Wiley & Sons.

Tracy, A.E., Maroney, D.I., Berbaum, J.C., & Groothius, J. (Eds.). (1999). *Your premature baby and child: Helpful answers and advice for parents.* New York: Berkley Publishing Group.

CHAPTER 6: UNDERSTANDING EARLY INTERVENTION

Bricker, D.D. (with Pretti-Frontczak, K., & McComas, N.). (1998). *An activity-based approach to early intervention* (2nd ed.). Baltimore: Paul H. Brookes Publishing Co.

Butler, K.G. (1994). *Early intervention II: Working with parents and families.* Gaithersburg, MD: Aspen Publishers.

Cantor, J.A., & Cantor, R.F. (1995). *Parents' guide to special needs schooling.* Westport, CT: Greenwood Publishing Group.

Coleman, J.G. (1999). *The early intervention dictionary: A multidisciplinary guide to terminology.* Bethesda, MD: Woodbine House.

Cripe, J.J.W. (Producer), & Crabtree, J. (Director). (1995). *Family-guided activity-based intervention for infants & toddlers* [Videotape]. Baltimore: Paul H. Brookes Publishing Co.

Education of the Handicapped Act Amendments of 1986, PL 99-457, 20 U.S.C. §§ 1400 *et seq.*

Hanlon, G.M. (1999). *Successfully parenting your baby with special needs: Early intervention for ages birth to three* [Videotape]. Fair Haven, NJ: Edvantage Media. (Available from Paul H. Brookes Publishing Co., 800-638-3775, http://www.brookespublishing.com)

Ramey, C.T., & Ramey, S.L. (1999). *Right from birth: Building your child's foundation for life*. New York: Goddard Press.

Ramey, S.L., & Ramey, C.T. (1999). Early educational intervention with disadvantaged children: To what effect? *Applied and Preventive Psychology, 1*, 131–140.

Ramey, S.L., & Ramey, C.T. (1999). Early experience and early intervention for children "at risk" for developmental delay and mental retardation. *Mental Retardation and Developmental Disabilities Research Reviews, 5*, 1–10.

Ramey, S.L., & Ramey, C.T. (1999). *Going to school: How to help your child succeed in school. A handbook for parents of children ages 3–8*. New York: Goddard Press.

Shackelford, J. (1998). *State and jurisdictional eligibility definitions for infants and toddlers with disabilities under IDEA*. Chapel Hill: University of North Carolina, National Early Childhood Technical Assistance System.

American Association of University Affiliated Programs, 8630 Fenton Street, Suite 410, Silver Spring, MD 20910 (http://www.aaup.org)

Division of Early Childhood (DEC) of the Council for Exceptional Children (CEC), 1920 Association Drive, Reston, VA 20191, (888-CEC-SPED; TTY [text only]: 703-264-9446; http://www.dec-sped.org)

International Society on Early Intervention (ISEI), University of Washington, Center on Human Development and Disability, Box 357920, Seattle, WA 98195 (http://www.depts.washington.edu/isei)

Technical Assistance Alliance for Parent Centers, PACER Center, Inc. (Parent Advocacy Coalition for Education Rights), 4826 Chicago Avenue, S., Minneapolis, MN 55417 (888-248-0822; http://www.taalliance.org; alliance@taalliance.org)

ZERO TO THREE: National Center for Infants, Toddlers and Families, 734 15th Street, NW, Suite 1000, Washington, DC 20005 (202-638-1144; http://www.zerotothree.org)

CHAPTER 7: NUTRITION AND FEEDING

Dietz, W.H., & Stern, L. (1999). *American Academy of Pediatrics' guide to your child's nutrition*. New York: Villard Books.

Kedesdy, J.H., & Budd, K.S. (1998). *Childhood feeding disorders: Assessment and intervention*. Baltimore: Paul H. Brookes Publishing Co.

Morris, S.E. (1987). *Pre-feeding skills*. Tucson, AZ: Therapy Skill Builders.

Queen, P.M. (1993). *Handbook of pediatric nutrition*. Gaithersburg, MD: Aspen Publishers.

Roberts, S.B., & Heyman, M.B. (1999). *Feeding your child for lifelong health: Birth through age six*. New York: Bantam Doubleday Dell.

Satter, E. (1987). *How to get your kid to eat . . . but not too much*. Palo Alto, CA: Bull Publishing.

Sears, W., & Sears, M. (1999). *The family nutrition book: Everything you need to know about feeding your children from birth through adolescence.* Boston: Little, Brown.

Sullivan, P.B., & Rosenbloom, L. (1996). *Feeding the disabled child: Clinics in developmental medicine.* New York: Cambridge University Press.

Food Pyramid Guide, http://www.nal.usda.gov/fnic/Fpyr/pyramid.html

Recommended Dietary Allowances, http://www.nutritionhealthreports.com/RDA.html

CHAPTER 8: DENTAL CARE FOR YOUR CHILD WITH SPECIAL NEEDS

McDonald, R.E., & Avery, D.R. (Eds.). (1999). *Dentistry for the child and adolescent.* St. Louis: Mosby.

Nowak, A.J. (1976). *Dentistry for the handicapped patient.* St. Louis: Mosby.

American Academy of Pediatric Dentistry, 211 E. Chicago Avenue, #700, Chicago, IL 60611 (312-337-2169; http://www.aapd.org)

American Dental Association (ADA), 211 E. Chicago Avenue, Chicago, IL 60611 (312-440-2500; http://www.ada.org)

CHAPTER 9: UNDERSTANDING REHABILITATION THERAPIES

Campbell, S.K. (1994). *Physical therapy for children.* Philadelphia: W.B. Saunders.

Case-Smith, J., Allen, A.S., & Pratt, P.N. (1996). *Occupational therapy for children* (3rd ed.). St. Louis: Mosby.

Cook, A., & Hussey, S. (1995). *Assistive technologies: Principles and practices.* St. Louis: Mosby.

DeFeo, A. (Ed.). (1995). *Parent articles 2.* Tucson, AZ: Communication Skill Builders.

Finnie, N.R. (1997). *Handling the young child with cerebral palsy at home* (3rd ed.). Woburn, MA: Butterworth-Heinemann.

Kelker, K., Holt, R., & Sullivan, J. (1998). *Family guide to assistive technology.* Cambridge, MA: Brookline Books.

Lawrence, K.E., & Niemeyer, S. (Eds.). (1994). *Caregiver education guide for children with developmental disabilities.* Gaithersburg, MD: Aspen Publishers.

Manolson, A. (1992). *It takes two to talk: A parent's guide to helping children communicate.* Toronto: Hanen Centre Publications.

McCormick, S., & Schiefelbusch, R.L. (1990). *Early language intervention: An introduction* (2nd ed.). Columbus, OH: Charles E. Merrill.

Schrader, M. (Ed.). (1992). *Parent articles 1.* Tucson, AZ: Communication Skill Builders.

American Occupational Therapy Association (AOTA), 4720 Montgomery Lane, Post Office Box 31220, Bethesda, MD 20824 (301-652-2682; http://www.aota.org)

American Physical Therapy Association (APTA), 1111 North Fairfax Street, Alexandria, VA 22314 (703-684-2782; http://www.apta.org)

National Lekotek Center, 2100 Ridge Avenue, Evanston, IL 60201 (800-366-PLAY; http://www.lekotek.org)

National Rehabilitation Information Center (NARIC), 8455 Colesville Road, Suite 935, Silver Spring, MD 20910 (800-346-2742; http://www.abledata.com)

CHAPTER 10: COMMONLY USED MEDICATIONS

Agins, A.P. (1999). *Parent & educators drug reference: A guide to common medical conditions & drugs used in school-aged children.* Cranston, RI: PRN Press. (Available from Paul H. Brookes Publishing Co., 800-638-3775, http://www.brookespublishing.com)

American National Red Cross. (1992). *Standard first aid.* St. Louis: Mosby Year Book.

Ammerman, R.T., Hersen, M., & Last, C.G. (Eds.). (1999). *Handbook of prescriptive treatments for children and adolescents* (2nd ed.). Needham Heights, MA: Allyn & Bacon.

Griffith, H.W. (1989). *Complete guide to pediatric symptoms, illness, and medications: Parent's guide for treating sick children from infancy through adolescence.* New York: HPBooks.

Peirce, A. (1997). *American Pharmaceutical Association's parent's guide to childhood medications.* Kansas City, MO: Andrews McMeel Publishing.

Physicians' desk reference (54th ed.). (2000). Montvale, NJ: Medical Economics.

Physicians' desk reference for nonprescription drugs (21st ed.). (2000). Montvale, NJ: Medical Economics.

The Johns Hopkins Hospital. (1996). *The Harriet Lane handbook* (14th ed.). St. Louis: Mosby.

Van Gilder, M., & Masline, S.R. (1997). *Prescription and nonprescription medications for children: What parents need to know.* New York: Pocket Books.

U.S. Food and Drug Administration (FDA) Center for Drug Evaluation and Research (CDER) (Information on FDA-approved drugs and FDA links), http://www.fda.gov/cder/drug.htm

CHAPTER 11: ENCOURAGING APPROPRIATE CHILD BEHAVIOR

Anderson, D.R., Hodson, G.D., & Jones, W.G. (1975). *Instructional programming for the handicapped student.* Springfield, IL: Charles C Thomas.

Baker, B.L., & Brightman, A.J. (1997). *Steps to independence: Teaching everyday skills to children with special needs* (3rd ed.). Baltimore: Paul H. Brookes Publishing Co.

Baker, B.L., Brightman, A.J., Heifetz, L.J., & Murphy, D.M. (1990). *Behavior problems.* Champaign, IL: Research Press.

Becker, W.C. (1990). *Parents are teachers: A child management program.* Champaign, IL: Research Press.

Blechman, E.A. (1985). *Solving child behavior problems at home and at school.* Champaign, IL: Research Press.

Carr, E.G., Levin, L., McConnachie, G., Carlson, J.I., Kemp, D.C., & Smith, C.E. (1994). *Communication-based intervention for problem behavior: A user's guide for producing positive change.* Baltimore: Paul H. Brookes Publishing Co.

Christophersen, E.R. (1977). *Little people: Guidelines for common sense child rearing* (2nd ed.). Austin, TX: PRO-ED.

Durand, V.M. (1990). *Severe behavior problems: A functional communication training approach.* New York: Guilford Press.

Durand, V.M. (1998). *Sleep better: A guide to improving sleep for children with special needs.* Baltimore: Paul H. Brookes Publishing Co.

Green, C. (1990). *Toddler training: The guide to your child from one to four.* Sydney, Australia: Doubleday.

Martin, G., & Pear, J. (1996). *Behavior modification: What it is and how to do it* (5th ed.). Upper Saddle River, NJ: Prentice-Hall.

Mrazek, D., Garrison, W., & Elliot, L. (1993). *A to Z guide to your child's behavior: A parent's easy and authoritative reference to hundreds of everyday problems and concerns from birth to 12 years.* New York: Penguin Putnam.

Miller, L.K. (1980). *Principles of everyday behavior analysis* (2nd ed.). Pacific Grove, CA: Brooks/Cole Publishing Co.

Nelsen, J. (Ed.). (1996). *Positive discipline* (2nd rev. ed.). New York: Ballantine Books.

Patterson, G.R. (1990). *Families: Applications of social learning to family life.* Champaign, IL: Research Press.

Association for the Advancement of Behavior Therapy (AABT), 305 Seventh Avenue, 16th Floor, New York, NY 10001 (212-647-1890; http://www.aabt.org)

Association for Behavior Analysis (ABA), Department of Psychology, Western Michigan University, Kalamazoo, MI 49008 (616-387-4494; http://www.wmich.edu/aba)

American Psychological Association (APA), 750 First Street, NE, Washington, DC 20002 (202-336-5500; http://www.apa.org)

CHAPTER 12: YOUR CHILD'S EDUCATIONAL RIGHTS

Anderson, W., Chitwood, S., & Hayden, D. (1997). *Negotiating the special education maze: A guide for parents and teachers.* Bethesda, MD: Woodbine House.

Barr, V.M. (1997). *Heath national resource directory on postsecondary education and disability.* Upland, PA: DIANE Publishing Company.

Giangreco, M.F. (1997). *Quick guides to inclusion.* Baltimore: Paul H. Brookes Publishing Co.

Giangreco, M.F. (1998). *Quick guides to inclusion 2.* Baltimore: Paul H. Brookes Publishing Co.

Hanlon, G.M. (Producer). (1998). *The 3 R's for special education: Rights, resources, results: A guide for parents, a tool for educators* [Videotape]. Fair Haven, NJ: Edvantage Media. (Available from Paul H. Brookes Publishing Co., 800-638-3775, http://www.brookespublishing.com)

Individuals with Disabilities Education Act (IDEA) of 1990, PL 101-476, 20 U.S.C. §§ 1400 *et seq.*

Individuals with Disabilities Education Act Amendments of 1997: Report of the Committee on Education and the Workforce, House of Representatives, on H.R. 5 together with additional and dissenting views (House of Representatives Report 105-95). (1997, May 13). Washington, DC: U.S. Government Printing Office.

Moore, L.O. (1996). *Inclusion: A practical guide for parents: Tools to enhance your child's success in learning.* Minnetonka, MN: Peytral Publications.

Moore, L.O. (1997). *Inclusion: Strategies for working with young children: A resource guide for teachers, childcare providers, and parents.* Minnetonka, MN: Peytral Publications.

The Council for Exceptional Children (CEC), 1920 Association Drive, Reston, VA 20191 (888-CEC-SPED; TTY [text only]: 703-264-9446; http://www.cec.sped.org)

LDResources, 202 Lake Road, New Preston, CT 06777 (800-868-3214; http://www
.ldresources.com)

The National Parent Network on Disabilities (NPND), 1130 17th Street, NW, Suite 400,
Washington, DC 20036 (202-463-2299; http://www.npnd.org)

National School Boards Association, 1680 Duke Street, Alexandria, VA 22314 (703-838-
6722; http://www.nsba.org)

Office of Special Education and Rehabilitative Services (OSERS), Communication and
Information Services, U.S. Department of Education, 330 C Street, SW, Room 3132,
Washington, DC 20202 (202-205-8241; http://www.ed.gov/offices/OSERS)

TASH (formerly The Association for Persons with Severe Handicaps), 29 W. Susque-
hanna Avenue, Suite 210, Baltimore, MD 21204 (410-828-8274; http://www.tash
.org)

CHAPTER 13: IDENTIFYING
LEGAL RIGHTS AND BENEFITS

Americans with Disabilities Act (ADA) of 1990, PL 101-336, 42 U.S.C. §§ 12101 *et seq.*
Also available on-line: http://www.usdoj.gov/crt/ada/pubs/ada.txt

Consolidated Omnibus Budget Reconciliation Act (COBRA) of 1985, PL 99-272, 42
U.S.C. §§ 300 *et seq.* Also available on-line: http://www.ssa.gov

Developmental Disabilities Assistance and Bill of Rights Act Amendments of 1996, PL
104-719, 42 U.S.C. §§ 6000 *et seq.* Also available on-line: http://www.igc.apc.org/
NADDC/ddact.html

Developmental Disabilities Assistance and Bill of Rights Act of 1975, PL 94-103, 100
Stat. 840, 42 U.S.C. §§ 6000 *et seq.*

Education for All Handicapped Children Act of 1975, PL 94-142, 20 U.S.C. §§ 1400 *et
seq.*

Family Voices. (1998). *Facts about Medicaid and children with special health care needs* [On-
line]. Algodones, NM: Author. Available: http://www.familyvoices.org/fs/mafacts
.html

Fee, R.W. (1994). The letter of intent. *NICHCY News Digest* [On-line], 2(1). Available:
http://www.nichcy.org/pubs/newsdig/nd18txt.htm

Fee, R.W. (1994). The special needs trust. *NICHCY News Digest* [On-line], 2(1). Available: http://www.nichcy.org/pubs/newsdig/nd18txt.htm

Frolick, L.A. (1994). Overview of estate planning issues. *NICHCY News Digest* [On-
line], 2(1). Available: http://www.nichcy.org/pubs/newsdig/nd18txt.htm

Henderson, K. (1995, June). Overview: ADA, IDEA, and Section 504 of the Rehabilitation Act. *ERIC Digest* (E537; ERIC Document Reproduction Service No. ED 389
142).

Individuals with Disabilities Education Act Amendments of 1997, PL 105-17, 20 U.S.C.
§§ 1400 *et seq.* Also available on-line: http://www.ed.gov/offices/OSERS/IDEA

Malone, D.M., & Orthner, D.K. (1988). Infant care as a parent education resource:
Recent trends in care issues. *Family Relations, 37*, 367–372.

Medicaid, 42 U.S.C. §§ 1397 *et seq.*

Personal Responsibility and Work Opportunity Reconciliation Act of 1996 (Supplemental Security Income Program for Children), PL 104-193, 42 U.S.C. §§ 211 *et seq.*

Rehabilitation Act Amendments of 1998, PL 105-220, 29 U.S.C. §§ 791 *et seq.*

Rehabilitation Act of 1973, PL 93-112, 29 U.S.C. §§ 701 *et seq.*

Rothman, S.M., & Ostrosky, M.M. (1998, August). Six recommendations to consider when choosing an advocate for your special needs child. *National Parent Information Network: Parent News* [On-line], 4(8). Available: http://npin.org/pnews/1998/pnew898.htm

Social Security Administration. (1997). *Benefits for children with disabilities* (SSA Publication No. 05-10026). Washington, DC: Author.

Social Security Administration. (1997). *Supplemental security income* (SSA Publication No. 05-11000). Washington, DC: Author.

Social Security Administration. (1998). *What you need to know when you get SSI* (SSA Publication No. 05-11011). Washington, DC: Author.

Administration on Developmental Disabilities (ADD), Administration for Children and Families, U.S. Department of Health and Human Services, Mail Stop: HHH 300-F, 370 L'Enfant Promenade, SW, Washington, DC, 20447 (202-690-6590; http://www.acf.dhh.gov/programs/add)

American Bar Association, Commission on Mental and Physical Disabilities Law (202-662-1570; http://www.abanet.org/disability/subcm.html)

Children's Defense Fund, 25 E Street, NW, Washington, DC 20001 (800-233-1200; http://www.childrensdefense.org)

Disabilities Rights Education and Defense Fund (DREDF), 2212 Sixth Street, Berkeley, CA 94710 (510-644-2555; http://www.dredf.org)

Social Security Administration (800-772-1213; TTY except in Missouri: 800-325-0778; TTY in Missouri: 800-392-0812; http://www.ssa.gov)

U.S. Department of Education, 400 Maryland Avenue, SW, Washington, DC 20202 (800-USA-LEARN; http://www.ed.gov)

Regional Resource Centers

Six federally funded regional resource centers (RRCs) across the United States assist state education agencies in building capacity to improve programs for children with disabilities:

Great Lakes Area Regional Resource Center, Ohio State University, 700 Ackerman Road, Suite 440, Columbus, OH 43202 (614-447-0844). States served: IL, IN, MI, MN, OH, PA, and WI.

Mid-South Regional Resource Center, University of Kentucky, Interdisciplinary Human Development Institute, 126 Mineral Industries Building, Lexington, KY 40506 (606-257-4921). States served: DC, DE, KY, MD, NC, SC, TN, VA, and WV.

Mountain Plains Regional Resource Center, Utah State University, 1780 N. Research Parkway, Suite 112, Logan, UT 84321 (801-752-0238). Areas served: CO, IA, KS, MO, MT, ND, NE, SD, UT, WY, and the Bureau of Indian Affairs.

Northeast Regional Resource Center, Trinity College of Vermont, Institute for Program Development, McCauley Hall, 208 Colchester Avenue, Burlington, VT 05401 (802-658-5036). States served: CT, MA, ME, NH, NJ, NY, RI, and VT.

South Atlantic Regional Resource Center, Florida Atlantic University, 1236 University Drive North, Plantation, FL 33322 (305-473-6106). Areas served: AL, AR, FL, GA, LA, MS, NM, OK, TX, Puerto Rico, and the U.S. Virgin Islands.

Western Regional Resource Center, University of Oregon, Clinical Services Building, Eugene, OR 97403 (503-346-5641). Areas served: AK, AZ, CA, HI, ID, NV, OR, WA, American Samoa, Federated States of Micronesia, Guam, Republic of the Marshall Islands, the Republic of Palau, and the Commonwealth of the Northern Marianas.

CHAPTER 14: MENTAL RETARDATION

Brace, J.A., Hodapp, R.M., & Seigneur, E. (Eds.). (1998). *Handbook of mental retardation and development.* New York: Cambridge University Press.

Field, M.A., & Sanchez, V.A. (2000). *Equal treatment for people with mental retardation: Having and raising children.* Cambridge, MA: Harvard University Press.

Gill, B. (1998). *Changed by a child: Companion notes for parents of a child with a disability.* New York: Bantam Doubleday Dell.

Kaufman, S.Z. (1999). *Retarded isn't stupid, Mom!* (Rev. ed.). Baltimore: Paul H. Brookes Publishing Co.

McNey, M., & Fisch, L. (1996). *Leslie's story: A book about a girl with mental retardation.* Minneapolis, MN: Lerner Publications Co.

Smith, R. (Ed.). (1993). *Children with mental retardation: A parents' guide.* Bethesda, MD: Woodbine House.

American Association on Mental Retardation (AAMR), 444 North Capitol Street, NW, Suite 846, Washington, DC 20001 (800-424-3688; http://www.aamr.org)

The Arc (formerly The Association for Retarded Citizens of the United States), 500 East Border Street, Suite 300, Arlington, TX 76010 (817-261-6003; http://www.thearc.org)

CHAPTER 15: DOWN SYNDROME

Bruni, M. (1998). *Fine motor skills in children with Down syndrome: A guide for parents and professionals.* Bethesda, MD: Woodbine House.

Bryan, J. (1999). *Living with Down syndrome.* Austin, TX: Raintree/Steck-Vaughn.

Cunningham, C. (1996). *Understanding Down syndrome: An introduction for parents.* Cambridge, MA: Brookline Books.

Hassold, T., & Patterson, D. (1998). *Down syndrome: A promising future, together.* New York: Wiley-Liss.

Kumin, L. (1994). *Communication skills in children with Down syndrome: A guide for parents.* Bethesda, MD: Woodbine House.

Levitz, M., & Kingsley, J. (1994). *Count us in: Growing up with Down syndrome.* San Diego: Harcourt, Brace & Co.

Oelwein, P.L. (1995). *Teaching reading to children with Down syndrome: A guide for parents and teachers.* Bethesda, MD: Woodbine House.

Pueschel, S.M. (2001). *Parents' guide to Down syndrome: Toward a brighter future* (2nd ed.). Baltimore: Paul H. Brookes Publishing Co.

Pueschel, S.M., & Šuštrová, M. (1997). *Adolescents with Down syndrome: Toward a more fulfilling life.* Baltimore: Paul H. Brookes Publishing Co.

Selikowitz, M. (1997). *Down syndrome: The facts.* New York: Oxford Medical Publications.

Stray-Gundersen, K. (1995). *Babies with Down syndrome.* Bethesda, MD: Woodbine House.

Targ-Brill, M. (1993). *Barron's parenting keys series: Keys to parenting a child with Down's syndrome.* Hauppage, NY: Barron's Educational Series.

Van Dyke, D.C., Mattheis, P., Eberly, S.S., & Williams, J. (Eds.). (1995). *Medical and surgical care for children with Down syndrome: A guide for parents.* Bethesda, MD: Woodbine House.

Winders, P.C. (1997). *Gross motor skills in children with Down syndrome: A guide for parents and professionals*. Bethesda, MD: Woodbine House.

National Down Syndrome Congress (NDSC), 7000 Peachtree-Dunwoody Road, NE, Lakeridge, 400 Office Park, Building #5, Suite 100, Atlanta, GA 30328 (800-232-NDSC; http://www.members.carol.net/~ndsc/index_fr.html)

National Down Syndrome Society (NDSS), 666 Broadway, New York, NY 10012 (212-460-9330; http://www.ndss.org)

CHAPTER 16: GENETIC SYNDROMES

Dykens, E.M., Hodapp, R.M., & Finucane, B.M. (2000). *Genetics and mental retardation syndromes: A new look at behavior and interventions*. Baltimore: Paul H. Brookes Publishing.

Gilbert, P. (1998). *The A–Z reference book of syndromes and inherited disorders*. San Diego: Singular Publishing Group.

McKusick, V.A. (1994). *Mendelian inheritance in man: A catalog of human genes and genetic disorders* (11th ed.). Baltimore: The Johns Hopkins University Press.

Wilson, G., & Cooley, W.C. (2000). *Preventive management of children with congenital anomalies and syndromes*. New York: Cambridge University Press.

National Organization for Rare Disorders (NORD), Post Office Box 8923, New Fairfield, CT 06812 (203-746-6518; http://www.rarediseases.org)

National Alliance of Genetic Support Groups, 4301 Connecticut Avenue, NW, Suite 404, Washington, DC 20008 (800-336-GENE; http://www.geneticalliance.org)

Online Mendelian Inheritance in Man (OMIM), Center for Medical Genetics, The Johns Hopkins University, Baltimore, MD, and National Center for Biotechnology Information, National Library of Medicine, Bethesda, MD (http://www.ncbi.nlm.nih.gov/omim)

CHAPTER 17: SPINA BIFIDA

Bannister, C.M., & Tew, B. (1991). *Current concepts in spina bifida and hydrocephalus*. London: MacKeith Press.

Bloom, B., & Seljeskog, E.L. (1988). *A parent's guide to spina bifida*. Minneapolis: University of Minnesota Press.

Lutkenhoff, M., & Oppenheimer, S.G. (1997). *SPINAbilities: A young person's guide to spina bifida*. Bethesda, MD: Woodbine House.

Sandler, A. (1997). *Living with spina bifida: A guide for families and professionals*. Chapel Hill: University of North Carolina Press.

Shaer, C.M. (1995). *Answering your questions about spina bifida*. Washington, DC: Children's National Medical Center.

Sloan, S.L., Leibold, S.R., & Atkinson, J.H. (1995). *Sexuality and the person with spina bifida*. Washington, DC: Spina Bifida Association of America.

Spina Bifida Association of America, 4590 MacArthur Boulevard, NW, Suite 250, Washington, DC 20007 (800-621-3141; http://www.sbaa.org)

CHAPTER 18: EPILEPSY

Anderson, R. (1995.). *Black water.* New York: Henry Holt.

Devinsky, O. (1994). *A guide to understanding & living with epilepsy.* Philadelphia: F.A. Davis Company.

Dudley, M.E., & Spencer, S.S. (1997). *Healthwatch series: Epilepsy.* Parsippany, NJ: Crestwood House.

Freeman, J.M., Kelly, M., & Freeman, J. (1996). *The epilepsy diet treatment: An introduction to the ketogenic diet* (2nd ed.). New York: Demos Medical Publishing.

Freeman, J.M., Vining, E., & Pillas, D. (1997). *Seizures and epilepsy in childhood: A guide for parents* (2nd ed.). Baltimore: The John Hopkins University Press.

Gino, C. (1997). *Rusty's story* (Rev. ed.). New York: Aah-ha! Books.

Gosselin, K., & Freedman, M. (1996). *Special kids in school series: Vol. 3. Taking seizure disorders to school: A story about epilepsy.* Valley Park, MO: JayJo Books.

Grumnit, R.J. (1995). *Your child and epilepsy: A guide to living well.* New York: Demos Medical Publishing.

Landau, E. (1995). *Understanding illness series: Epilepsy.* New York: Twenty First Century Books.

Lechtenberg, R. (1999). *Epilepsy and the family.* Cambridge, MA: Harvard University Press.

Marshall, F. (1998). *The natural way series: Epilepsy.* Boston: Element Books.

Richard, A., & Reiter, J. (1995). *Epilepsy: A new approach* (Rev. paperback ed.). New York: Walker & Co.

Sander, J., & Hart, Y. (1997). *Epilepsy: Questions and answers.* Coral Springs, FL: Merit Publishing International.

Schachter, S., Montouris, G., & Pollack, J. (1996). *The brainstorms family: Epilepsy on our terms. Stories by children with seizures and their parents.* Philadelphia: Lippincott, Williams & Wilkins.

Schachter, S., & Schomer, D. (1998). *The comprehensive evaluation and treatment of epilepsy: A practical guide.* New York: Academic Press.

Smith, T. (1999). *Epilepsy.* New York: DK Publishing.

Wilner, A. (1996). *Epilepsy: 199 answers. A doctor responds to his patients' questions.* New York: Demos Medical Publishing.

Epilepsy Foundation of America (EFA), 4351 Garden City Drive, Landover, MD 20785 (800-EFA-1000; http://www.efa.org)

CHAPTER 19: CEREBRAL PALSY

Bridge, G. (1999). *Parents as care managers: The experiences of those caring for young children with cerebral palsy.* Brookfield, VT: Ashgate.

Dormans, J.P., & Pellegrino, L. (Eds.). (1998). *Caring for children with cerebral palsy: A team approach.* Baltimore: Paul H. Brookes Publishing Co.

Finnie, N.R., Bavin, J., Bax, M., Browne, M., & Gardner, M. (1997). *Handling the young child with cerebral palsy at home.* Woburn, MA: Butterworth-Heinemann Medical.

Geralis, E. (Ed.). (1998). *Children with cerebral palsy: A parents' guide.* Bethesda, MD: Woodbine House.

Leonard, J.F., Myers, M.E., & Cadenhead, S.L. (1997). *Barron's parenting keys series: Keys to parenting a child with cerebral palsy.* Hauppage, NY: Barron's Educational Series.

Miller, F., & Bachrach, S.J. (1998). *Cerebral palsy: A complete guide for caregiving.* Baltimore: The Johns Hopkins University Press.

Schleichkorn, J. (1993). *Coping with cerebral palsy: Answers to questions parents often ask* (2nd ed.). Austin, TX: PRO-ED.

American Academy for Cerebral Palsy and Developmental Medicine (AACPDM), 6300 North River Road, Suite 727, Rosemont, IL 60018 (847-698-1635; http://www .aacpdm.org)

United Cerebral Palsy Associations (UCPA), 1660 L Street, NW, Suite 700, Washington, DC 20036 (800-872-5827; http://www.ucpa.org)

CHAPTER 20: HEARING LOSS

Adams, J.W. (1997).*You and your deaf child: A self-help guide for parents of deaf and hard of hearing children.* Washington, DC: Clerc Books.

Cohen, L.H. (1994). *Train go sorry: Inside a deaf world.* Boston: Houghton Mifflin.

Families with deaf children: Discovering your needs, exploring your choices [Videotape]. (Available from The Boys Town Press, 13603 Flanagan Boulevard, Boys Town, NE 68010; 800-282-6657)

For a deaf son [Videotape]. (Available from KERA/Channel 13, 300 Harry Hines Boulevard, Dallas, TX 75201; 214-871-1390)

Frazier-Maiwald, V., & Williams, L.M. (1999). *Barron's parenting keys series: Keys to raising a deaf child.* Hauppage, NY: Barron's Educational Series.

Kelley-King, J., & King, J.F. (1995). *American sign language basics for hearing parents of deaf children.* Hillsboro, OR: Butte Publications.

Knight, P., & Swanwick, R. (1999). *The care and education of a deaf child: A book for parents.* Clevedon, Avon, England: Multilingual Matters Ltd. (Available from the publisher, Frankfurt Lodge, Clevedon Hall, Victoria Road, Clevedon, Avon BS21 7HH, England; http://www.multilingual-matters.com)

Marschark, M. (1997). *Raising and educating a deaf child.* New York: Oxford University Press.

Ogden, P.W. (1996). *The silent garden: Raising your deaf child.* Washington, DC: Gallaudet University Press.

Oral Deaf Education. *Dreams spoken here* [Free videotape]. Palo Alto, CA: Author. (Available from Oral Deaf Education, Post Office Box 50215, Palo Alto, CA 94303; 877-ORALDEAF; http://www.oraldeafed.org)

Schwartz, S. (1996). *Choices in deafness: A parents' guide to communication options.* Bethesda, MD: Woodbine House.

Schleper, D.R. (1997). *Reading to deaf children.* Washington, DC: Gallaudet University Pre-College Products.

Spradley, T.S., & Spradley, J.P. (1985). *Deaf like me.* Washington, DC: Gallaudet University Press.

Winefield, R. (1996). *Never the twain shall meet: Bell, Gallaudet, and the communications debate.* Washington, DC: Gallaudet University Press.

Alexander Graham Bell Association for the Deaf, 3417 Volta Place, NW, Washington, DC 20007 (202-337-5220; http://www.agbell.org)

American Society for Deaf Children, 1820 Tribute Road, Suite A, Sacramento, CA 95815 (800-942-2732; http://www.deafchildren.org)

National Association for the Deaf (NAD), 814 Thayer Avenue, Silver Spring, MD 20910-4500 (301-587-1788; http://www.nad.org)

National Information Center on Deafness, Gallaudet University, 800 Florida Avenue, NE, Washington, DC 20002-3695 (202-651-5051; http://www.gallaudet.edu/~nicd)

CHAPTER 21: COMMUNICATION DISORDERS

Bernstein, D.K., & Tiegerman, E. (1997). *Language and communication disorders in children* (4th ed.). Needham Heights, MA: Allyn & Bacon.

Hamaguchi, P.M. (1995). *Childhood speech, language, and listening problems: What every parent should know.* New York: John Wiley & Sons.

Klein, H.B., & Moses, N. (1998). *Intervention planning for children with communication disorders* (2nd ed.). Paramus, NJ: Prentice-Hall Direct.

Krepelin, E. (1996). *Sound and articulation activities for children with speech-language problems.* Paramus, NJ: Center for Applied Research in Education.

Martin, K.L. (1997). *Does my child have a speech problem?* Chicago: Chicago Reviewer Press.

Ownes, R.E., & Metz, D. (2000). *Introduction to communication disorders.* Needham Heights, MA: Allyn & Bacon.

Schwartz, S., & Miller, J. (1996). *The new language of toys: Teaching communication skills to special needs children* (2nd ed.). Bethesda, MD: Woodbine House.

Treiber, P. (1993). *Barron's parenting keys series: Keys to dealing with stuttering.* Hauppage, NY: Barron's Educational Series.

American Speech-Language-Hearing Association (ASHA), 10801 Rockville Pike, Rockville, MD 28852 (800-498-2071; http://www.asha.org)

International Society for Augmentative and Alternative Communication (ISAAC), 49 The Donway West, Suite 308, Toronto, Ontario M3C 3M9, Canada (416-385-0351; http://www.isaac-online.org)

CHAPTER 22: EYE DISORDERS AND VISUAL IMPAIRMENTS

Ferrell, K.A. (1985). *Reach out and teach: Meeting the training needs of parents of visually and multiply handicapped young children.* New York: American Foundation for the Blind.

Fraiberg, S. (1977). *Insights from the blind: Comparative studies of blind and sighted infants.* New York: Basic Books.

Freeman, R.D., Goetz, E., Richards, D.P., Groenveld, M., Blockberger, S., Jan, J.E., & Sykanda, A.M. (1989). Blind children's early emotional development: Do we know enough to help? *Child: Care, Health and Development, 15,* 3–28.

Greenwald, M.J. (1983). Visual development in infancy and childhood. *Pediatric Clinics of North America, 30,* 977–993.

Holbrook, M.C., (1996). *Children with visual impairments: A parents' guide.* Bethesda, MD: Woodbine House.

Isenberg, S.J. (1994). *The eye in infancy* (2nd ed.). St. Louis: Mosby.

Jaafar, M.S. (1996). Evaluation of the visually impaired infant. *Ophthalmology Clinics of North America, 9,* 299–308.

Paul, W. (1999). The role of computer assistive technology in rehabilitation of the visually impaired: A personal perspective. *American Journal of Ophthalmology, 127,* 75–76.

Pogrund, R.L. (1995). *Teaching age-appropriate purposeful skills: An orientation and mobility curriculum for students with visual impairments.* Austin: Texas School for the Blind.

Prevention of Blindness Society of the Metropolitan Area. *Coping with visual impairment: A resource directory for parents with children who are visually impaired.* Washington, DC: Author. (Available from the author, 1775 Church Street, NW, Washington, DC 20036)

Rogers, J. (1998, November 30). Yellow skies, blue trees? I'm colorblind, but that doesn't mean my world is psychedelic—just confusing. *Newsweek,* 14.

Sacks, S., Kekelis, L., & Gaylord-Ross, R. (1992). *The development of social skills by blind and visually impaired students: Exploratory studies and strategies.* New York: American Foundation for the Blind.

Sacks, S.Z., & Silberman, R.K. (Eds.). (1998). *Educating students who have visual impairments with other disabilities.* Baltimore: Paul H. Brookes Publishing Co.

Scott, E.P., Jan, J.E., & Freeman, R.D. (1994). *Can't your child see?: A guide for parents and professionals about young children who are visually impaired* (3rd ed.). Austin, TX: PRO-ED.

Swallow, R.M., & Huebner, K.M. (1987). *How to thrive, not just survive : A guide to developing independent life skills for blind and visually impaired children and youths.* New York: American Foundation for the Blind.

Warren, D.H. (1994). *Blindness and children: An individual differences approach.* Cambridge, England: Cambridge University Press.

Wolffe, K.E. (1988). *Skills for success: A career education handbook for children and adolescents with visual impairments.* New York: American Foundation for the Blind.

American Council of the Blind (ACB), 1155 15th Street, NW, Suite 720, Washington, DC 20005 (800-424-8666; http://www.acb.org)

American Foundation for the Blind (AFB), 11 Penn Plaza, Suite 300, New York, NY 10001 (800-232-5463; http://www.afb.org/afb)

American Printing House for the Blind (APH), Post Office Box 6085, Louisville, KY 40206 (502-895-2405; http://www.aph.org)

Associated Services for the Blind, 919 Walnut Street, Philadelphia, PA 19107 (215-627-0600; http://www.libertynet.org/asbinfo)

Association for Education and Rehabilitation of the Blind and Visually Impaired, 4600 Duke Street, Suite 430, Post Office Box 22397, Alexandria, VA 22304 (703-823-9690; http://www.aerbvi.org)

International Institute for the Visually Impaired, 1975 Rutgers, East Lansing, MI 48823

The Lighthouse National Center for Vision and Child Development, 111 E. 59th Street, New York, NY 10126 (http://www.lighthouse.org)

National Association for the Visually Handicapped, 22 W. 21st Street, 6th Floor, New York, NY 10010 (212-889-3141; http://www.navh.org)

National Library Service for the Blind and Physically Handicapped, Library of Congress, 1291 Taylor Street, NW, Washington, DC 20542 (http://lcweb.loc.gov/nls)

Prevent Blindness America, 500 E. Remington Road, Schaumburg, IL 60173 (http://www.prevent_blindness.org)

CHAPTER 23: AUTISM SPECTRUM DISORDERS

Attwood, T. (1997). *Asperger's syndrome: A guide for parents and professionals.* London, England: Jessica Kingsley Publishers.

Baron-Cohen, S., & Bolton, P. (1993). *Autism: The facts.* Oxford, England: Oxford University Press.

Cohen, S. (1999). *Targeting autism: What we know, don't know, and can do to help young children with autism and related disorders.* Berkeley: University of California Press.

Dillon, K.M. (1995). *Living with autism: The parents' stories.* Boone, NC: Parkway.

Frith, U. (Ed.). (1992). *Autism and Asperger syndrome.* Cambridge, England: Cambridge University Press.

Gerlach, E.K. (1998). *Autism treatment guide.* Eugene, OR: Four Leaf Press.

Grandin, T. (1996). *Thinking in pictures and other reports from my life with autism.* New York: Vintage Books.

Greenspan, S.I., & Weider, S. (1998). *The child with special needs: Encouraging intellectual and emotional growth.* Reading, MA: Addison Wesley Longman.

Harris, S.L., & Powers, M.D. (Ed.). (1994). *Siblings of children with autism: A guide for families.* Bethesda, MD: Woodbine House.

Harris, S.L., & Weiss, M.J. (1998). *Right from the start: Behavioral intervention for young children with autism. A guide for parents and professionals.* Bethesda, MD: Woodbine House.

Kephardt, B. (1998). *A slant of sun: One child's courage.* New York: W.W. Norton.

Kozloff, M.A. (1998). *Reaching the autistic child: A parent training program.* Cambridge, MA: Brookline Books.

Maurice, C., Green, G., & Luce, S.C. (1996). *Behavioral intervention for young children with autism: A manual for parents and professionals.* Austin, TX: PRO-ED.

Peeters, T. (1997). *Autism: From understanding to educational intervention.* San Diego: Singular Publishing Group.

Powers, M.D. (2000). *Children with autism: A parents' guide* (2nd ed.). Bethesda, MD: Woodbine House.

Quill, K.A. (1995). *Teaching children with autism: Strategies to enhance communication and socialization.* Albany, NY: Delmar Publishers, Inc.

Quill, K.A. (2000). *Do-watch-listen-say: Social and communication intervention for children with autism.* Baltimore: Paul H. Brookes Publishing Co.

Schopler, E. (Ed.). (1995). *Parent survival manual: A guide to crisis resolution in autism and related developmental disabilities.* New York: Plenum.

Siegel, B. (1998). *The world of the autistic child: Understanding and treating autistic spectrum disorders.* Oxford, England: Oxford University Press.

Simpson, R.L. (1997). *Asperger syndrome: A guide for educators and parents.* Austin, TX: PRO-ED.

Sperry, V.W. (2000). *Fragile success: Ten autistic children, childhood to adulthood* (2nd ed.). Baltimore: Paul H. Brookes Publishing Co.

Williams, D. (1994). *Nobody nowhere: The extraordinary autobiography of an autistic.* New York: Avon Books.

Autism Society of America, 7910 Woodmont Ave, Suite 300, Bethesda, MD 20814 (800-3AUTISM x150; http://www.autism-society.org)

Center for the Study of Autism (CSA), Post Office Box 4539, Salem, OR 97302 (503-336-9110; http://www.autism.org)

CHAPTER 24: ATTENTION-DEFICIT/ HYPERACTIVITY DISORDER

Accardo, P., Blondis, T., Whitman, B.Y., & Stein, M. (2000). *Attention deficits and hyperactivity in children and adults: Diagnosis, treatment, management* (2nd ed.). New York: Marcel Dekker.

Alexander-Roberts, C. (1994). *The ADHD parenting handbook: Practical advice for parents from parents.* Dallas, TX: Taylor Publishing.

Alexander-Roberts, C. (1995). *ADHD and teens: A parent's guide to making it through the tough years.* Dallas, TX: Taylor Publishing.

Barkley, R.A. (1995). *Taking charge of ADHD: The complete, authoritative guide for parents.* New York: Guilford Press.

Dendy, C.A.Z. (1995). *Teenagers with ADD: A parents' guide.* Bethesda, MD: Woodbine House.

Ferraro, S. (1995). *Otto learns about his medicine: A story about medication for children with AD/HD.* Washington, DC: American Psychological Association.

Flick, G.L. (1998). *ADD/ADHD behavior-change resource kit: Ready-to-use strategies & activities for helping children with attention deficit disorder.* Paramus, NJ: Center for Applied Research in Education.

Flick, G.L., & Parker, H.C. (1996). *Power parenting for ADD/ADHD children: A practical parent's guide to managing difficult behaviors.* Paramus, NJ: Prentice-Hall Direct.

Gordon, M. (1991). *Jumpin' Johnny get back to work!: A child's guide to ADHD/hyperactivity.* Dewitt, NY: GSI Publications.

Gordon, M. (1992). *My brother's a world-class pain: A sibling's guide to AD/HD-hyperactivity.* Dewitt, NY: GSI Publications.

Green, C., & Chee, K. (1998). *Understanding AD/HD: Attention deficit hyperactivity disorder.* New York: Fawcett Columbine.

Hannah, J. (1999). *Parenting a child with attention-deficit hyperactivity disorder.* Austin, TX: PRO-ED.

Ingersoll, B.D. (1995). *Distant drums, different drummers: A guide for young people with AD/HD.* Bethesda, MD: Cape Publications.

Janover, C. (1997). *Zipper: The kid with AD/HD.* Bethesda, MD: Woodbine House.

Jordan, D.R. (1998). *Attention deficit disorder: AD/HD and ADD syndromes* (3rd ed.). Austin, TX: PRO-ED.

Morrison, J. (1997). *Coping with ADD/AD/HD.* Center City, MN: Hazelden Informational and Educational Services.

Quinn, P.O. (Ed.). (1994). *ADD and the college student: A guide for high school and college students with attention deficit disorder.* Washington, DC: Magination.

Rief, S.F. (1998). *The ADD/AD/HD checklist.* Paramus, NJ: Prentice-Hall Trade.

Silver, L.B. (1999). *Dr. Larry Silver's advice to parents on attention-deficit hyperactivity disorder* (2nd ed.). New York: Times Books.

Stevens, S.H. (1997). *Classroom success for the LD and AD/HD child.* Winston-Salem, NC: John F. Blair.

Weiss, G., & Hechtman, L.T. (Eds.). (1993). *Hyperactive children grown up: AD/HD in children, adolescents, and adults* (2nd ed.). New York: Guilford Press.

Wodrich, D.L. (2000). *Attention deficit/hyperactivity disorder: What every parent wants to know* (2nd ed.). Baltimore: Paul H. Brookes Publishing Co.

Children and Adults with Attention Deficit Hyperactivity Disorder (CHADD), 8181 Professional Place, Suite 201, Landover, MD 20785 (800-233-4050; http://www .chadd.org)

National Attention Deficit Disorder Association (ADDA), 1788 Second Street, Suite 200, Highland Park, IL 60035 (847-432-ADDA)

CHAPTER 25: LEARNING DISABILITIES

American Academy of Pediatrics (Committee on Children with Disabilities), American Association for Pediatric Ophthalmology and Strabismus, & American Academy of Ophthalmology. (1992). Learning disabilities, dyslexia, and vision. *Pediatrics, 90,* 124–125.

Capute, A.J., Accardo, P.J., & Shapiro, B.K. (1994). *Learning disability spectrum: ADD, ADHD, and LD.* Timonium, MD: York Press.

Hall, S.L., & Moats, L.C. (1999). *Straight talk about reading: How parents can make a difference during the early years.* Lincolnwood, IL: NTC/Contemporary Publishing Company.

Hallahan, D.P., & Kauffman, J.M. (1998). *Introduction to learning disability.* New York: Simon & Schuster.

Harwell, J. M. (1995). *Complete learning disabilities resource library.* Paramus, NJ: Center for Applied Research in Education.

Kravets, M. (1999). *The K & W guide to colleges for the learning disabled: A resource guide for students, parents, and professionals.* New York: Random House.

Mangrum, C.T. (Ed.). (1997). *Peterson's colleges with programs for students with learning disabilities or attention deficit disorders* (5th ed.). Lawrenceville, NJ: Peterson's.

McNamara, F.J., & McNamara, B.E. (1995). *Barron's parenting keys series: Keys to parenting a child with a learning disability.* Hauppage, NY: Barron's Educational Series.

Rief, S. (1997). *How to help your child succeed in school: strategies and guidance for parents of children with ADHD and/or learning disabilities* [Videotape]. San Diego: National Professional Resources. (Available from Paul H. Brookes Publishing Co., 800-638-3775, http://www.brookespublishing.com)

Schatzow, M. (1999). *Learning disability.* New York: Viking Penguin.

Shapiro, B.K., Accardo, P.J., & Capute, A.J. (1998). *Specific reading disability: A view of the spectrum.* Timonium, MD: York Press.

Silver, L.B. (1998). *Misunderstood child: Understanding and coping with your child's learning disabilities.* New York: Times Books.

Smith, C., & Strick, L. (1997). *Parent's guide to learning disabilities.* New York: Free Press.

Wong, B.Y. (1996). *The ABCs of learning disabilities.* San Diego: Academic Press.

The International Dyslexia Association (IDA), 8600 LaSalle Road, Chester Building, Suite 382, Baltimore, MD 21286-2044 (messages: 800-ABCD123; http://www .interdys.org)

Learning Disabilities Association of America (LDA), 4156 Library Road, Pittsburgh, PA 15234-1349 (412-341-1515; http://www.ldanatl.org)

CHAPTER 26: WHAT ABOUT OUR NEXT CHILD?

Baker, D.L., Schuette, J.L., & Uhlmann, W.R. (1998). *A guide to genetic counseling.* New York: John Wiley & Sons.

Gardener, R.J.M., & Sutherland, G.R. (1996). *Chromosome abnormalities and genetic counseling.* New York: Oxford University Press.

Gonick, L. (1991). *The cartoon guide to genetics.* New York: HarperCollins.

Teichler-Zallen, D.T. (1997). *Does it run in the family?: A consumer's guide to DNA testing for genetic disorders.* New Brunswick, NJ: Rutgers University Press.

American College of Medical Genetics, 9650 Rockville Pike, Bethesda, MD 20814 (301-530-7127; http://www.faseb.org/genetics)

National Society of Genetic Counselors, 233 Canterbury Drive, Wallingford, PA 19086 (610-872-7608; http://www.nsgc.org)

CHAPTER 27: KEEPING UP WITH CHANGES IN HEALTH CARE

Keene, N. (1998). *Working with your doctor: Getting the healthcare you deserve.* Cambridge, MA: O'Reilly & Associates.

Families USA, 1334 G Street, NW, Washington, DC 20005 (202-628-3030; http://www.familiesusa.org)

Family Voices National Office, Post Office Box 769, Algodones, NM 87001 (888-835-5669; http://www.familyvoices.org; kidshealth@familyvoices.org)

CHAPTER 28: SUCCESS ON THE ROAD TO ADULTHOOD

Antonello, S.J. (1995). *Social skills development: Practical strategies for adolescents and adults with developmental disabilities.* Needham Heights, MA: Allyn & Bacon.

Brown, D.S. (1999). *Learning a living.* Bethesda, MD: Woodbine House.

Goldstein, S. (1996). *Managing attention and learning disorders in late adolescence and adulthood.* New York: John Wiley & Sons.

Powers, L.E., Singer, G.H.S., & Sowers, J.-A. (Eds.). (1996). *On the road to autonomy: Promoting self-confidence in children and youth with disabilities.* Baltimore: Paul H. Brookes Publishing Co.

Rehabilitation Act Amendments of 1992, PL 102-569, 29 U.S.C. §§ 701 *et seq.*

Schwier, K.M., & Hingsburger, D. (2000). *Sexuality: Your sons and daughters with intellectual disabilities.* Baltimore: Paul H. Brookes Publishing Co.

Adolescent Employment Readiness Center, Children's National Medical Center, 111 Michigan Avenue, NW, Washington, DC 20010 (202-884-3202; http://www.cnmc.org)

The Association on Higher Education and Disability (AHEAD), Post Office Box 21192, Columbus, OH 43221 (614-488-4972; http://www.ahead.org)

Council of State Administrators of Vocational Rehabilitation, Post Office Box 3776, Washington, DC 20007 (202-638-4634)

HEATH Resource Center, American Council on Education, One Dupont Circle, NW, Suite 800, Washington, DC 20036 (202-939-9320)

National Center for Youth with Disabilities, University of Minnesota, 420 Delaware Street, SW, Box 721, Minneapolis, MN 55455 (800-333-6293; http://www.cyfc.umn.edu/Youth/ncyd.html)

National Council on Independent Living, 1916 Wilson Boulevard, Suite 209, Arlington, VA 22201 (703-525-3406)

National School for Work Learning and Information Center, 400 Virginia Avenue, SW, Room 210, Washington, DC 20024 (800-251-7236)

The National Transition Alliance for Youth with Disabilities, University of Illinois, Transition Research Institute, 51 Gerty Drive, Champaign, IL 61820 (217-333-2325; http://www.aed.org/Transition/Alliance/NTA.html)

PACER Center, Inc. (Parent Advocacy Coalition for Education Rights), 4826 Chicago Avenue, S., Minneapolis, MN 55417 (612-827-2966; http://www.pacer.org)

Index

Page numbers followed by *f* indicate figures; those followed by *t* indicate tables.

Sources of Reprinted Material

Table 6.1 from 34 Code of Federal Register (CFR) 303.12(d).

Table 6.2 from 34 Code of Federal Register (CFR) 300.5, 300.6, and 300.17.

Table 10.11 adapted from Batshaw, M.L., & Perret, Y.M. (1981). *Children with handicaps: A medical primer* (p. 412). Baltimore: Paul H. Brookes Publishing Co.

Tables 14.1, 23.1, and 24.1 adapted with permission from the *Diagnostic and Statistical Manual of Mental Disorders, Fourth Edition.* Copyright 1994 American Psychiatric Association.

Table 14.2 from Batshaw, M.L., & Shapiro, B.K. (1997). Mental retardation. In M.L. Batshaw (Ed.), *Children with disabilities* (4th ed., p. 350). Baltimore: Paul H. Brookes Publishing Co.

Tables 17.1–3 from The Spina Bifida Program, Department of General Pediatrics. (1995). *Answering your questions about spina bifida: A guide from The Spina Bifida Program, Department of General Pediatrics* (pp. 11, 19, 33). Washington, DC: Children's National Medical Center; adapted by permission.

Table 18.1 from Kuntz, K.R. (1996). Seizures. In L.A. Kurtz, P.W. Dowrick, S.E. Levy, & M.L. Batshaw (Eds.), *Handbook of developmental disabilities: Resources for interdisciplinary care* (p. 398). Gaithersburg, MD: Aspen Publishers; adapted by permission.

Table 25.1 adapted from Shapiro, B.K., & Gallico, R.P. (1993). Learning disabilities. *Pediatric Clinics of North America, 40*(3), 491–506.

Table 27.1 from Family Voices. *Family voices discusses: Managed care* [On-line]; adapted by permission. Algodones, NM: Author. Available: http://www.familyvoices.org/MANCARE1.html

Figures 4.1 and 9.3 from Pellegrino, L. (1997). Cerebral palsy. In M.L. Batshaw (Ed.), *Children with disabilities* (4th ed., pp. 505, 521). Baltimore: Paul H. Brookes Publishing Co.

Figure 5.1 from Evans, J.R. (1997). The first weeks of life. In M.L. Batshaw (Ed.), *Children with disabilities* (4th ed., p. 103). Baltimore: Paul H. Brookes Publishing Co. (Courtesy of Dr. Roger Saunders, Department of Radiology, the Johns Hopkins Hospital, Baltimore.)

Figure 7.2 from Eicher, P.S. (1997). Feeding. In M.L. Batshaw (Ed.), *Children with disabilities* (4th ed., p. 636). Baltimore: Paul H. Brookes Publishing Co.

Figure 9.1 from Blanchet, D., & McGee, M. (1996). Principles of splint design and use. In L.A. Kurtz, P.W. Dowrick, S.E. Levy, & M.L. Batshaw (Eds.), *Handbook of developmental disabilities: Resources for interdisciplinary care* (pp. 468, 478). Gaithersburg, MD: Aspen Publishers.

Figure 9.2 from Deitz Curry, J.E. (1998). Promoting functional mobility. In J.P. Dormans & L. Pellegrino (Eds.), *Caring for children with cerebral palsy: A team approach* (pp. 315). Baltimore: Paul H. Brookes Publishing Co.

Figure 9.4 from Burstein, J.R., Wright-Drechsel, M.L., & Wood, A. (1998). Assistive technology. In J.P. Dormans & L. Pellegrino (Eds.), *Caring for children with cerebral palsy: A team approach* (p. 378). Baltimore: Paul H. Brookes Publishing Co.

Figure 10.1 from American Academy of Pediatrics (2000). *Recommended childhood immunization schedule: United States, January–December 2000* [On-line]. Elk Grove Village, IL: Author. Available: http://www.aap.org/family/parents/immunize.htm

Figure 15.1 from Roizen, N.J. (1997). Mental retardation. In M.L. Batshaw (Ed.), *Children with disabilities* (4th ed., pp. 362). Baltimore: Paul H. Brookes Publishing Co.

Figure 15.3 courtesy of Beverly Emanuel, Ph.D., Division of Genetics, Children's Hospital of Philadelphia.

Figure 17.1 from The Spina Bifida Program, Department of General Pediatrics. (1995). *Answering your questions about spina bifida: A guide from The Spina Bifida Program, Department of General Pediatrics* (p. 5). Washington, DC: Children's National Medical Center; reprinted by permission.

Figure 19.1 from Pellegrino, L. (1997). Cerebral palsy. In M.L. Batshaw (Ed.), *Children with disabilities* (4th ed., p. 502). Baltimore: Paul H. Brookes Publishing Co.

Figure 19.2 from Ried, S., Pellegrino, L., Albinson-Scull, S., & Dormans, J.P. (1998). The management of spasticity. In J.P. Dormans & L. Pellegrino (Eds.), *Caring for children with cerebral palsy: A team approach* (p. 106). Baltimore: Paul H. Brookes Publishing Co.

Figures 20.4 and 20.5 from Steinberg, A.G., & Knightly, C.A. (1997). Hearing: Sounds and silences. In M.L. Batshaw (Ed.), *Children with disabilities* (4th ed., pp. 265, 266). Baltimore: Paul H. Brookes Publishing Co.

Figures 22.2–22.4 from Menacker, S.J., & Batshaw, M.L. (1997). Vision. In M.L. Batshaw (Ed.), *Children with disabilities* (4th ed., pp. 217, 223, 225). Baltimore: Paul H. Brookes Publishing Co.

Figure 22.5 from Fraiberg, S. (1977). *Insights from the blind: Comparative studies of blind and sighted infants.* New York: Basic Books, Inc.; reprinted by permission of Perseus Books Group.

Figure 26.1 adapted from National Institutes of Health/National Cancer Institute. (1997, January). *Understanding gene testing* (NIH Publication 97-3905) [On-line]. Rockville, MD: Author. Available: http://rex.nci.nih.gov/PATIENTS/INFO_TEACHER/bookshelf/NIH_gene_testing/gene02.html

Figure 26.2 courtesy of Dr. Stephen Schonberg, American Medical Laboratories.

Figure 26.9 courtesy of Dr. Dorothy Bulas, Department of Diagnostic Imaging, Children's National Medical Center.

as a "game" that requires your child to name objects in pictures. Other techniques may seem more like play than like work and can occur in a natural environment. These are often used with children too young to do well in more structured activities. For example, the therapist might coax a 2-year-old to name objects while playing with toy figures.

Stimulation is the second approach to therapy. There are two basic types of stimulation: speech-language stimulation (also called *developmental stimulation*) and oral-motor stimulation. Speech-language stimulation programs use play activities to encourage your child to use language appropriately and to learn better communication skills. An example would be a therapist's playing Peekaboo with a 9-month-old who has cerebral palsy. Peekaboo teaches the child that communication is enjoyable, that people take turns in conversation, and that speaking is a means of interacting with others. Speech-language stimulation is usually used in early intervention programs before your child is developmentally advanced enough to engage in more structured therapy activities.

If your child has difficulty with the physical act of speaking, his or her therapy will probably involve oral-motor stimulation. Physical stimulation of the mouth, face, and throat can improve oral-motor abilities that are used in producing speech. For example, a 22-month-old girl with cerebral palsy might receive oral-motor stimulation that consists of feeding and rubbing her cheek with a soft object. If oral-motor movements improve, the speech will naturally be better. (See Chapter 7 for a discussion of oral-motor therapy and feeding problems.)

The goal of parent–teacher consultation is usually to facilitate an understanding of your child's disabilities so that you and the teacher can learn specific techniques to assist in your child's speech-language development. As part of this approach, for example, a therapist might show you how to teach your baby to make babbling noises and give you a pamphlet on the importance of babbling to the development of speech. In fact, especially when your child is young or newly diagnosed, parent–teacher training may be the most important aspect of therapy.

Therapy Environments

Therapy is usually performed in one of three locations: a therapy room, a classroom, or your home. Of these three, the treatment room is the most commonly used. It is likely to be located in a hospital, a school, or a clinic; however, the trend in the United States to work with children in natural environments is changing the location of therapy. The room should be quiet and uncluttered, so your child will not become distracted. Although the treatment room may be the ideal location for teaching new skills, it is less appropriate when teaching your child to apply skills to daily activities. In such instances, your child will benefit from therapy in a more natural environment, such as the classroom.